ANNALS *of* THE NEW YORK ACADEMY OF SCIENCES

VOLUME
1290

ISBN-10: 1-57331-897-3; **ISBN-13:** 978-1-57331-897-6

ISSUE

Resveratrol and Health

2nd International Scientific Conference on Resveratrol and Health

ISSUE EDITORS
Karen Brown[a] and Ole Vang[b]

[a]University of Leicester and [b]Roskilde University

T0344665

TABLE OF CONTENTS

Annals of the New York Academy of Sciences (ISSN: 0077-8923 [print]; ISSN: 1749-6632 [online]) is published 30 times a year on behalf of the New York Academy of Sciences by Wiley Subscription Services, Inc., a Wiley Company, 111 River Street, Hoboken, NJ 07030-5774.

Mailing: *Annals of the New York Academy of Sciences* is mailed standard rate.

Postmaster: Send all address changes to ANNALS OF THE NEW YORK ACADEMY OF SCIENCES, Journal Customer Services, John Wiley & Sons Inc., 350 Main Street, Malden, MA 02148-5020.

Disclaimer: The publisher, the New York Academy of Sciences, and the editors cannot be held responsible for errors or any consequences arising from the use of information contained in this publication; the views and opinions expressed do not necessarily reflect those of the publisher, the New York Academy of Sciences, and editors, neither does the publication of advertisements constitute any endorsement by the publisher, the New York Academy of Sciences and editors of the products advertised.

Publisher: *Annals of the New York Academy of Sciences* is published by Wiley Periodicals, Inc., Commerce Place, 350 Main Street, Malden, MA 02148; Telephone: 781 388 8200; Fax: 781 388 8210.

Journal Customer Services: For ordering information, claims, and any inquiry concerning your subscription, please go to www.wileycustomerhelp.com/ask or contact your nearest office. *Americas:* Email: cs-journals@wiley.com; Tel:+1 781 388 8598 or 1 800 835 6770 (Toll free in the USA & Canada). *Europe, Middle East, Asia:* Email: cs-journals@wiley. com; Tel: +44 (0) 1865 778315. *Asia Pacific:* Email: cs-journals@wiley.com; Tel: +65 6511 8000. *Japan:* For Japanese speaking support, Email: cs-japan@wiley.com; Tel: +65 6511 8010 or Tel (toll-free): 005 316 50 480. Visit our Online Customer Get-Help available in 6 languages at www.wileycustomerhelp.com.

Information for Subscribers: *Annals of the New York Academy of Sciences* is published in 30 volumes per year. Subscription prices for 2013 are: Print & Online: US$6,053 (US), US$6,589 (Rest of World), €4,269 (Europe), £3,364 (UK). Prices are exclusive of tax. Australian GST, Canadian GST, and European VAT will be applied at the appropriate rates. For more information on current tax rates, please go to www.wileyonlinelibrary.com/tax-vat. The price includes online access to the current and all online back files to January 1, 2009, where available. For other pricing options, including access information and terms and conditions, please visit www.wileyonlinelibrary.com/access.

Delivery Terms and Legal Title: Where the subscription price includes print volumes and delivery is to the recipient's address, delivery terms are Delivered at Place (DAP); the recipient is responsible for paying any import duty or taxes. Title to all volumes transfers FOB our shipping point, freight prepaid. We will endeavour to fulfill claims for missing or damaged copies within six months of publication, within our reasonable discretion and subject to availability.

Back issues: Recent single volumes are available to institutions at the current single volume price from cs-journals@wiley.com. Earlier volumes may be obtained from Periodicals Service Company, 11 Main Street, Germantown, NY 12526, USA. Tel: +1 518 537 4700, Fax: +1 518 537 5899, Email: psc@periodicals.com. For submission instructions, subscription, and all other information visit: www.wileyonlinelibrary.com/journal/nyas.

Production Editors: Kelly McSweeney and Allie Struzik (email: nyas@wiley.com).

Commercial Reprints: Dan Nicholas (email: dnicholas@wiley.com).

Membership information: Members may order copies of *Annals* volumes directly from the Academy by visiting www. nyas.org/annals, emailing customerservice@nyas.org, faxing +1 212 298 3650, or calling 1 800 843 6927 (toll free in the USA), or +1 212 298 8640. For more information on becoming a member of the New York Academy of Sciences, please visit www.nyas.org/membership. Claims and inquiries on member orders should be directed to the Academy at email: membership@nyas.org or Tel: 1 800 843 6927 (toll free in the USA) or +1 212 298 8640.

Printed in the USA by The Sheridan Group.

View *Annals* online at www.wileyonlinelibrary.com/journal/nyas.

Abstracting and Indexing Services: *Annals of the New York Academy of Sciences* is indexed by MEDLINE, Science Citation Index, and SCOPUS. For a complete list of A&I services, please visit the journal homepage at www. wileyonlinelibrary.com/journal/nyas.

Access to *Annals* is available free online within institutions in the developing world through the AGORA initiative with the FAO, the HINARI initiative with the WHO, and the OARE initiative with UNEP. For information, visit www. aginternetwork.org, www.healthinternetwork.org, www.oarescience.org.

Annals of the New York Academy of Sciences accepts articles for Open Access publication. Please visit http://olabout.wiley.com/WileyCDA/Section/id-406241.html for further information about OnlineOpen.

Wiley's Corporate Citizenship initiative seeks to address the environmental, social, economic, and ethical challenges faced in our business and which are important to our diverse stakeholder groups. Since launching the initiative, we have focused on sharing our content with those in need, enhancing community philanthropy, reducing our carbon impact, creating global guidelines and best practices for paper use, establishing a vendor code of ethics, and engaging our colleagues and other stakeholders in our efforts. Follow our progress at www.wiley.com/go/citizenship.

Ann. N.Y. Acad. Sci. ISSN 0077-8923

What is new for resveratrol? Is a new set of recommendations necessary?

Ole Vang

Department of Science, System, and Models, Roskilde University, Roskilde, Denmark

Address for correspondence: Ole Vang, Department of Science, System and Models, Roskilde University, Universitetsvej 1, DK-4000 Roskilde, Denmark. ov@ruc.dk

Numerous scientific papers have suggested health-promoting effects of resveratrol, including claims in the prevention of diseases such as coronary heart disease, diabetes, and cancer. Therefore, it was proposed that the scientific community needed to express recommendations on the human use of resveratrol. Such recommendations were formulated after the first international resveratrol conference in Denmark, Resveratrol2010. The working group stated that the evidence was "not sufficiently strong to justify recommendation for the chronic administration of resveratrol to human beings, beyond the dose which can be obtained from dietary sources." It was a disappointing conclusion relative to the positive claims about the therapeutic potential of resveratrol made by the media. However, since 2010, results from the first clinical trials on resveratrol have been made available. Because of these emerging results, it is necessary to formulate updated versions of the recommendations.

Keywords: resveratrol; clinical trials; human use; human health

Introduction

Resveratrol is a naturally occurring stilbene, colloquially known as "red wine medicine." Resveratrol is a chemically simple compound, but various resveratrol derivatives, as well as dimeric, trimeric, and tetrameric forms, are found in nature. Although recent studies have explored these resveratrol derivatives, the present review is focusing on resveratrol only.

Resveratrol has received much attention in public and scientific communities, and a set of recommendations in relation to human consumption was formulated at Resveratrol2010, the 1st International Conference on Resveratrol and Health (Helsingør, Denmark). The aim of the present review is to show the relevance of these recommendations in 2010 and to discuss the necessity of formulating a new set of recommendations at the Resveratrol2012 meeting in Leicester, December 2012.

When Takaoka first published the existence of resveratrol in *Veratrum grandiflorum*,[1] very few noticed this observation, until some biological effects observed from extracts of *Polygonum cuspidatum* were linked to its high content of resveratrol[2] and resveratrol was found in edible sources such as grapes and wine.[3] The major findings of biological responses to resveratrol (Fig. 1) can be characterized as (1) Frankel *et al.* found in 1993 that resveratrol modulates LDL levels, indicating a potential reduced risk for development of coronary heart disease;[4] (2) the chemo-preventive effect of reseveratrol in a mouse skin cancer model was shown by Jang *et al.*[5] in 1997; (3) a major focus was prompted by the observation that resveratrol extends the life span of yeast;[6] (4) the effect of resveratrol on obesity and diabetes was identified by two groups in 2006.[7,8] A few phase I clinical trials focusing on the pharmacokinetics of resveratrol were published before 2010, but since then, the number of clinical trials exploring the biological effects of resveratrol has increased significantly.

Scientific focus on resveratrol

The scientific focus on resveratrol has followed the profile of curcumin and, to a lesser extent quercetin (Fig. 1), whereas several other naturally

doi: 10.1111/nyas.12173

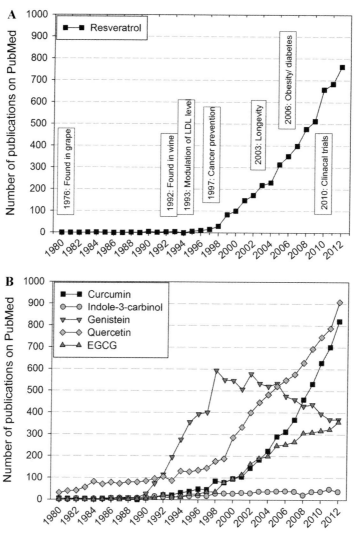

Figure 1. Increasing scientific interest on the biological effects of resveratrol and other naturally occurring bioactive substances. The number of hits obtained by searching (A) "resveratrol" and (B) "curcumin," "indole-3-carbinol," "genistein," "quercetin," or "epigallocatechin-3-gallate" (EGCG) for each year from 1980 to 2012 on PubMed (http://www.ncbi.nlm.nih.gov/pubmed?db=pubmed) is shown.

occurring bioactive substances, such as indole-3-carbinol (from cruciferous vegetables) or genistein (mainly from soybeans) have shown quite different profiles of interest. The chemopreventive effect of indole-3-carbinol was proposed in animal models in 1978 by Wattenberg *et al.*,[9] but the annual number of scientific publications has been quite constant over the years. The scientific interest in the flavonoid quercetin was also significant in the 1980s and 1990s, with an increased interest during the first decade of 2000. Comparisons of publication frequency indicate a more specific increased

scientific interest in resveratrol and curcumin relative to many other potentially health-promoting naturally occurring compounds. Further, the interest for resveratrol and curcumin has not yet reached a plateau, as observed for genistein.

The total number of scientific publications indexed in PubMed has increased in the period analyzed (from about 280,000 in 1980 to about 910,000 in 2012). Even when taking this total increase of publications into consideration, the increase in publications focusing on resveratrol or curcumin is very significant. The scientific focus on

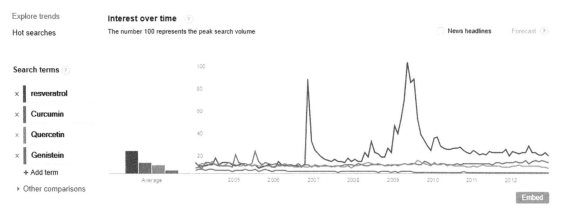

Figure 2. Relative search activity on the Internet using Google. The search activity is displayed by using Google Trends (http://www.google.com/trends/explore) in the period of January 2004–December 2012. The search words were "resveratrol," "curcumin," "genistein," and "quercetin."

resveratrol is high relative to other naturally occurring compounds. By December 2012, the accumulated number of PubMed-identified publications focused on resveratrol was comparable with curcumin (both around 5400 publications), nearly half as many as genistein or quercetin (both around 9600 publications), and significantly more than well-known bioactive compounds like apigenin, epigallocatechin-3-gallate, lycopene, ellagic acid, naringin, sulforaphane, and dialylsulfide (ranging between 300 and 3000 publications).

Resveratrol claims

Nearly all data concerning the biological effects of resveratrol up to 2010 were generated *in vitro* or in animal models. Therefore, the health significance of resveratrol in humans has been unclear, even though the substance has been popularly claimed as a treatment agent for a range of cancers and as an antiaging compound. Such claims are not supported by strong scientific evidence. Translating specific scientific messages from experimental laboratories to the general public is a very difficult and complex task. It is in general a major challenge that most of the statements concerning the health effects of resveratrol are based on animal studies and mechanistic studies (*in vitro*), and details relevant to experimental setup and models are often lost in translation from the scientific literature to the mass media.

In addition, there are a number of examples where the outcome from *in vitro* experiments differs from the response in experimental animals or from the

effects observed in humans. As one recent example, resveratrol inhibited cell proliferation and invasiveness of ovarian cancer cells *in vitro,* but did not exhibit this effect on the same cancer cells *in vivo.*[10] Therefore, one has to be careful when translating data from *in vitro* experiments or animal experiments to humans. On the other hand, as will be discussed later, the options for performing the optimal or correct experiments in humans to prove the effect of substances like resveratrol are rather limited.

The focus on resveratrol in the public domain

Scanning Internet search activities can provide a relevant parameter of interest in the public domain. A search using Google Trends (http://www.google.com/trends/) provides the relative search activities using Google search machinery since 2004 (Fig. 2). In the public domain as well as in the scientific community, there is a large interest for information on resveratrol, which peaked in late 2006 and during 2009. The peak in interest in 2006 can be related to the scientific breakthroughs that year by Baur *et al.*[7] and Lagouge *et al.,*[8] whereas the peak in 2009 was likely because of a high public focus on resveratrol by trendsetters like Oprah Winfrey. The interest has, since 2009, generally been at a much higher level compared to curcumin, genistein, or quercetin. In the same time period, the number of websites dedicated to resveratrol has increased exponentially, with significantly more sites focusing on resveratrol than curcumin.

Overall conclusions from the working group at Resveratrol 2010

By 2010, in light of the increasingly large number of publications, the growing hype around resveratrol, and the large number of unsupported claims about its health benefits propagated by the media, there was a need to sum up all the available scientific data on resveratrol and to formulate recommendations for the human use of resveratrol and for research in the coming years. As a follow-up from Resveratrol2010, the 1st International Conference on Resveratrol and Health (Helsingør, Denmark), such recommendations were formulated and published in *PLoS One* in 2011.[11] By considering the knowledge gained as a result of the formulation of these recommendations, we can evaluate their significance and consider whether the recommendations need to be updated.

The overall conclusion from the Resveratrol2010 working group was presented as a double statement: "The published evidence is not sufficiently strong to justify a recommendation for the administration of resveratrol to humans, beyond the dose which can be obtained from dietary sources," but "animal data are promising in prevention of various cancer types, coronary heart diseases, and diabetes, which strongly indicate the need for human clinical trials."[11] The major challenge at the time of formulation of the recommendations was that no human clinical trials were available, even though a few were published in the few months after the conference. On the basis of the animal data alone, the working group could not support recommendations for resveratrol use in humans at higher concentrations than those obtained through the diet. The translation from animal to human is not straightforward because of potential differences between experimental animals (rodents) and humans in the bioavailability and mechanisms of action of resveratrol. A careful statement was chosen, which was supported by the animal experiments completed and published at that time.

The evaluation was based on the following five test questions:[11]

1. Can resveratrol be recommended in the prevention or treatment of human diseases?
2. Are there observed side effects caused by the intake of resveratrol in humans?
3. What is the relevant dose of resveratrol?
4. What valid data are available regarding an effect in various species of experimental animals?
5. Which relevant (overall) mechanisms of action of resveratrol have been documented?

Questions 1–3 focus on the effects of resveratrol in humans, whereas question 4 concerns the effects of resveratrol in animal models. The first part of the overall conclusion addressed 1–3, stating that administration of extended levels of resveratrol to humans cannot be recommended. As long-term exposure trials with resveratrol had not been performed at that time; there were neither direct data on side effects nor data from humans that could support an estimated dose of resveratrol for human use. No-observed-adverse-effect levels for maternal toxicity and embryo–fetal development are around 750 mg resveratrol/kg/day in rats, which has been translated to a safe daily dose of 450 mg for a 60 kg person.[12] This estimate was based on one long-term study in one species and a study in a second species is necessary.

Although the working group could not recommend a specific dose of resveratrol for human intake because health-promoting effects had not been investigated in humans, it was also necessary to state that no significant side effects have been observed in animal studies or in short-term human studies when very high doses of resveratrol were used (e.g., 2.5–5 g/day).

Advantages and challenges of the recommendations

These formal recommendations on the human use of resveratrol summarize the existing body of knowledge in a few lines, assuming that the members of the working group have done their best to compile the most valid data in the recommendations. The conclusions may be used directly by medical doctors to address questions from their patients about whether dietary supplementation with resveratrol may prevent lifestyle diseases. The recommendations may be used also by a well-oriented layperson, relevant target person, or member of the media who needs a source for presenting valid scientific information on resveratrol. The recommendations also provide goals for the future of research needed in the field of resveratrol to answer the question of human use.

Ann. N.Y. Acad. Sci. 1290 (2013) 1–11 © 2013 New York Academy of Sciences.

On the other hand, such short brief statements may well be too simple to express the nuances relevant to the diversity of biological effects of resveratrol. Resveratrol seems to have numerous cellular targets. Not all of these targets are likely to be equally relevant to any one disease. Problems relevant to issues like resveratrol administration may also be masked by such brevity. In the attempt to make clear recommendations, the working group may have made the same error of oversimplification of which we accuse the media in relation to the effects of resveratrol.

How was the message received in the scientific and general societies?

Scientific relevance can be measured by the number of citations of the publication in *PLoS One*.[11] Using the metric analysis at the *PLoS One* article homepage (http://www.plosone.org/article/info%3Adoi%2F 10.1371%2Fjournal.pone.0019881), where the paper was ranked among the top five resveratrol papers published in *PLoS One* (December 2012) in relation to number of citations and the usage of the article (number of downloads), $1\frac{1}{2}$ years after publication. In contrast, the recommendations have only rarely been cited on the Internet outside of scientific publications. However, claims found on the Internet in relation to the health effects of resveratrol appear to be much more balanced at present, indicating that the formulation of the recommendations has had an effect on the delivery of the information on resveratrol.

Clinical trials testing the health-promoting effect of resveratrol: what has happened since September 2010?

One of the central recommendations from the working group at the Resveratrol2010 conference was to initiate clinical trials to evaluate the health effects of resveratrol in humans, and many such trials have been published since September 2010. Table 1 lists the published trials up to the end of 2012 testing the effect of pure resveratrol, whereas Table 2 lists trials of resveratrol as part of a mixture with other potentially bioactive compounds. Translating the effects of resveratrol from studies using a mixture containing resveratrol is not possible without data from experiments where resveratrol is used in a pure form. On the other hand, exclusively evaluating trials with pure resveratrol will not reveal relevant combina-

tory effects of resveratrol with other bioactive compounds.

The specific doses of resveratrol used in the various experiments differ dramatically. Using pure resveratrol, daily doses as low as 5 mg twice daily for four weeks showed an effect on insulin sensitivity,[13] and 10 mg/day for three months produced increased flow-mediated dilation.[14] Daily doses up to 2.5 or 5 g resveratrol have been used in several trials for up to 29 days with effects on the relevant biochemical parameters.[15,16] Adverse effects have been observed using such high resveratrol levels: therefore the daily dose during long-term exposure to pure resveratrol should be kept below 1–1.5 g.

Both sexes have been included in the trials. Only a few trials have included young healthy subjects,[17] as most trials have focused on subjects with a disease or increased risk for the development of the disease. Designing trials using subjects with pre-disease status introduces difficulties in demonstrating preventive effects, as several disease stages may have already initiated even though the disease is not manifest. Therefore, long-term clinical trials including young subjects will need to be performed to assess preventive effects, but it will be challenging to demonstrate relevant effects of resveratrol in such low-risk cohorts.

The duration of the trials varies from acute exposure,[18,19] to a few days (5–8) of exposure,[20,21] to up to one year.[22] Most trials expose the subjects to resveratrol in time frames of 1–3 months. The relatively short duration of the trials is a challenge, as they permit analysis of therapeutic but not preventive potential. Without taking the practical and economical aspects of such studies into consideration, a trial to show a preventive effect of resveratrol should run for a minimum of one year. It is obvious that such trials are expensive and not easily funded, but they will be necessary to obtain relevant information about the preventive potential of resveratrol.

Most of the clinical trials, particularly the larger ones, have focused on the effects of resveratrol on cardiovascular disease and diabetes and on inflammation status. The strongest effects were observed in subjects with enhanced levels of disease-related markers,[13,14,19,23–25] but some trials did not show any effect of resveratrol,[26] even though study participants had high-risk profiles.[27] Trials examining resveratrol in relation to cancer have been small in

Table 1. Clinical trials analyzing biological effects of resveratrol. The biological effects of resveratrol (Resv) alone have been studied in the trials shown in the table. The various effects are divided into groups depending on the major scope of the trial

Number of subjects	Type of study	Dose and duration	Effect of Resv	Reference
		Cognitive/brain function/emotional		
22	Double-blind, placebo-controlled, crossover study	250 or 500 mg Resv in a single dose	Cerebral blood flow ↑ Oxygen extraction ↑	18
		Cancer		
20 colorectal cancer patients	Open-label study	0.5 or 1.0 g daily doses of Resv for 8 days	Tumor cell proliferation ↓	21
40: 18♀, 22♂	Open-label study	0.5, 1, 2.5, or 5 g Resv/day for 29 days	IGF-I ↓ IGF-binding protein-3 ↓	15
42: 31 ♀, 11 ♂	Open-label study	1 g Resv/day for 4 weeks	Level of specific cytochrome P450 enzymes ↓ GST activity and GST-π →	28
9 subjects, stage IV colo-rectal cancer, w. hepatic metastases	Randomized (2:1) double-blind study	5 g Resv/day for 10–21 days	Hepatic apoptosis ↑	16
		Metabolic syndrome/insulin sensitivity/NAFLD/diabetes		
11 overweight ♂	Randomized, double-blinded crossover study	150 mg Resv/day in 30 days	Sleeping and metabolic rate ↓ Fat in liver ↓ Circulating glucose ↓ Triglycerides ↓ Inflam. markers ↓ Systolic blood press. ↓ Lipolysis in adipose tissue ↓ Plasma fatty acids ↓ Glycerol in the postprandial state ↓	23
Nonobese, postmenopausal ♀	Randomized, double-blind, placebo-controlled study	75 mg Resv/day for 12 weeks	Body composition → Resting metabolic rate → Plasma lipids → Inflammatory markers → Adipose tissue insulin sensitivity →	26
24 obese, healthy ♂	Randomized, double-blinded, placebo-controlled, and parallel-group design	3 × 500 mg Resv/day for 4 weeks	Insulin sensitivity → Endogenous glucose production → Turnover and oxidation rates of glucose → No effect on blood pressure → Resting energy expenditure → Oxidation rates of lipid → Ectopic or visceral fat content → Inflammatory and metabolic biomarkers →	27

Continued

Ann. N.Y. Acad. Sci. 1290 (2013) 1–11 © 2013 New York Academy of Sciences.

Table 1. *Continued*

Number of subjects	Type of study	Dose and duration	Effect of Resv	Reference
19 type 2 diabetic patients	Randomized, double-blinded, and placebo-controlled study	5 mg Resv b.i.d. for 4 weeks	Insulin sensitivity ↑ Oxidative stress ↓	13
10 older people w/ moderately insulin resistance	Randomized, open-label study	Daily dose of 1, 1.5, or 2 g Resv for 4 weeks	Peak post-meal glucose ↓ 3 hour glucose ↓ Post-meal insulin ↓ Insulin sensitivity ↑	24
		Cardiovascular		
40	Randomized, double-blinded and placebo-controlled study	10 mg Resv/day in 3 months	Flow-mediated dilation ↑ Left ventricular diastolic function ↑ LDLc ↓	14
19	Randomized, double-blinded, placebo-controlled, and crossover study	A single acute dose of 0, 30, 90, and 270 mg Resv	Flow-mediated dilation ↑, dose dependent	19
87 in three groups	Randomized, double-blinded, active-controlled,	20 mg Resv/day ± calcium fructoborate for 60 days	Inflam. markers ↓ LDLc ↓ HDLc ↑ Triacylglycerols ↓ Quality of life ↑	25
		Skin		
20 patients (8♀, 12♂) with facial acne vulgaris	Single-blinded, placebo-controlled study	10 μg/g of gel. Applied daily for 60 days	GAGS score: ↓	29

GAGS, global acne grading system; GST, glutathione S-transferase; HDLc, high-density lipoprotein-cholesterol; IGF-I, insulin-like growth factor-1; LDLc, low-density lipoprotein-cholesterol; ↑, increased response; ↓, decreased response; →, no significant effect.

size and have focused on the therapeutic effect of resveratrol in relation to cancer markers. Ironically, such therapeutic studies have not really been performed in experimental animals, where studies have focused on the preventive effect of resveratrol.

To some extent, is it more meaningful to estimate the effect of resveratrol when it is part of a dietary matrix. It is likely also easier to get such trials accepted, as supplementations are more natural and the exposure to resveratrol is generally lower in these trials. Among the published trials where resveratrol is part of a matrix, medium-high levels of resveratrol have been used, but these have not shown statistically significant effects: in one trial, a 100–400 mg resveratrol exposure reduced inflammation[30] and increased flow-mediated dilation,[31] but these parameters were not found changed in other trials

using the same levels of resveratrol.[20,31] However, a set of trials where the subjects were exposed to low amounts of resveratrol for six months and one year did show significant effects on cardiovascular biochemical markers.[22,32]

Beyond these major diseases, the effect of resveratrol on cognitive or brain function has been only marginally investigated,[17,18] while a significant effect of resveratrol on skin was found in two studies.[29,33]

Do we need a new set of recommendations for the use of resveratrol?

On the basis of the human trials focused on the health-promoting effects of resveratrol conducted during the last two years, the set of recommendations formulated in September 2010 have to be updated. The clinical trials are still small relative to

Table 2. Clinical trials analyzing biological effects of resveratrol as part of a mix. The biological effects of resveratrol (Resv) as part of a mixture have been studied in the trials shown in the table. The various effects are divided into the major groups depending on the major scope of the trial

Number of subjects	Type of study	Dose and duration	Effect of Resv	Reference
Cognitive/brain function/emotional				
40 subjects in two groups	Randomized, double blinded, placebo-controlled study	Daily 46 g grape powder with 1.75 mg Resv/kg (0.08 mg/day) for 45 days	Mood $\rightarrow$	17
Cancer				
8 colon cancer patients	Open-label study	3.9 or 15.6 mg/day Resv with quercetin	Wnt signaling in colon cancer cells $\rightarrow$	34
8 colon cancer patients	Open-label study	Freeze-dried grape powder with Resv (corresponding to 0.073 and 0.114 mg Resv/day)	Wnt signaling in colon cancer cells $\rightarrow$ In normal cells $\downarrow$	34
12: 7 ♀, 5 ♂	Open-label study	Food supplement containing 2 mg Resv + 100 mg grape extract 3 times daily for 5 days	DNA stability $\rightarrow$ Redox status $\rightarrow$ Inflammation $\rightarrow$	20
36 ♀	Randomized crossover study	237 mL red or white wine for 21 days. The level of Resv is not shown	Red relative to white wine: Testosterone $\uparrow$ Sex hormone binding globulin $\uparrow$ Luteinizing hormone $\uparrow$	35
30 healthy subjects	Open-label study	1/3, 2/3, or 1 lb of red grapes per day for 2 weeks, but the level of Resv was not shown	Colonic mucosal cell proliferation $\downarrow$ Cyclin D1 and CD133 $\downarrow$	36
Inflammation				
20	Randomized, placebo controlled study	*Polygonum cuspidatum* extract containing 40 mg Resv/day for 6 weeks	ROS $\downarrow$ Inflammatory markers $\downarrow$ HDL, LDL $\rightarrow$ Insulin, glucose $\rightarrow$	37
10 subjects (31 ♀, 11 ♂) given a high-fat, high-carbohydrate diet	Crossover and placebo-controlled study	100 mg of Resv + 75 mg polyphenols from a grape extract/single administration	TLR4 $\downarrow$, CD14 $\downarrow$, SOCS3 $\downarrow$, IL-1β $\downarrow$, Keap-1 $\downarrow$ Nrf-2 binding activity $\uparrow$, expression of NQO-1 and GST-P1 $\uparrow$	30
36 ♂, with BMI between 25.5 and 35.0 and a low-grade inflammation	Randomized, double-blind, placebo-controlled, crossover study	Anti-inflammatory dietary mix (AIDM) containing Resv (25.2 mg/day for 5 weeks	Inflammatory markers $\rightarrow$ Adiponectin $\uparrow$ Adipose tissue inflammation $\downarrow$ Endothelial function $\downarrow$ Liver fatty acid Oxidation $\uparrow$	38

Continued

Ann. N.Y. Acad. Sci. 1290 (2013) 1–11 © 2013 New York Academy of Sciences.

Table 2. *Continued*

Number of subjects	Type of study	Dose and duration	Effect of Resv	Reference
Metabolic syndrome/insulin sensitivity/NAFLD/diabetes				
34 people with metabolic syndrome	Randomized	100 mg Resv (Longevinex®) daily for 0–3 or 3–6 months	Insulin resistance → Lipid profile → Inflamm. markers →	31
32 obese in 3 groups (17♀, 15♂)	Randomized, single-blinded, with sequential design	1 capsule/day of 150 mg Resv, 400 mg catechin-rich grape seed extract (CGSE), or 300 mg RTP for 28 days	GSH ↓ Anti-oxid. enzymes → Lipid perxid → oxLDL → 8-OH-dG →	39
Cardiovascular				
75 in 3 groups	Triple-blinded randomized study	Placebo, 350 mg grape extract (GE), 350 Resv-enriched GE (8 mg Resv) for 6 months	LDLc ↓, ApoB ↓, oxLDL ↓ oxLDL/ApoB; ↓ non-HDLc /ApoB ↑	32
150 in 3 groups	Randomized double-blinded placebo-controlled study	Placebo, 350 mg grape extract (GE), 350 Resv-enriched GE (8 mg Resv) for 6 months + double amount for next 6 months	Inflamm. markers ↓ Adiponectin ↑	22
34 subjects with metabolic syndrome	Randomized	100 mg Resv (Longevinex) daily for 0–3 or 3– 6 months	Flow-mediated dilatation ↑ Blood pressure →	31
67 subjects w/ high risk for atherosclerosis	Randomized, placebo-controlled crossover study	272 mL red wine/day (0.82 mg Resv) for 4 weeks	ICAM-1 ↓, E-selectin ↓, IL-6 ↓ Lymphocyte function-associated antigen 1 ↓ Macrophage-1 Receptor ↓ Sialyl-Lewis X ↓ C-C chemokine receptor type 2 ↓	40
Skin				
50: 35♀, 15♂	Randomized, placebo-controlled study	133 mg grape extract (8 mg Resv) /day for 60 days	Moisturization index ↑ Skin elasticity ↑ Skin roughness ↓ Wrinkle depth ↓	33
Fitness and muscle injury				
40 active young adults in two groups	Randomized, double blinded, placebo-controlled study	Daily 46 g grape powder with 1.75 mg Resv/kg (0.08 mg/day) for 45 days	VO$_2$max → Work capacity → Perceived health status → Inflammation → Pain → Physical function responses →	17

8-OH-dG, 8-deoxy-guanine; ApoB, apolipoprotein B; GSH, glutathione; GST, glutathion S-transferase; HDL, high density lipoprotein; ICAM-1, intercellular adhesion molecule 1; IL, interleukin; oxLDL, oxidized LDL; LDL, low density lipoprotein; ROS, reactive oxygen species; TLR4, Toll-like receptor 4; SOCS3, suppressor of cytokine signaling 3; ↑, increased response; ↓, decreased response; →, no significant effect.

the sample sizes used for testing drugs, and analysis of the possible disease-preventive effect is facing several challenges. To determine potential preventive effects of a dietary compound like resveratrol, long-term exposures of large cohorts of participants in stages of low risk of disease development are needed. The dietary bioactive compounds do not work like typically man-made drugs that have a single high-affinity target, but rather modulate a range of cellular targets with only low affinity. Therefore, the effects of a single compound at low levels are rather small, and one may expect that the biological effects are caused by combined effects of several (or many) dietary bioactive compounds ingested simultaneously. Therefore, the effect of resveratrol may be underestimated when analyzed as a single compound under investigation.

Conclusions: what has been learned from working with the recommendations?

Resveratrol has been the focus of considerable hype in both the general and scientific communities. This hype has propelled research on the compound, but it has also stimulated the propagation of many unsupported claims concerning the putative health benefits of the compound. Therefore, it was necessary in 2010 to formulate a set of recommendations on the use of resveratrol. These have, in general, been accepted well and have contributed to the establishment of a series of clinical trials focusing on the health effects of resveratrol. This high number of clinical trials analyzing the effect of resveratrol demand a new set of recommendations.

Most of these clinical trials have been designed to evaluate the therapeutic effect of resveratrol rather than the disease-preventive effect of the compound. A preventive study needs to expose test subjects before they show any sign of the disease, and then the cohort members have to be treated for a sufficiently long time that a significant amount of subjects in the control group will develop the disease. To get substantial power in the analysis, the number of participants has to be high. Therefore, these trials will be very expensive, and the number of such studies in the future will be low: other models for prevention studies have to be included. The use of the pig as a reliable model will support the prevention experiments in rodents and provide us with necessary knowledge that may not be available in humans.

Acknowledgments

O.V. would like to thank Prof. Ole Andersen (Roskilde University) for valuable input during preparation of this manuscript.

Conflicts of interest

The author declares no conflicts of interest.

References

1. Takaoka, M. 1939. Resveratrol, a new phenolic compound from Veratrum grandiflorum. *Nippon Kagaku Kaichi* **60:** 1090–1100.
2. Arichi, H., Y. Kimura, H. Okuda, *et al.* 1982. Effects of stilbene components of the roots of *Polygonum cuspidatum* Sieb. et Zucc. on lipid metabolism. *Chem. Pharm. Bull.* **30:** 1766–1770.
3. Siemann, E.H. & L.L. Creasy. 1992. Concentration of the phytoalexin resveratrol in wine. *Amer. J. Enol. Viticult.* **43:** 49–52.
4. Frankel, E.N., A.L. Waterhouse & J.E. Kinsella. 1993. Inhibition of human LDL oxidation by resveratrol. *Lancet* **341:** 1103–1104.
5. Jang, M., L. Cai, G.O. Udeani, *et al.* 1997. Cancer chemopreventive activity of resveratrol, a natural product derived from grapes. *Science* **275:** 218–220.
6. Howitz, K.T., K.J. Bitterman, H.Y. Cohen, *et al.* 2003. Small molecule activators of sirtuins extend Saccharomyces cerevisiae lifespan. *Nature* **425:** 191–196.
7. Baur, J. A., K.J. Pearson, N.L. Price, *et al.* 2006. Resveratrol improves health and survival of mice on a high-calorie diet. *Nature* **444:** 337–342.
8. Lagouge, M., C. Argmann, Z. Gerhart-Hines, *et al.* 2006. Resveratrol improves mitochondrial function and protects against metabolic disease by activating SIRT1 and PGC-1alpha. *Cell* **127:** 1109–1122.
9. Wattenberg, L.W. & W.D. Loub. 1978. Inhibition of polycyclic aromatic hydrocarbon-induced neoplasia by naturally occurring indoles. *Cancer Res.* **38:** 1410–1413.
10. Stakleff, K.S., T. Sloan, D. Blanco, *et al.* 2012. Resveratrol exerts differential effects in vitro and in vivo against ovarian cancer cells. *Asian Pac. J. Cancer Prev.* **13:** 1333–1340.
11. Vang, O., N. Ahmad, C.A. Baile, *et al.* 2011. What is new for an old molecule? Systematic review and recommendations on the use of resveratrol. *PLoS ONE* **6:** e19881.
12. Williams, L.D., G.A. Burdock, J.A. Edwards, *et al.* 2009. Safety studies conducted on high-purity trans-resveratrol in experimental animals. *Food Chem. Toxicol.* **49:** 2170–2182.
13. Brasnyo, P., G.A. Molnar, M. Mohas, *et al.* 2011. Resveratrol improves insulin sensitivity, reduces oxidative stress and activates the Akt pathway in type 2 diabetic patients. *Br. J. Nutr.* **106:** 383–389.
14. Magyar, K., R. Halmosi, A. Palfi, *et al.* 2012. Cardioprotection by resveratrol: a human clinical trial in patients with stable coronary artery disease. *Clin. Hemorheol. Microcirc.* **50:** 179–187.
15. Brown, V.A., K.R. Patel, M. Viskaduraki, *et al.* 2010. Repeat dose study of the cancer chemopreventive agent resveratrol

in healthy volunteers: safety, pharmacokinetics, and effect on the insulin-like growth factor axis. *Cancer Res.* **70:** 9003–9011.

16. Howells, L.M., D.P. Berry, P.J. Elliott, *et al.* 2011. Phase I randomised double-blind pilot study of micronized resveratrol (SRT501) in patients with hepatic metastases—safety, pharmacokinetics andpharmacodynamics. *Cancer Prev. Res.* **4:** 1419–1425.

17. O'Connor, P.J., A.L. Caravalho, E.C. Freese & K.J. Cureton. 2013. Grape consumption effects on fitness, muscle injury, mood and perceived health. *Int. J. Sport Nutr. Exerc. Metab.* **23:** 57–64.

18. Kennedy, D.O., E.L. Wightman, J.L. Reay, *et al.* 2010. Effects of resveratrol on cerebral blood flow variables and cognitive performance in humans: a double-blind, placebo-controlled, crossover investigation. *Am. J. Clin. Nutr.* **91:** 1590–1597.

19. Wong, R.H.X., P.R.C. Howe, J.D. Buckley, *et al.* 2011. Acute resveratrol supplementation improves flow-mediated dilatation in overweight/obese individuals with mildly elevated blood pressure. *Nutr. Metab. Cardiovasc. Dis.* **21:** 851–856.

20. Heger, A., F. Ferk, A. Nersesyan, *et al.* 2012. Intake of a resveratrol-containing dietary supplement has no impact on DNA stability in healthy subjects. *Mutat. Res.* **749:** 82–86.

21. Patel, K.R., V.A. Brown, D.J. Jones, *et al.* 2010. Clinical pharmacology of resveratrol and its metabolites in colorectal cancer patients. *Cancer Res.* **70:** 7392–7399.

22. Tome-Carneiro, J., M. Gonzalvez, M. Larrosa, *et al.* 2012. Consumption of a grape extract supplement containing resveratrol decreases oxidized LDL and ApoB in patients undergoing primary prevention of cardiovascular disease: A triple-blind, 6-month follow-up, placebo-controlled, randomized trial. *Mol. Nutr. Food Res.* **56:** 810–821.

23. Timmers, S., E. Konings, L. Bilet, *et al.* 2011. Calorie restriction-like effects of 30 days of resveratrol supplementation on energy metabolism and metabolic profile in obese humans. *Cell Metab.* **14:** 612–622.

24. Crandall, J.P., V. Oram, G. Trandafirescu, *et al.* 2010. Resveratrol improves glucose metabolism in older adults with IGT [abstract]. *Diabetes* **59:** A201.

25. Militaru, C., I. Donoiu, A. Craciun, *et al.* 2013. Oral resveratrol and calcium fructoborate supplementation in subjects with stable angina pectoris: effects on lipid profiles, inflammation markers, and quality of life. *Nutrition* **29:** 178–183.

26. Yoshino, J., C. Conte, L. Fontana, *et al.* 2012. Resveratrol supplementation does not improve metabolic function in nonobese women with normal glucose tolerance. *Cell Metab.* **15:** 658–664.

27. Poulsen, M.M., P.F. Vestergaard, B.F. Clasen, *et al.* 2013. High-dose resveratrol supplementation in obese men: an investigator-initiated, randomized, placebo-controlled clinical trial of substrate metabolism, insulin sensitivity, and body composition. *Diabetes* DOI: 10.2337/db12-0975.

28. Chow, H.H., L.L. Garland, C.H. Hsu, *et al.* 2010. Resveratrol modulates drug- and carcinogen-metabolizing enzymes in a healthy volunteer study. *Cancer Prev. Res.* **3:** 1168–1175.

29. Fabbrocini, G., S. Staibano, G. De Rosa, *et al.* 2011. Resveratrol-containing gel for the treatment of acne vulgaris: a single-blind, vehicle-controlled, pilot study. *Am. J. Clin. Dermatol.* **12:** 133–141.

30. Ghanim, H., C.L. Sia, K. Korzeniewski, *et al.* 2011. A resveratrol and polyphenol preparation suppresses oxidative and inflammatory stress response to a high-fat, high-carbohydrate meal. *J. Clin. Endocrinol. Metab.* **96:** 1409–1414.

31. Fujitaka, K., H. Otani, F. Jo, *et al.* 2011. Modified resveratrol Longevinex improves endothelial function in adults with metabolic syndrome receiving standard treatment. *Nutr. Res.* **31:** 842–847.

32. Tome-Carneiro, J., M. Gonzalvez, M. Larrosa, *et al.* 2012. One-year consumption of a grape nutraceutical containing resveratrol improves the inflammatory and fibrinolytic status of patients in primary prevention of cardiovascular disease. *Am. J. Cardiol.* **110:** 356–363.

33. Buonocore, D., A. Lazzeretti, P. Tocabens, *et al.* 2012. Resveratrol-procyanidin blend: nutraceutical and antiaging efficacy evaluated in a placebocontrolled, double-blind study. *Clin Cosmet. Investig. Dermatol.* **5:** 159–165.

34. Nguyen, A.V., M. Martinez, M.J. Stamos, *et al.* 2009. Results of a phase I pilot clinical trial examining the effect of plant-derived resveratrol and grape powder on Wnt pathway target gene expression in colonic mucosa and colon cancer. *Cancer Manag. Res.* **1:** 25–37.

35. Shufelt, C., C.N. Merz, Y. Yang, *et al.* 2012. Red versus white wine as a nutritional aromatase inhibitor in premenopausal women: a pilot study. *J. Womens Health (Larchmt.)* **21:** 281–284.

36. Martinez, M., C. Hope, K. Planutis, *et al.* 2010. Dietary grape-derived resveratrol for colon cancer prevention [abstract]. *J. Clin. Oncol.* **28,** 15S, Abstr. 3622.

37. Ghanim, H., C.L. Sia, S. Abuaysheh, *et al.* 2010. An antiinflammatory and reactive oxygen species suppressive effects of an extract of *Polygonum cuspidatum* containing resveratrol. *J. Clin. Endocrinol. Metab.* **95:** E1–E8.

38. Bakker, G.C.M., M.J. van Erk, L. Pellis, *et al.* 2010. An antiinflammatory dietary mix modulates inflammation and oxidative and metabolic stress in overweight men: a nutrigenomics approach. *Am. J. Clin. Nutr.* **91:** 1044–1059.

39. De Groote, D., K. Van Belleghem, J. Deviere, *et al.* 2012. Effect of the intake of resveratrol, resveratrol phosphate, and catechin-rich grape seed extract on markers of oxidative stress and gene expression in adult obese subjects. *Ann. Nutr. Metab.* **61:** 15–24.

40. Chiva-Blanch, G., M. Urpi-Sarda, R. Llorach, *et al.* 2012. Differential effects of polyphenols and alcohol of red wine on the expression of adhesion molecules and inflammatory cytokines related to atherosclerosis: a randomized clinical trial. *Am. J. Clin. Nutr.* **95:** 326–334.

Ann. N.Y. Acad. Sci. ISSN 0077-8923

ANNALS OF THE NEW YORK ACADEMY OF SCIENCES

Issue: *Resveratrol and Health*

Resveratrol in the management of human cancer: how strong is the clinical evidence?

Andreas Gescher, William P. Steward, and Karen Brown

Cancer Chemoprevention Group, Department of Cancer Studies and Molecular Medicine, University of Leicester, Leicester, United Kingdom

Address for correspondence: Karen Brown, Department of Cancer Studies and Molecular Medicine, University of Leicester, Leicester, LE2 7LX, UK. kb20@le.ac.uk

Among the plethora of biochemical mechanisms engaged by resveratrol in preclinical systems, its anticarcinogenic effects represent some of the most convincing and intriguing. As outlined in this review, there is considerable interest in developing resveratrol for cancer prevention and treatment. The plasma pharmacokinetics of resveratrol in humans are now reasonably well defined, and studies have shown that repeated daily doses up to 1 g are safe and well tolerated, although gastrointestinal toxicity is observed at higher intakes. However, care is needed regarding underlying conditions in specific patient groups, and there is potential for drug interactions at doses greater than 1 gram. Little is known regarding the pharmacodynamic effects of resveratrol in humans, but the observation that it modulates components of the insulin-like growth factor system in the plasma of volunteers is encouraging. While the knowledge base that helps determine whether resveratrol may be useful in cancer management has increased substantially in recent years, important questions remain.

Keywords: resveratrol; cancer; clinical trial; pharmacokinetics; biomarkers; colon

Introduction

Resveratrol (*trans*-3,5,4′-trihydroxystilbene), which is found in red grapes, wine, nuts, and common or garden plants such as Japanese knotweed (*Polygonum cuspidatum*), is one of the most intensely investigated of all phytochemicals with putative beneficial effects on human health. Over the past 20 years, a plethora of publications have described a multitude of biochemical mechanisms engaged by resveratrol in preclinical systems, which may explain its pharmacological effects pertinent to cardiovascular health, obesity, diabetes, and cancer (for review, see Ref. 1). In contrast, relatively few reports of human intervention studies using resveratrol as a single agent exist in the literature (reviewed in Refs. 2–4). To date, the majority of these trials have been devoted to unraveling the systemic availability and metabolism of resveratrol, which is a particularly important issue since its three phenolic hydroxy moieties render the molecule exquisitely sensitive to conjugative metabolism and thus avid removal from plasma and tissues.

Among the pharmacological properties of resveratrol seen in preclinical systems, its anticarcinogenic effects represent some of the most convincing and intriguing.[5,6] Therefore, intervention studies of resveratrol targeted at cancer management are being received and discussed with particular eagerness by the nutraceutical research community. In the light of this interest, the aim of the present paper is to review clinical intervention studies of resveratrol that address questions pertinent to cancer prevention and treatment. This short review encompasses published studies and recent and ongoing trials listed on the clinicaltrials.gov website; the latter are referenced by the NCT trial identifier.

Preclinical evidence for the potential role of resveratrol in cancer management

In cells and subcellular systems, resveratrol has been convincingly shown to engage mechanisms that can interfere with certain hallmarks of cancer, common traits that govern the transformation of normal cells to malignancy. Prominent among

doi: 10.1111/nyas.12205

Ann. N.Y. Acad. Sci. 1290 (2013) 12–20 © 2013 New York Academy of Sciences.

these mechanisms are antioxidation, interference with cytochrome p450 isoenzymes, modulation of arachidonic acid metabolism through inhibition and downregulation of cyclooxygenase enzymes, and effects on transcription factors such as NF-κB.[7] More recent evidence has demonstrated the ability of resveratrol to act as a calorie restriction mimetic and protect against metabolic disease, via activation of the histone deacetylase SIRT1 and the adenosine monophosphate–activated protein kinase (AMPK), a critical energy sensor that maintains cellular energy balance and regulates metabolic function.[8,9] These pathways are also important in the development of malignancy and may therefore contribute to the anticancer activity of resveratrol.

When added to the diet of rodents, resveratrol has been shown to impede the development of cancer at multiple sites, including the colorectum, skin, pancreas, breast, and prostate.[6,10] Taken together, the preclinical evidence for anticarcinogenic effects exerted by resveratrol is sufficiently persuasive to consider early phase clinical intervention studies aimed at cancer management.

Design of early clinical trials to explore resveratrol for cancer management

The design of trials for exploring the potential usefulness of resveratrol in cancer management depends on whether the aim is related to chemoprevention or chemotherapy. In the case of chemoprevention, the long-term safety and acceptability of the chosen formulation to the trial subjects is an issue of prime importance, since it is ultimately likely that the agent will have to be taken for a very long period of time. A major objective of early chemoprevention trials is therefore to define the minimal dose that may be beneficial, while obviating any adverse effects.[11] In the case of early trials evaluating the potential chemotherapeutic benefit derived from resveratrol, either alone or more likely in combination with or following a standard treatment regimen, the emphasis needs to be on efficacy, and small to moderate untoward effects are acceptable. Administration is usually for relatively short periods, for weeks rather than the years required for chemopreventive interventions, and the predominant aim is to define the maximal, hopefully efficacious, nontoxic dose. Germane to both trial paradigms is the inclusion of potential pharmacodynamic biomarkers, that is, measurable changes

in biological processes intrinsically associated with antineoplastic mechanisms elicited by resveratrol. Such biomarkers would give an early indication of potential efficacy, and are of absolute crucial importance in the chemoprevention setting, where it is not feasible to wait for a clinically detectable outcome because of the time frames involved and size of trials needed to detect significant intervention-related differences in tumor development.[11,12] Furthermore, measures of activity in humans are also needed for initial dose titration, to identify the optimum dose to take forward into larger prevention trials.

The clinical studies of resveratrol that have hitherto been published and are described below are pilot studies (so-called phase 0 or phase I trials), involving a relatively small number of subjects and short duration, typically several days up to a few weeks.[2,3] The aim of these pilot trials has been to increase our knowledge of the absorption, distribution, metabolism, and elimination of resveratrol and of its pharmacodynamic effects in humans. A greater understanding of resveratrol pharmacodynamics will facilitate the discovery of potential biomarkers that are intrinsically linked to the key mechanisms of action.[13] These data are exceedingly useful, because they will help optimize the rational design of future large trials in which the putative efficacy of resveratrol is to be studied (phase II or phase III trials).

Clinical pharmacokinetics of resveratrol

In the trials performed to date aimed at elucidating its clinical pharmacokinetics, resveratrol has been taken either as a single-agent supplement or as part of a dietary mixture, with doses spanning a 1000-fold range (reviewed in Refs. 2–4). Overall, these studies suggest that resveratrol is rapidly metabolized in humans to conjugates with activated sulfate or UDP-glucuronic acid, which drastically curtails bioavailability of the parent, as consistently predicted from preclinical rodent experiments (for a summary of resveratrol metabolic conjugation in humans, see Fig. 1). The following section outlines the findings from selected trials of high dose resveratrol supplementation in healthy volunteers and cancer patients; the results presented are broadly representative of the body of clinical pharmacokinetic data currently available.

To define the single-dose plasma pharmacokinetics of resveratrol, healthy volunteers (10 per

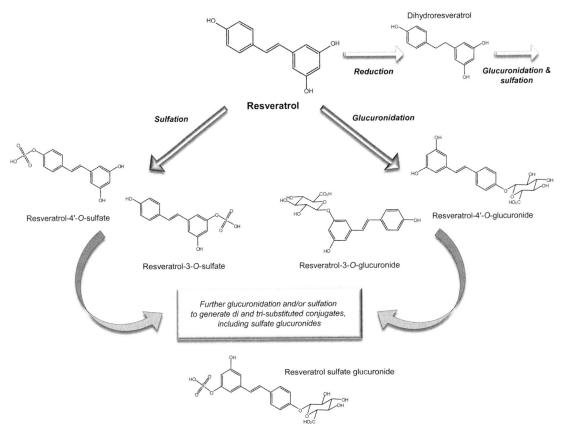

Figure 1. Overview of the major resveratrol conjugates detected in human samples.

group) received either 0.5, 1.0, 2.5, or 5.0 g, then resveratrol and its metabolites were quantified over 24 h by HPLC-UV analysis.[14] The maximal-mean plasma concentration of resveratrol achievable in these individuals was 2.3 ± 1.2 μM, which was achieved 1.5 h after ingestion of the highest dose. Peak levels of two monoglucuronides and resveratrol-3-*O*-sulfate were three- to eightfold higher than that of the parent. The area under the curve (AUC) values, which represent total exposure to a compound, for the 3-*O*-sulfate and resveratrol monoglucuronides were up to 23-fold greater than those of resveratrol itself. Renal excretion of resveratrol and its metabolites was rapid, with 77% of all urinary agent–derived species excreted within 4 h after the lowest dose. While metabolites dominated the urinary profile, they accounted for less than 1% of resveratrol species in fecal samples, which may be explained by the transit of appreciable amounts of nonabsorbed material or by conjugate hydrolysis within the gastrointestinal tract. In a subsequent

trial using the same protocol but for a period of 29 days, the pharmacokinetic consequence of multiple dosing was examined.[15] The maximal plasma concentration and area under the plasma concentration versus time curve in volunteers after 3–4 weeks of intervention were broadly similar to the values determined after a single exposure for any given dose. However, there was evidence of some resveratrol accumulation in those individuals receiving 5.0 g daily, with the average peak plasma level (4.2 μM) being about twice that achieved with an equivalent single dose. Maximal plasma levels of the two monoglucuronide metabolites in the highest dose group were twice as high as in the single-dose study, and AUC values for resveratrol and its metabolites consistently exceeded those observed after single dosing. Another subtle difference was apparent at the lowest dose (0.5 g), after which the greatest plasma concentrations attained for resveratrol-3-*O*-sulfate and the two monoglucuronides were 50–60% of those reached after a single dose; this is consistent with multiple administration causing inhibition of resveratrol conjugation or augmentation of metabolite elimination. The pattern of metabolites generated following repeated ingestion mirrored that produced by a single dose, with the 3-*O*-sulfate and the 4′- and 3-*O*-glucuronides being the major derivatives formed. These conjugates occurred at concentrations vastly exceeding the parent, by as much as 13-fold. Resveratrol undergoes metabolic reduction in humans to dihydroresveratrol through the action of intestinal bacteria, and this derivative can also be conjugated.[16] Furthermore, 3,4′-dihydroxy-*trans*-stilbene and 3,4′-dihydroxybibenzyl (lunularin) have very recently been described as novel dehydroxylated resveratrol metabolites generated by the gut microbiota, and it is conceivable that they may affect its pharmacological activities.[17]

In order to exert efficacy, resveratrol must be capable of reaching the target organ in sufficient concentrations to elicit molecular changes consistent with anticancer activity. Tissue levels of resveratrol have been studied in the colon, one of its potential targets for cancer chemoprevention in humans. Colorectal cancer patients earmarked for surgical resection received resveratrol for 8 days at either 0.5 g or 1.0 g daily (10 patients per group). HPLC-UV and LC-MS/MS analysis of the tumor and adjacent nonmalignant tissue revealed the presence of the parent as a predominant species, plus six conjugated metabolites, resveratrol-3-*O*-sulfate, resveratrol-4′-*O*-sulfate, resveratrol-3-*O*-glucuronide, resveratrol-4′-*O*-glucuronide, resveratrol disulfate, and resveratrol sulfate glucuronide.[18] Resveratrol concentrations measured within the colon at around 6 h after the last dose was taken were noticeably higher than those attained in the plasma for an equivalent dose, but were extremely variable; values ranged from nondetectable in some samples originating from the left side of the colorectum to as high as ∼3800 nmol/g in patients on the 1-g dose. Interestingly, higher concentrations were consistently achieved in tissue taken from the right side of the colon. A somewhat similar pilot study was conducted using SRT501 (Sirtris Pharmaceuticals Inc., Cambridge, MA), a proprietary formulation of micronized resveratrol designed to improve resveratrol absorption. Patients with metastatic colorectal cancer scheduled to undergo hepatectomy received fourteen daily doses of 5.0 g SRT501.[19] Detectable concentrations of resveratrol in hepatic tissues were found in five out of six patients. Mean concentrations were ∼5 nmol/g and ∼2 nmol/g in tumor and normal tissue, respectively, which is at least 134-fold lower than average levels previously detected in colon tissue after ingestion of one-fifth of the dose of nonmicronized resveratrol.[18] In contrast, SRT501 generated higher parent plasma concentrations (∼8.5 μM) than a comparable dose of nonmicronized resveratrol.[19] This study intimates that resveratrol can reach tissues distant to the gastrointestinal tract at potentially pharmacologically relevant concentrations. Thus far, resveratrol tissue pharmacokinetics have only been investigated in the colon and liver; further characterization in other target organs such as the prostate and pancreas is required to help assess the potential value of resveratrol in the management of these malignancies before conducting trials with activity/efficacy endpoints.

Safety of resveratrol

Preclinical toxicology data on resveratrol suggest that it possesses an excellent safety record. Daily intake of up to 700 mg/kg body weight has been found to be nontoxic in standard rodent tests.[20] A subchronic oral toxicity study in dogs demonstrated no treatment-related mortality, clinical signs of toxicity, or gross pathology up to doses of 1200 mg/kg/day.[21] There was, however, a significant reduction in mean body weight for both male and female animals at the highest intake level, which was associated with decreased food consumption. On the basis of body-weight effects, the no-observed-adverse-effect level for resveratrol in dogs was 600 mg/kg/day.[21] To date, safety and tolerability has been assessed in just a small number of human studies.[14,15,18,22–24] Only a fraction of these incorporated a placebo control group, so it is difficult to unequivocally ascribe the adverse effects observed to resveratrol. When taken as a single oral dose, resveratrol (0.5–5.0 g) was well tolerated by healthy volunteers.[14] In the follow-up study involving daily ingestion of resveratrol over the same dose range but for 29 days, 28 of the 40 volunteers experienced one or more adverse events while on the trial. The majority of these occurred in subjects on the two highest doses (2.5 and 5.0 g).[15] The most common side effects were gastrointestinal, particularly diarrhea, nausea, and abdominal pain, which were only reported in individuals consuming more than 1.0 g per day. Consistent with these findings, in another trial resveratrol (2.0 g) taken twice daily for two periods of eight days was also well tolerated by healthy subjects with no clinically relevant changes in serum biochemistry or hematological parameters. However, mild diarrhea was observed in three-fourths of the volunteers.[23]

The safety of resveratrol and its micronized formulation SRT501 has been assessed in patients with primary colorectal cancer and hepatic metastases, respectively. Ingestion of 0.5 or 1.0 g resveratrol for eight days before resection did not cause any resveratrol-related side effects and was well tolerated, consistent with observations in volunteers.[15] In the small placebo-controlled pilot study of SRT501,[19] in which six patients received 5.0 g of SRT501 daily for ~14 days before surgery, adverse events possibly attributable to the intervention were primarily gastrointestinal and mild. Other adverse reactions included skin irritation, rash, chills, and vascular flushing, which all resolved without consequences. SRT501 was also studied in a phase II trial in patients with multiple myeloma who had relapsed or were refractory to prior therapy.[25] Patients received SRT501 (5.0 g) with or without bortezumib daily for 20 days per treatment cycle. The trial was suspended in early 2010 due to safety concerns, as five of the 24 patients recruited developed unexpected renal failure.[25] The authors noted that nephrotoxicity was not reported in other trials of SRT501 and that renal impairment is commonly associated with multiple myeloma and can occur in up to 50% of patients; this specific group may therefore be at an increased risk of renal failure due to their underlying condition.

Another aspect of the safety of resveratrol concerns its putative potential to interfere with the pharmacokinetics of other drugs, thus eliciting unwanted and potentially harmful drug interactions. Chow *et al.*[24] investigated the effects of resveratrol on the activity and/or expression of a series of drug-metabolizing enzymes, including the phase I mono-oxygenases CYP1A2, CYP2D6, CYP2C9, and CYP3A4 in healthy volunteers. Intervention with resveratrol (1.0 g daily) for four weeks inhibited the phenotypic indices of CYP3A4, CYP2D6, and CYP2C9 compared to predose activity, while inducing CYP1A2. Since CYP3A4, CYP2D6, and CYP2C9 are responsible for metabolizing the majority of drug classes, the findings intimate that resveratrol may reduce the clearance and increase plasma levels of many coadministered drugs, which may in turn lead to toxicity. A similar hypothesis is currently being tested in a clinical study at the University of Washington (NCT01173640). The aim is to explore whether resveratrol can inhibit human intestinal and hepatic CYP3A4 enzymes, as reflected by the clearance of the prototypic CYP3A4 probe drug, midazolam. Individuals receive a single or multiple (seven) daily doses of 1 g resveratrol before oral midazolam, and concentrations of midazolam and its metabolites are measured in blood and urine then compared to baseline kinetic profiles in each volunteer to identify alterations associated with resveratrol ingestion.

The safety data accumulated so far have engendered the recommendation that resveratrol doses lower than 1.0 g should be employed in future clinical trials.[25] Furthermore, caution is needed when new resveratrol formulations with enhanced bioavailability are studied, as the potential for interactions is likely to be greater than for the equivalent dose of unformulated resveratrol.

Clinical pharmacodynamics of resveratrol germane to anticarcinogenesis

Considering the abundance of preclinical data on anticarcinogenic mechanisms engaged by resveratrol, there is relatively little information on corresponding pharmacodynamic effects in humans. Published pharmacodynamic trial endpoints germane to cancer relate to signaling via the insulin system or Wnt, redox status, and cellular energy metabolism. Most of these studies have been conducted in healthy individuals or patients suffering from conditions other than cancer.

The effect of resveratrol (0.5–5.0 g daily) on components of the insulin-like growth factor (IGF) system has been investigated in healthy volunteers following ingestion for four weeks.[15] This signaling system influences malignant development in that IGFs, which are antiapoptotic and mitogenic[26,27] can affect neoplastic transformation, cell differentiation, and metastasis.[26,28,29] The system is regulated by IGF-binding proteins, particularly IGFBP-3, which sequester IGFs in the extracellular milieu, decreasing circulating concentrations and the possibility for interaction with IGF receptors. The potential importance of IGF-1 in cancer is illustrated by several studies describing a direct relationship between levels of IGF-1 and risk of lung, prostate, colorectal, or breast cancer.[30] Current information on the role of IGFBP-3 is conflicting. Conventionally, this peptide is thought to have a protective effect due to IGF-1 binding; however, there are also data indicating that higher concentrations are associated with an increased, rather than reduced, risk of breast cancer in premenopausal women.[31] Moreover, although high levels inversely correlated with lung cancer risk in a meta-regression analysis, there was no such relationship with other cancers, including colon and prostate.[31] In the volunteer trial, when results from all participants were combined regardless of dose, consumption of resveratrol was associated with a significant but small reduction in both IGF-1 and IGFBP-3 compared to preintervention baseline levels.[15] However, when each dose group was considered separately, the most prominent and consistent reductions in plasma IGF-1 occurred in those ingesting 2.5 g resveratrol, whereas the other doses (0.5, 1.0, 5.0 g) had no significant effect. Average IGFBP-3 concentrations were also significantly decreased in volunteers taking 1.0 or 2.5 g resveratrol, but no changes were evident in the remaining dose groups.

The Wnt signaling cascade is critically important in the development of colon cancer and is activated in >85% of sporadic cases. Constitutive activation of the pathway promotes cell growth and proliferation while inhibiting normal patterns of colonic stem cell differentiation. On the back of preclinical data revealing that resveratrol can inhibit Wnt signaling, Nguyen *et al.* conducted a recent phase I pilot study to ascertain whether these effects might translate to humans.[32] Eight patients with colon cancer received up to ~16 mg of resveratrol per day as a plant-derived formulation that also contained quercetin, or as a grape seed extract containing numerous other potentially bioactive constituents, for two weeks before surgical resection. Neither intervention was found to inhibit the Wnt pathway in malignant colon tissue, assessed using a gene expression array for Wnt ligands and their receptors, intracellular signaling molecules, and representative target genes. However, alterations between pre- and postintervention samples were evident in normal colonic mucosa, although the most significant reduction in Wnt target gene expression was seen with the grape seed extract, which actually contained the lowest amount of resveratrol. Drawing conclusions from this study

with respect to resveratrol is extremely difficult owing to its small size and the presence of other active compounds in both formulations used; further investigations are needed to ascertain whether resveratrol affects Wnt signaling in humans.

Other evidence in support of resveratrol activity in target tissues comes from a study by Patel *et al.*, in which the effect of resveratrol on colorectal epithelial cell proliferation was examined in tumor tissue from patients that ingested resveratrol (0.5 or 1.0 g/daily) for eight days before surgery.[18] Resveratrol exposure was associated with reduced proliferation compared to predose levels, as assessed by Ki-67 positivity detected by immunohistochemistry. Although the effect was small and only significant when data were combined from patients in both dose groups, it suggests resveratrol has the potential to favorably alter cell proliferation in humans.

In a current trial (NCT01476592) the hypothesis is being tested that resveratrol can alter Notch-1 signaling in patients with neuroendocrine tumors. Emerging data indicate that Notch signaling pathways play important roles in the development and progression of a variety of cancers.[33] In this trial, patients receive 2.5 g resveratrol twice daily for up to three months, and expression of Notch-related proteins is compared in pre- and post-treatment tumor specimens. Secondary outcome measures include assessment of resveratrol toxicity and tolerability in this patient population and the effect of resveratrol on tumor growth, as demonstrated by standard cross-sectional imaging and levels of tumor markers. Results have thus far not been communicated.

One of the properties of resveratrol that has received considerable scientific and media attention is its ability to mimic calorie restriction in preclinical models.[1] This feature is important for the potential usefulness of resveratrol in the prevention and treatment of obesity and age-related diseases such as diabetes. It is also attractive and intriguing from the standpoint of cancer management in the light of preclinical investigations supporting the notion that calorie restriction is a feasible cancer prevention strategy.[34] Although the precise biochemical mechanisms involved are still rather obscure, it is now accepted that modulation of cellular energy metabolism can affect the process of carcinogenesis. In a recent trial in obese men, a daily dietary supplement of 150 mg resveratrol ingested for 30 days decreased total energy expenditure and improved measures of metabolism and overall health to the extent that the trial participants appeared to have similar metabolic changes as people subjected to severe calorie restriction.[35] One can only speculate as to the potential tantalizing implications of this finding in relation to the putative cancer chemopreventive activity of resveratrol. One must also bear in mind that the beneficial effects on energy metabolism indicated in this trial may well be restricted to obese individuals. In this respect, Yoshino *et al.* recently reported that resveratrol supplementation (75 mg/day) failed to exert beneficial metabolic effects in nonobese, postmenopausal women with normal glucose tolerance.[36]

Oxidative stress has long been considered a carcinogenic trigger; it therefore seems to follow that strategies to reduce reactive oxygen species may potentially contribute to the prevention of cancer. In a placebo-controlled trial in type 2 diabetics, men were randomized to resveratrol (2 × 5 mg daily) or placebo for four weeks.[37] At the end of the intervention period, those patients on active treatment had significantly decreased insulin resistance and urinary ortho-tyrosine excretion, which is a measure of oxidative stress. Moreover, the ratio of phosphorylated protein kinase B to protein kinase B (pAkt/Akt) in platelets was increased. It was postulated that the effects observed may be attributed to resveratrol decreasing oxidative stress, which subsequently leads to more efficient insulin signaling via the Akt pathway.[37]

Another study providing evidence that resveratrol may act as an antioxidant in humans was designed to establish whether a preparation containing resveratrol (100 mg) plus other polyphenols (75 mg) from *P. cuspidatum* and grape extracts can protect against the oxidative and inflammatory stress caused by consumption of a high-carbohydrate, high-fat meal.[38] Intake of the supplement by ten healthy volunteers interfered with postprandial circulating indicators of inflammatory and oxidative stress, also stimulating activity of the transcription factor Nrf-2 and increasing the expression of its target antioxidant genes NQO1 and GST-π1 in blood cells. As with other trials utilizing mixtures, the presence of additional polyphenols in the test preparation confounds the interpretation of these data, but the observations suggest it may reduce acute oxidative and inflammatory responses in the postprandial state. These general properties may have implications for

the management of a variety of diseases, including cancer.

A trial conceived specifically to investigate the antioxidant and anti-inflammatory effects of resveratrol in otherwise healthy, tobacco-smoking adults has recently been completed at the University of Turin (NCT01492114). The underlying hypothesis is that resveratrol may protect against the inflammatory and oxidative mediators that characterize the low-grade systemic inflammatory state and the oxidant/antioxidant imbalance of tobacco users. In this randomized, placebo-controlled, crossover study, resveratrol (500 mg daily) was administered to 40 participants for 30 days, with a total study duration, including wash-out period, of three months. Parameters under investigation include intervention-induced changes in circulating concentrations of C-reactive protein, total antioxidant status, and levels of 4-hydroxynonenal and nitrotyrosine. The results from this trial have yet to be published.

Conclusion

The studies of resveratrol outlined above have employed a wide range of doses. For example, in the pharmacokinetic trial in healthy volunteers[15] the maximum daily dose employed was 5 grams. In contrast, just 10 mg per day was required to elicit antioxidant effects in diabetic men.[37] This discrepancy suggests that rationalizing the ideal dose of resveratrol is complicated. One must also remember that the dose of resveratrol when ingested in the diet is at most a few milligrams, suggesting that effects of such low doses are certainly worthy of investigation. However, experiments using such tiny doses of resveratrol pose considerable experimental challenges, not least on the analytical chemistry front.[11] The traditionally designed clinical studies have attempted to define the highest safe dose. The objective here was driven by the desire to achieve levels in the plasma and tissues that mimic concentrations of resveratrol shown to elicit biochemical changes in cells or isolated biomatrices *in vitro*, which are typically in the order of 10^{-5} M or more. The issue is made even more complex by the suspicion that the pharmacological effects exerted by resveratrol—as is probably the case for many other diet-derived agents—may be governed by a bell-shaped concentration–response curve, meaning that low concentrations may be more active than higher ones for certain molecular targets.[13,39]

In summary, the trials reviewed here suggest that the clinical knowledge base to help determine whether resveratrol may be useful in cancer management, and if so how, has increased substantially over the past few years. The overall evidence seems to suggest that ingestion of resveratrol at daily doses of up to 1 g is safe, and that the molecule can reach tissues remote from the site of absorption. There are also several tantalizing indications of mechanistic changes in human biomatrices. Nevertheless, crucial gaps in insight remain, and they need to be bridged before large clinical trials of resveratrol in the chemoprevention or chemotherapy of particular malignancies can be convincingly advocated. Prominent among the important questions that need to be addressed are the optimal efficacious dose and the discovery and validation of suitable mechanism-based biomarkers indicative of efficacy.

Acknowledgments

We thank Cancer Research UK for funding (program Grant C325/A6691; ECMC C325/A15575, in conjunction with the UK Department of Health) and the United Kingdom Environmental Mutagen Society for sponsorship of Resveratrol 2012, the 2nd International Scientific Conference on Resveratrol and Health.

Conflicts of interest

The authors declare no conflicts of interest.

References

1. Baur, J.A. & D.A. Sinclair. 2006. Therapeutic potential of resveratrol: the *in vivo* evidence. *Nat. Rev. Drug Discover.* **5:** 493–506.
2. Smoliga, J.M., J.A. Baur & H.A. Hausenblas. 2011. Resveratrol and health—a comprehensive review of clinical trials. *Mol. Nutr. Food Res.* **55:** 1129–1141.
3. Patel, K.R., E. Scott, V.A. Brown, *et al.* 2011. Clinical trials of resveratrol. *Ann. N.Y. Acad. Sci.* **1215:** 161–169.
4. Patel, K.R., W.P. Steward, A.J. Gescher & K. Brown. 2012. Clinical development of resveratrol. In *Resveratrol: Sources, Production and Health Benefits.* Chapter 23, Delmas, D., Ed.: 511–532. Nova Science Publishers, Huntington, NY.
5. Jang, M., L. Cai, G.O. Udeani, *et al.* 1997. Cancer chemopreventive activity of resveratrol, a natural product derived from grapes. *Science* **275:** 218–220.
6. Bishayee, A. 2009. Cancer prevention and treatment with resveratrol: from rodent studies to clinical trials. *Cancer Prev. Res.* **2:** 409–418.
7. Pezzuto, J.M. 2008. Resveratrol as an inhibitor of carcinogenesis. *Pharmaceutical Biol.* **46,** 443–457.
8. Baur, J.A., K.J. Pearson, N.L. Price, *et al.* 2006. Resveratrol improves health and survival of mice on a high-calorie diet. *Nature* **444:** 337–342.
9. Price, N.L., A.P. Gomes, A.J.Y. Ling, *et al.* 2012. SIRT1 is required for AMPK activation and the beneficial effects of resveratrol on mitochondrial function. *Cell Metab.* **15:** 675–690.
10. Vang, O., N. Ahmad, C.A. Baile, *et al.* 2011. What is new for an old molecule? Systematic review and recommendations on the use of resveratrol. *PLoS One* **6,** e19881.
11. Scott, E.N., A.J. Gescher, W.P. Steward & K. Brown. 2009. Development of dietary phytochemical chemopreventive agents: biomarkers and choice of dose for early clinical trials. *Cancer Prev. Res.* **2:** 525–530.
12. Kelloff, G.J., S.M. Lippman, A.J. Dannenberg, *et al.* 2006. Progress in chemoprevention drug development: the promise of molecular biomarkers for prevention of intraepithelial neoplasia and cancer–a plan to move forward. *Clin. Cancer Res.* **12:** 3661–3697.
13. Scott, E., W.P. Steward, A.J. Gescher & K. Brown. 2011. Resveratrol in human cancer chemoprevention – choosing the "right" dose. *Mol. Nutr. Food Res.* **56:** 7–13.
14. Boocock, D.J., G.E. Faust, K.R. Patel, *et al.* 2007. Phase I dose escalation pharmacokinetic study in healthy volunteers of resveratrol, a potential cancer chemopreventive agent. *Cancer Epidemiol. Biomarkers Prev.* **16:** 1246–1252.
15. Brown, V., K. Patel, M. Viskaduraki, *et al.* 2010. Repeat dose study of the cancer chemopreventive agent resveratrol in healthy volunteers: safety, pharmacokinetics and effect on the insulin-like growth factor axis. *Cancer Res.* **70:** 9003–9011.
16. Rotches Ribalta, M., C. Andres-Lacueva, R. Estruch, *et al.* 2012. Pharmacokinetics of resveratrol metabolic profile in healthy humans after moderate consumption of red wine and grape extract tablets. *Pharmacol. Res.* **66:** 375–382.
17. Bode, L.M., D. Bunzel, M. Huch, *et al.* 2013. In vivo and in vitro metabolism of trans-resveratrol by human gut microbiota. *Am. J. Clin. Nutr.* **97:** 295–309.
18. Patel, K.R., V.A. Brown, D.J.L. Jones, *et al.* 2010. Clinical pharmacology of resveratrol and its metabolites in colorectal cancer patients. *Cancer Res.* **70:** 7392–7399.
19. Howells, L.M., D.P. Berry, P.J, Elliott, *et al.* 2011. Phase I randomized, double-blind pilot study of micronized resveratrol (SRT501) in patients with hepatic metastases—safety, pharmacokinetics, and pharmacodynamics. *Cancer Prev. Res.* **4:** 1419–1425.
20. Williams, L.D., G.A. Burdock, J.A. Edwards, *et al.* 2009. Safety studies conducted on high-purity trans-resveratrol in experimental animals. *Food Chem. Toxicol.* **47:** 2170–2182.
21. Johnson, W.D., R.L. Morrissey, A.L. Usborne, *et al.* 2011. Subchronic oral toxicity and cardiovascular safety pharmacology studies of resveratrol, a naturally occurring polyphenol with cancer preventive activity. *Food Chem. Tox.* **49:** 3319–3327.
22. Almeida, L., M. Vaz-da-Silva, A. Falcao, *et al.* 2009. Pharmacokinetic and safety profile of trans-resveratrol in a rising multiple-dose study in healthy volunteers. *Mol. Nutr. Food Res.* **53**(Suppl 1): S7–S15.

23. la Porte, C., N. Voduc, G. Zhang, *et al.* 2010. Steady-State pharmacokinetics and tolerability of trans-resveratrol 2000 mg twice daily with food, quercetin and alcohol (ethanol) in healthy human subjects. *Clin. Pharmacokinet.* **49:** 449–454.

24. Chow, H.H., L.L. Garland, C.H. Hsu, *et al.* 2010. Resveratrol modulates drug- and carcinogen-metabolizing enzymes in a healthy volunteer study. *Cancer Prev. Res.* **3:** 1168–1175.

25. Popat, R., T. Plesner, F. Davies, *et al.* 2013. A phase 2 study of SRT501 (resveratrol) with bortezomib for patients with relapsed and or refractory multiple myeloma. *Br. J. Haematol.* **160:** 714–717.

26. Butt, A.J., S.M. Firth & R.C. Baxter. 1999. The IGF axis and programmed cell death. *Immunol. Cell Biol.* **77:** 256–262.

27. Ibrahim, Y.H. & D. Yee. 2004. Insulin-like growth factor-1 and cancer risk. *Growth Horm. IGF Res.* **14:** 261–269.

28. Lopez, T. & D. Hanahan. 2002. Elevated levels of IGF-1 receptor convey invasive and metastatic capability in a mouse model of pancreatic isle tumorigenesis. *Cancer Cell* **1:** 339–353.

29. Samani, A.A., E. Chevet, L. Fallavollita, *et al.* 2004. Loss of tumorigenicity and metastatic potential in carcinoma cells expressing the extracellular domain of the type 1 insulin-like growth factor receptor. *Cancer Res.* **64:** 3380–3385.

30. Sandhu, M.S., D.B. Dunger & E.L. Giovannucci. 2002. Insulin, insulin-like growth factor-I (IGF-I), IGF binding proteins, their biologic interactions, and colorectal cancer. *J. Natl. Cancer Inst.* **94:** 972–980.

31. Renehan, A.G., M. Zwahlen, C. Minder, *et al.* 2004. Insulin-like growth factor (IGF)-1, IGF binding protein-3, and cancer risk: systematic review and meta-regression analysis. *Lancet* **363:** 1346–1353.

32. Nguyen, A.V., M. Martinez, M.J. Stamos, *et al.* 2009. Results of a phase I pilot clinical trial examining the effect of plant-derived resveratrol and grape powder on Wnt pathway target gene expression in colonic mucosa and colon cancer. *Cancer Manag. Res.* **1:** 25–37.

33. Jun, H.T., J. Stevens & P. Kaplan-Lefko. 2008. Top NOTCH targets: notch signaling in cancer. *Drug Develop. Res.* **69:** 319–328.

34. Grifantini, K. 2008. Understanding pathways of calorie restriction: a way to prevent cancer? *J. Natl. Cancer Inst.* **100:** 619–621.

35. Timmers, S., E. Konings, L. Bilet, *et al.* 2011. Calorie restriction-like effects of 30 days of resveratrol supplementation on energy metabolism and metabolic profile in obese humans. *Cell Metab.* **14:** 612–622.

36. Yoshino, J., C. Conte, L. Fontana, *et al.* 2012. Resveratrol supplementation does not improve metabolic function in non-obese women with normal glucose tolerance. *Cell Metab.* **16:** 658–664.

37. Brasnyo, P., G.A. Molnar, M. Mohas, *et al.* 2011. Resveratrol improves insulin sensitivity, reduces oxidative stress and activates the Akt pathway in type 2 diabetic patients. *Br. J. Nutr.* **106:** 383–389.

38. Ghanim, H., C.L. Sia, K. Korzeniewski, *et al.* 2011. A resveratrol and polyphenol preparation suppresses oxidative and inflammatory stress response to a high-fat, high-carbohydrate meal. *J. Clin. Endocrinol. Metab.* **96:** 1409–1414.

39. Calabrese, E.J., M.P. Mattson & V. Calabrese. 2010. Resveratrol commonly displays hormesis: occurrence and biomedical significance. *Hum. Exp. Toxicol.* **29:** 980–1015.

Ann. N.Y. Acad. Sci. ISSN 0077-8923

ANNALS OF THE NEW YORK ACADEMY OF SCIENCES

Issue: *Resveratrol and Health*

Resveratrol analogs: promising chemopreventive agents

Talysa Ogas, Tamara P. Kondratyuk, and John M. Pezzuto

Daniel K. Inouye College of Pharmacy, University of Hawaii at Hilo, Hilo, Hawaii

Address for correspondence: John M. Pezzuto, Daniel K. Inouye College of Pharmacy, University of Hawaii at Hilo, 34 Rainbow Drive, Hilo, HI 96720. pezzuto@hawaii.edu

Although resveratrol can modulate multiple stages of carcinogenesis, by most common standards it is not a good drug candidate. Resveratrol lacks potency, high efficacy, and target specificity; it is rapidly metabolized and serum concentrations are low. Using resveratrol as a scaffold, we produced over 100 derivatives, some of which have target specificity in the nanomolar range. Aromatase inhibition was enhanced over 6000-fold by using 1,3-thiazole as the central ring of resveratrol. Optimizing the substitution pattern of the two phenyl rings and the central heterocyclic linker led to selective QR1 induction with a CD value of 87 nM. Several derivatives have been selected for evaluation of synergistic effects. Preliminary results with pairs of compounds are promising and further experiments, in a constant multidrug manner, will allow us to create polygonograms for larger combinations of derivatives. The objective is to develop a highly efficacious cocktail of derivatives based on the structure of resveratrol.

Keywords: chemoprevention; combination; derivatives; metabolites; resveratrol; synergy

Resveratrol has been reported to exert a variety of biological activities. Some of these include antioxidant, anti-inflammatory, anti-infective, anti-ischemic, cardioprotective, neuroprotective, anti-aging (prolongs life span), antiobesity, antiviral, and cancer chemopreventive effects.[1–4] We have primarily focused on cancer chemoprevention, an approach to decrease cancer morbidity and mortality through inhibition of carcinogenesis and prevention of disease progression. Although the *trans*-stilbene resveratrol has chemopreventive properties, its action is compromised by weak nonspecific effects on many biological targets. Resveratrol is known to exhibit low oral bioavailability with high absorption but rapid metabolism and low tissue concentrations.[5–8] In human studies, when given an oral dose of 25 mg, 70% absorption was observed; peak plasma (C_{max}) levels of resveratrol and metabolites combined were about 490 ng/mL, with a C_{max} of unchanged resveratrol less than 5 ng/mL and a half-life ($t_{1/2}$) of 9 h. The bioavailability of unchanged resveratrol was close to nil.[5] The most abundant metabolites of resveratrol result from first-pass metabolism yielding sulfate and glucuronic acid conjugates.[5–7]

The efficient absorption of resveratrol upon oral administration, followed by rapid metabolism, casts doubt on the physiological relevance of high resveratrol concentrations typically used for *in vitro* studies. It may be suggested that at least some, if not most, of the biological effects elicited by resveratrol may be attributed to resveratrol metabolites.[8] Not surprisingly, the activities of the sulfate metabolites decrease in general as the degree of sulfation increases, although there are exceptions. For example, the 3-sulfate was more potent than resveratrol as an inhibitor of COX-1[9] and 12-*O*-tetradecanoylphorbol 13-acetate (TPA)–induced ornithine decarboxylase (ODC),[10] whereas the other sulfate metabolites were all less potent. However, all of the sulfates retained some degree of activity. Because serum concentrations of sulfated metabolites are higher than the serum concentrations of resveratrol, the ability of the metabolites to typically retain some degree of activity may be of relevance.[9,11]

The C_{max} of unchanged resveratrol can be increased with the administration of high doses, for example, 0.5–5 g given orally once or twice daily, which appear to be well tolerated in healthy human subjects with minimal adverse side effects.[7,12] At a 5 g

doi: 10.1111/nyas.12196

oral dose of resveratrol, peak plasma concentration of unchanged resveratrol reached 538 ng/mL, with rapid absorption and low bioavailability.[7] Other factors, such as a high-fat diet, have been taken into account in order to determine the effects on resveratrol steady-state pharmacokinetics. It was found that a high-fat breakfast significantly decreased the C_{max} of a 2-g twice-daily oral dose of resveratrol by up to 46%.[12]

Although it is common for polyphenols to be rapidly metabolized and have low bioavailability, derivatives of polyphenols can show increased *in vivo* stability (e.g., methylated polyphenols[13]). Pterostilbene, a dimethyl ether analog of resveratrol with the same peroxyl-radical scavenging activity as resveratrol, has a bioavailability of 80% in rats, as opposed to 20% for resveratrol.[6,14] Due to low bioavailability, the logical approach is to use derivatives as a storage pool for resveratrol.[5,6] Desirable targets of resveratrol would require the use of these derivatives to reach the site of action by increasing bioavailability, peak plasma concentrations, and the overall stability of the molecule.

Molecular targets for resveratrol analogs

As noted, by many common standards in the field of drug development, resveratrol is not a good candidate. Importantly, however, resveratrol can interact with numerous targets, albeit in a weak and nonspecific manner. Logic would thereby dictate this is a superb lead for serving as a scaffold for the production of structural derivatives that could show greater efficacy and improved characteristics. Based on this notion, we designed, synthesized, and evaluated the biological activity of over 100 resveratrol derivatives. The derivatives include compounds differing in the number, position, and type of substituents and the presence or absence of the stilbenic double bond. Sulfate derivatives were synthesized and tested as well, because serum concentrations of these metabolites are higher than those of resveratrol following ingestion of the parent compound. We used a battery of *in vitro* assays to monitor the activity of all the designed derivatives, and some preliminary absorption and metabolism studies were performed with promising leads.[10]

Aromatase
Aromatase is one attractive target for the development of new agents for the prevention or treatment of breast cancer. Selective inhibition of aromatase, the enzyme responsible for the final step of estrogen biosynthesis, will not interfere with the production of other steroids.[15] Resveratrol (compound 1, Fig. 1) has relatively weak activity against aromatase ($IC_{50} = 48$ μM), but a series of resveratrol analogs displayed much greater inhibition. First, the *trans*-stilbene with a *para*-amino group was found to exhibit multiple biological activities including inhibition of nitric oxide synthase and of TNF-α–induced NF-κB activity, and was selected as a lead compound for further optimization. In order to improve the potency and selectivity, a limited number of methoxylated compounds were synthesized and observed empirically to enhance aromatase inhibitory activity. In particular, compound 2 (Fig. 1) was found to possess significant aromatase-inhibitory activity, with an IC_{50} value of 0.59 μM, which is comparable to the clinically useful aromatase inhibitor 2-aminoglutethimide ($IC_{50} = 0.27$ μM).[16] However, this response was not selective, so molecular modeling was used to investigate the mode of interaction, and a variety of structurally related stilbenes were designed and synthesized based on the results.

The crystal structure of human aromatase (PDB 3eqm) was used to analyze the mechanism of action of the aromatase inhibitor 2 through docking, molecular mechanics energy minimization, and computer graphics molecular modeling, and the information was utilized to design several very potent inhibitors of aromatase activity with IC_{50} values in the sub-micromolar or nanomolar range, including compounds 3 ($IC_{50} = 70$ nM) and 4 ($IC_{50} = 36$ nM).[16] From the preliminary structure–activity relationships and molecular modeling results, it appears that the *para*-amino group on the *trans*-stilbene benzene ring is essential for aromatase inhibitory activity, and the introduction of an imidazole moiety improves the activity greatly.[16]

In addition, the moderate and nonselective aromatase inhibitory activity of resveratrol was improved about 100-fold by replacement of the ethylenic bridge with a thiadiazole and the phenyl rings with pyridines (e.g., compound 5). Using this new framework provided higher accessibility and a more feasible chemical pathway. Thiazole derivatives with different "A" ring *para* substitutions were prepared and tested for their aromatase inhibitory activity. Among this set of compounds, the 4-pyridyl

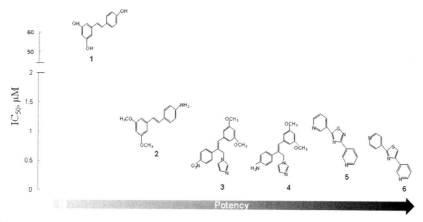

Figure 1. Inhibitory effect of resveratrol derivatives on aromatase. Aromatase activity was assayed as previously reported, with the necessary modifications to assay in a 384-well plate.[12] After termination of the reaction and shaking for 5 min, the plate was further incubated for 2 h at 37 °C. This enhances the ratio of signal to background. Fluorescence was measured at 485 nm (excitation) and 530 nm (emission). IC_{50} values were based on three independent experiments performed in duplicate using five concentrations of test substance. Naringenin (IC_{50} = 0.23 μM) was used as a positive control.

derivative (compound 6, Fig. 1) showed significantly greater inhibitory activity, with an IC_{50} value of 4 nM. These values are comparable with those of the clinically available nonsteroidal aromatase inhibitors letrozole, anastrozole, and fadrozole, suggesting this compound is a good drug candidate.

NF-κB signaling

As mentioned earlier, all compounds were subjected to a range of chemopreventive assays to test their target selectivity. Compound 6 had moderate NF-κB–inhibitory activity, with an IC_{50} of 2.5 μM. The aromatase-inhibitory activity was enhanced over 6000-fold by using 1,3-thiazole as the central ring and modifying the substituents on the "A" ring to target the Met374 residue of aromatase. On the other hand, targeting the hydroxyl group of Thr310 by a hydrogen-bond acceptor on the "B" ring did not improve the aromatase-inhibitory activity.[17]

Replacement of the stilbene ethylenic bridge of resveratrol with a 1,2,4-thiadiazole heterocycle and modification of the substituents on the two aromatic rings afforded potential chemopreventive agents with enhanced potencies not only for aromatase but for NF-κB and inducers of quinone reductase 1 (QR1).[18]

NAD(P)H:quinone reductase (QR1)

In principle, cancer chemoprevention can be achieved by terminating the effects of carcinogens through inhibiting or downregulating enzymes capable of generating cancer-promoting or car-

cinogenic species such as aromatase and inducible nitric oxide synthase (iNOS). On the other hand, cancer chemoprevention could also be achieved by activating or upregulating anticarcinogenic enzymes, which include electrophile-processing cytoprotective enzymes such as glutathione *S*-transferases, as well as superoxide dismutase and NAD(P)H:quinone reductase (QR1).[19] QR1 protects cells from the cytotoxic effects of free radicals by several different mechanisms. This enzyme catalyzes the NAD(P)H-dependent two-electron reduction pathway of quinones to hydroquinones, which are stable structures that bypass the radical pathway to semiquinones. QR1 inducers protect cells from oxidative stress mainly by diverting quinone metabolism away from the free radical–generating one-electron reduction pathway to the two-electron reduction pathway, which produces neutral hydroquinones. QR1 inducers can also generate α-tocopherolhydroquinone, which acts as a free radical scavenger.

A useful parameter employed to compare the QR1-induction activities of different compounds is the CD value, that is, the concentration that doubles QR1 activity. Because resveratrol is a weak QR1 inducer (CD = 21 μM), we investigated resveratrol derivatives that might show greater QR1-induction efficacy and selectivity. 3,5-Diphenyl-1,2,4-thiadiazole (compound 7, Fig. 2) provided a new scaffold for potent QR1 inducers. This new scaffold was derived from the natural product

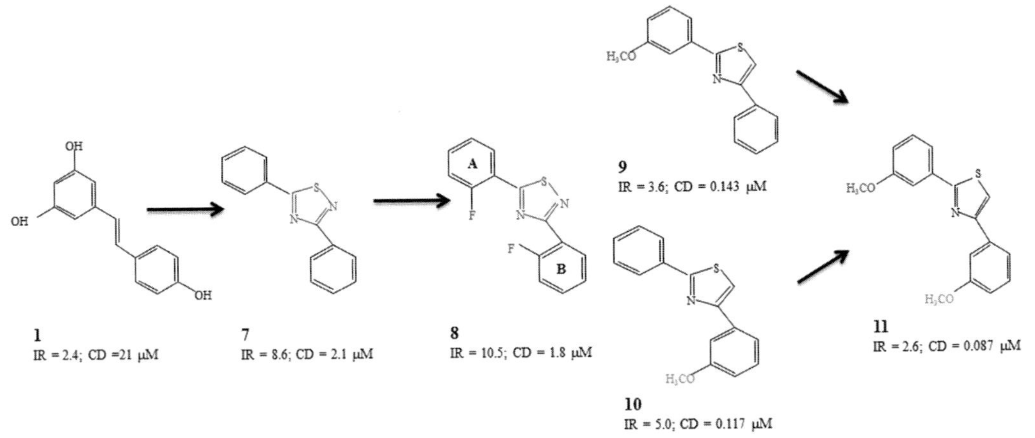

Figure 2. Using thiazole as a central ring and optimizing substitutions on the "A" and "B" rings provided potent QR1 inducers. IR: induction ratio. CD: compound concentration that doubles QR1 activity. CD values were determined for compounds with induction ratios >2. The two peripheral rings are arbitrarily denoted "A" and "B" in compound 3.

resveratrol by replacement of the ethylene linker with a five-membered heterocycle. Starting from the lead compound 7, its difluoro derivative 8 was obtained with a notable improvement in QR1-induction activity (CD = 1.8 μM) relative to resveratrol. Using thiazole as a central ring and optimizing substitutions on both the "A" and "B" rings provided very potent QR1 inducers such as compounds 9 (CD = 0.143 μM), 10 (CD = 0.117 μM), and 11 (CD = 0.087 μM) (Fig. 2).

Combinatorial analysis of resveratrol derivatives

The first step in our multifactorial approach requires the discovery and characterization of single resveratrol derivatives. It is necessary to test each agent singly in order to learn about the mechanism of action, metabolism, absorption, and behavior in animal models. As a result, these single agents may be viewed as promising candidates for further development. However, the ultimate goal of our work is to test combinations of chemical relatives in models with greater physiological complexity, such as breast cancer cells in culture. This is based on the notion that a strong synergistic response can be generated with unprecedented efficacy. In essence, this paradigm mimics empirical observations that mixtures of phytochemicals in the diet may mediate better responses than single pure isolates. But in contrast, our proposed multicomponent formulation based on the resveratrol scaffold will be rational, reproducible, and subject to well-defined

clinical protocols. Resveratrol is not a magic bullet. It is a promiscuous low molecular weight stilbene that has shown us the way to potentially create a magic bullet for the chemoprevention of cancer.

Along these lines, we have selected four promising compounds for more advanced testing and development. Compounds 12–15 (Table 1) show selective activity against aromatase, NF-κB, quinone reductase 2 (QR2), and ODC, respectively. In each case, potency was up to 125-fold greater than that mediated by resveratrol. In the first example, based on structure–activity relationships and molecular modeling results, it was determined that a *para*-amino group on the *trans*-stilbene benzene ring is essential for aromatase inhibitory activity, and the introduction of an imidazole moiety improved the activity significantly, resulting in compound 12, which showed an IC_{50} value of 0.2 μM against aromatase (resveratrol IC_{50} = 25 μM).

Inflammation is well known to play a casual role in progression and recurrence of cancer. NF-κB is a critical proinflammatory transcription factor. The NF-κB pathway is widely involved in the initiation and progression of breast cancer; NF-κB inhibitors can be useful in primary or adjuvant therapy.[20] Resveratrol is a moderate inhibitor of NF-κB (IC_{50} 8.5 μM), and as demonstrated by our group previously, NF-κB inhibition requires the planar conformation of resveratrol, preferring large, hydrophobic rings and a catechol at the R3 position.[21] In general, chemical modification does not greatly

Table 1. Novel resveratrol derivatives found to mediate specific biological responses

Compound tested	Aromatase IC_{50}	NF-κB IC_{50}	QR2 IC_{50}	ODC IC_{50}
1	25.0 ± 2.6	8.5 ± 0.3	6.9 ± 0.4	8.8 ± 1.2
12	0.20 ± 0.06	NA	NA	NA
13	NA	1.0 ± 0.22	NA	NA
14	NA	NA	3.3 ± 0.5	NA
15	NA	NA	NA	0.80 ± 0.14

All IC_{50} values are in μM.
NA, not active.

enhance NF-κB–inhibitory potential. However, several derivatives were identified that selectively inhibited NF-κB with IC_{50} values lower than that observed with resveratrol. One of the most active inhibitors was the dimethylated analog of resveratrol, compound 13 (pterostilbene), with an IC_{50} of 1.0 μM.

A high-affinity target of resveratrol is the enzyme quinone reductase 2 (QR2).[22] Inhibitors of QR2 can mediate antitumor activity or can function as chemoprevention agents by preventing the metabolic activation of toxic quinones, such as menadione. Although resveratrol inhibits QR2 effectively (IC_{50} 6.9 μM), compound 14 has a QR2 IC_{50} value of 3.3 μM and was chosen for further study in the chemopreventive formulation.

As a result of malignant transformation, metastasis is a major cause of mortality.[23] Cancer tissues have higher concentrations of polyamines than their corresponding normal tissues, and inhibitors of polyamine synthesis have the potential to inhibit tumor growth and metastasis.[24] Polyamine levels are controlled by ODC, which is the rate-limiting enzyme in polyamine biosynthesis. It is activated in different types of tumors and the discovery of highly specific inhibitors of ODC is a promising approach in the field of cancer chemoprevention. Of all derivatives tested, several compounds were found to actively inhibit the induction of ODC. They can be divided into two groups: those with IC_{50} values in the range 10–20 μM (eight compounds) and those in the range of 0.7–10 μM (15 compounds).

Resveratrol inhibits ODC modestly (IC$_{50}$ 8.8 μM) whereas compound 15 was identified as the most promising specific ODC inhibitor with an IC$_{50}$ of 0.80 μM (Table 1).

All of these derivatives are worthy of more advanced testing as cancer chemopreventive candidates. Notably, however, cocktails of drugs have been used clinically for many years, and a methodology for the quantitative analysis of dose–effect relationships for drug combinations has been devised. Chou and collaborators described the median-effect equation in the 1980s that is now considered the unified general theory for the four major equations in biomedical sciences: the Michaelis–Menten, Hill, Scatchard, and Henderson–Hasselbach equations. Although these four equations have very different physiochemical applications, the median-effect equation for single drugs can be derived from them all, thus, it is considered the general theory of dose and effect and can be extended to multiple (n) drugs.[25] With further derivations, the median-effect equation has resulted in the combination index plot, isobolograms, dose-reduction index plot, and polygonogram,[25] and establishes the mathematical means by which we base our combination studies with resveratrol derivatives.

Synergy results when two or more drugs, used simultaneously at doses lower than that required to achieve a given response when tested singly, result in a more efficacious therapeutic effect. The response is considered greater than additive. In contrast, antagonism results when two or more drugs result in an effect that is less than additive. The combination index (CI) and isobologram analysis has provided quantitative determination of drug interactions where CI < 1, =1, and >1 indicate synergism, additive effects, and antagonism, respectively.[25] For a classic isobologram, two drugs with their actual doses are on the x- and y-axes, as opposed to a normalized isobologram, where fractions of the two drugs are plotted on the axes, often used for nonconstant ratios. In both cases, a value that is plotted below, on, or above the line of additivity, is considered synergistic, additive, or antagonistic, respectively.[25]

In some experimental situations, a combination of agents may exhibit a superior response even if one agent, when tested alone, does not appear to be active. In our work, however, an agent must exhibit either an additive or a synergistic response among

specific resveratrol derivatives to be retained as a component for further study. We have elected to use growth inhibition with cultured breast cancer cells to monitor these effects. We feel this approach is valid even though it is obvious that on an individual or combinatorial basis the agents will be mediating responses at the molecular level that are not fully elucidated. In fact, although it may not be a comforting thought, we have argued that it is generally not possible to conclude any single mechanism is responsible for the physiological response mediated in the extraordinarily complex milieu of a human being.[26] Fortunately, these ethereal concepts will not interfere with the success of our studies. The cell culture studies will teach us what is most important to know—if the test agents function in an additive or synergistic manner, and lack the potential to mediate an antagonistic response. Moreover, as described by Chou, in order to determine synergism or antagonism, knowledge of the mechanism for each drug alone is not required.[25] Accordingly, the approach is entirely valid.

We have performed some preliminary combinatorial analyses with some of our resveratrol derivatives. For example, using Compusyn Software (ComboSyn, Inc., Paramus, NJ),[25] it was determined that when tested in combination, compounds 12 and 13 exhibit a synergistic response in cultured MCF-7 cells. When acting alone, compounds 12 and 13 inhibit the proliferation of MCF-7 cells with IC$_{50}$ values of 23.2 ± 0.12 and 4.3 ± 0.22 μM, respectively. When combined, these two compounds result in a synergistic response resulting in a CI value of 0.738 (CI < 1, synergy). Therefore, in order to achieve a combined IC$_{50}$ value, the amount of drug needed for compounds 12 and 13 would be reduced to 14.52 μM and 0.48 μM, respectively.

These results provide just a glimpse of the chemopreventive potential for these resveratrol derivatives, either alone or in combination with one another. In future work, the compounds will be tested in a constant 2-drug, 3-drug, and 4-drug manner, allowing us to create polygonograms for the combined resveratrol derivatives.[25]

Conclusions

Given the morbidity and mortality associated with cancer, as well as the significant economic burden, there continues to be a need for more effective strategies to cure or prevent this disease.

Cancer chemoprevention, the use of synthetic or natural agents to inhibit, retard, or reverse the process of carcinogenesis,[27] is one important approach for easing this formidable public health burden. Throughout history, natural products have played a dominant role in the treatment of human ailments. In the field of cancer chemoprevention, the most clinically relevant drug is the synthetic compound tamoxifen for the prevention of breast cancer, but dietary-derived natural products have been the subjects of much research. In particular, because many natural products are associated with low toxicity, they are prime candidates for use as chemopreventive agents.[28–30] Piceatannol, a naturally occurring analog of resveratrol, displays a wide spectrum of biological activity. The pharmacological properties of piceatannol, especially its antitumor, antioxidant, and anti-inflammatory activities, suggest that it might be a potentially useful nutritional and pharmacological biomolecule. Resveratrol itself demonstrates a broad spectrum of biological activities potentially capable of inhibiting carcinogenesis at the stages of initiation, promotion, and progression.[31] However, the molecule is unusually promiscuous.[4] Although at least one high-affinity target exists, quinone reductase 2,[22] it does not appear likely that resveratrol functions through one specific mechanism. We have taken the approach of exploring analogs capable of functioning with greater efficacy and specificity.

The structure–activity relationships that can be derived with resveratrol derivatives are extensive. A few highlights are given in the text, but these data can be generalized in a broader conceptual framework. First of all, relative to resveratrol, it is obvious that improvements in activity can be achieved. In some cases, as with resveratrol, pleiotropic activities can be observed with derivatives, albeit with greater potency. Perhaps of greater interest are chemical derivatives that demonstrate much greater specificity with much greater potency. In many cases, these novel compounds demonstrate activity even greater than the positive control compounds used for the respective assays, suggesting further exploration as therapeutic or preventative agents is reasonable.

A good example is the inhibition of aromatase. With the clinical success of synthetic aromatase inhibitors in the treatment of postmenopausal ER-positive breast cancer, aromatase inhibitors are proving to be an effective class of agents for the chemoprevention of breast cancer.[32] We demonstrated that replacement of the resveratrol *trans*-stilbene double bond with a thiadiazole ring and further chemical optimization of the lead compound furnished 3,5-dipyridyl-1,2,4-thiadiazoles, a new class of nonsteroidal aromatase inhibitors.[18] Optimization of the aromatase-inhibitory activities of pyridylthiazole analogs of resveratrol produced an inhibitor with over a 6000-fold enhancement in activity.[17] More attention has recently been given to improve the aromatase inhibitory activity of this newly discovered class of aromatase inhibitors, because aromatase is an established target in both breast cancer chemotherapy[33] and chemoprevention.[9]

Most of the effects reported with resveratrol are only achieved at levels which are difficult or impractical to obtain in humans. Although anti-inflammatory and antioxidant effects are found in the low micromolar range, other effects require higher concentrations ($>50\ \mu M$ to mM range).[34] Due to limited bioavailability and rapid metabolism, plasma concentrations of resveratrol in humans are usually much lower than the micromolar concentrations used in *in vitro* studies. Therefore, results from cell/animal studies with such high concentrations of resveratrol are not readily translated to human outcomes.[35] Several reviews have described the pharmacokinetics of resveratrol in animal model systems,[36] but additional preclinical work is needed for developing resveratrol as a standard clinical agent. Examples include further studies with animal models to address the tissue specificity of resveratrol, to determine sites where resveratrol may have the greatest potential for cancer prevention, establish the most efficacious delivery routes, modulate metabolism, and interact with other food components.[37] In our work, we have observed synergistic actions between resveratrol derivatives and downstream antiproliferative effects with cultured MCF-7 cells. These data demonstrate that either resveratrol or its derivatives may be combined at low concentrations to exert synergistic effects on proliferation-dependent outcomes. Ultimately, this approach may lead to more practical clinical protocols for the chemoprevention of cancer.

The National Cancer Institute (NCI) developed a chemoprevention-testing program in the late 1980s, in which over 40 drugs have since been selected for clinical evaluation. These compounds underwent thorough *in vitro* and *in vivo* toxicological and pharmacokinetic screening before entering phase I clinical trials and ultimately were chosen for clinical chemoprevention trials.[38] The most well-known compound to have undergone this process is the breast cancer chemopreventive agent, tamoxifen. Before being chosen for a chemoprevention trial, tamoxifen was well characterized as an FDA-approved anticancer therapy. The tamoxifen phase I clinical chemopreventive trial included over 13,000 patients and lasted for five years,[39] showcasing the large number of at-risk patients and the length of time needed to complete only a phase I chemopreventive trial. Emulating the NCI's preclinical testing of chemopreventive agents, the potential toxicity of analogs of resveratrol such as those described here would first need to be established, followed by well-characterized treatment protocols with specific targets for carcinogenesis/chemoprevention, such as antiproliferation, differentiation signals, or cell regulatory changes.[40] The entire clinical trial process could take 10–20 years before becoming available to the public for just a single agent, and further complications will arise in testing combinations. Clearly, the pathway to gaining approval for using resveratrol derivatives alone or in combination for the prevention of cancer in the healthy, high-risk public is a long and arduous process. Nonetheless, the eventual development of an effective protocol for the general population is essential.

Conflicts of interest

The authors declare no conflicts of interest.

References

1. Pezzuto, J.M., T.P. Kondratyuk & E. Shalaev. 2006. Cancer chemoprevention by wine polyphenols and resveratrol. In *Carcinogenic and Anticarcinogenic Food Components*. A. Baer-Dubowska, Bartoszek & D. Malejka-Giganti, Eds.: 239–282. Boca Raton, FL: CRC Press.
2. Calamini, B., K. Ratia, M. Malkowski, *et al.* 2010. Pleiotropic mechanisms facilitated by resveratrol and its metabolites. *Biochem. J.* **429**: 273–282.
3. Vang, O., N. Ahmad, C.A. Baile, *et al.* 2011. What is new for an old molecule? Systematic review and recommendations on the use of resveratrol. *PLoS One* **6**: e19881.
4. Pezzuto, J.M. 2011. The phenomenon of resveratrol: redefining the virtues of promiscuity. *Ann. N.Y. Acad. Sci.* **1215**: 123–130.
5. Walle, T., F. Hsieh, M.H. DeLegge, *et al.* 2004. High absorption but very low bioavailability of oral resveratrol in humans. *Drug Metab. Dispos.* **32**: 1377–1382.
6. Kapetanovic, I.M., M. Muzzio, Z. Huang, *et al.* 2011. Pharmacokinetics, oral bioavailability, and metabolic profile of resveratrol and its dimethylether analog, pterostilbene, in rats. *Cancer Chemother. Pharmacol.* **68**: 593–601.
7. Boocock, D.J., G.E. Faust, K.R. Patel, *et al.* 2007. Phase I dose escalation pharmacokinetic study in healthy volunteers of resveratrol, a potential cancer chemopreventive agent. *Cancer Epidemiol. Biomark. Prev.* **16**: 1246–1252.
8. Yu, C.W., Y.G. Shin, A. Chow, *et al.* 2002. Human, rat, and mouse metabolism of resveratrol. *Pharm. Res.* **19**: 1907–1914.
9. Hoshino, J., E.-J. Park, T.P. Kondratyuk, *et al.* 2010. Selective synthesis and biological evaluation of sulfate-conjugated resveratrol metabolites. *J. Med. Chem.* **53**: 5033–5043.
10. Kondratyuk, T.P., E.-J. Park, L.E. Marler, *et al.* 2011. Resveratrol derivatives as promising chemopreventive agents with improved potency and selectivity. *Mol. Nutr. Food Res.* **55**: 1249–1265.
11. Yu, C., Y.G. Shin, J.W. Kosmeder, *et al.* 2003. Liquid chromatography/tandem mass spectrometric determination of inhibition of human cytochrome P450 isozymes by resveratrol and resveratrol-3-sulfate. *Rapid Commun. Mass Spectrom.* **17**: 307–313.
12. la Porte, C., N. Voduc, G. Zhang, *et al.* 2010. Steady-state pharmacokinetics and tolerability of trans-resveratrol 2000 mg twice daily with food, quercetin and alcohol (ethanol) in healthy human subjects. *Clin. Pharmacokinet.* **49**: 449–454.
13. Wen, X. & T. Walle. 2006. Methylated flavonoids have greatly improved intestinal absorption and metabolic stability. *Drug Metab. Dispos.* **34**: 1786–1792.
14. Rimando, A.M., M. Cuendet, C. Desmarchelier, *et al.* 2002. Cancer chemopreventive and antioxidant activities of pterostilbene, a naturally occurring analogue of resveratrol. *J. Agric. Food Chem.* **50**: 3453–3457.
15. Maiti, A., M. Cuendet, V.L. Croy, *et al.* 2007. Synthesis and biological evaluation of (±)-abyssinone II and its analogues as aromatase inhibitors for chemoprevention of breast cancer. *J. Med. Chem.* **50**: 2799–2806.
16. Sun, B., J. Hoshino, K. Jermihov, *et al.* 2010. Design, synthesis, and biological evaluation of resveratrol analogues as aromatase and quinone reductase 2 inhibitors for chemoprevention of cancer. *Bioorg. Med Chem.* **18**: 5352–5366.
17. Mayhoub, A.S., L. Marler, T.P. Kondratyuk, *et al.* 2012. Optimization of the aromatase inhibitory activities of pyridylthiazole analogues of resveratrol. *Bioorg. Med. Chem.* **20**: 2427–2434.
18. Mayhoub, A.S., L. Marler, T.P. Kondratyuk, *et al.* 2012. Optimizing thiadiazole analogues of resveratrol versus three chemopreventive targets. *Bioorg. Med. Chem.* **20**: 510–520.
19. Abdelrahman, S.M., L. Marler, T.P. Kondratyuk, *et al.* 2012. Optimization of thiazole analogues of resveratrol for induction of NAD(P)H:quinone reductase 1 (QR1). *Bioorg. Med. Chem.* **20**: 7030–7039.
20. Hicks, C., R. Kumar, A. Pannuti & L. Miele. 2012. Integrative analysis of response to tamoxifen treatment in ER-positive breast cancer using GWAS information and transcription profiling breast cancer. *Basic Clin Res.* **6**: 47–66.

Ann. N.Y. Acad. Sci. 1290 (2013) 21–29 © 2013 New York Academy of Sciences.

21. Kang, S.S., M. Cuendet, D.C. Endringer, *et al.* 2009. Synthesis and biological evaluation of a library of resveratrol analogues as inhibitors of COX-1, COX-2 and NF-kappaB. *Bioorg. Med. Chem.* **17:** 1044–1054.

22. Buryanovskyy, L., Y. Fu, M. Boyd, *et al.* 2004. Crystal structure of quinone reductase 2 in complex with resveratrol. *Biochemistry.* **43:** 11417–11426.

23. Radice, D. & A. Redaelli. 2003. Breast cancer management: quality-of-life and cost considerations. *Pharmacoeconomics.* **21:** 383–396.

24. Arisan, E.D., P. Obakan, A. Coker & N. Palavan-Unsal. 2012. Inhibition of ornithine decarboxylase alters the roscovitine-induced mitochondrial-mediated apoptosis in MCF-7 breast cancer cells. *Mol. Med. Report.* **5:** 1323–1329.

25. Chou, T.C. 2006. Theoretical basis, experimental design, and computerized simulation of synergism and antagonism in drug combination studies. *Pharmacol. Rev.* **58:** 621–681.

26. Francy-Guilford, J. & J.M. Pezzuto. 2008. Mechanisms of cancer chemopreventive agents: a perspective. *Planta Med.* **74:** 1644–1650.

27. Pezzuto, J.M., J.W. Kosmeder, E.-J. Park, *et al.* 2005. Characterization of natural product chemopreventive agents. In *Cancer Chemoprevention, Volume 2: Strategies for Cancer Chemoprevention.* G.J. Kelloff, E.T. Hawk & C.C. Sigman, Eds.: 1–37. Totowa, New Jersey: Humana Press, Inc.

28. Pezzuto, J.M. 1997. Plant-derived anticancer agents. *Biochem. Pharmacol.* **53:** 121–133.

29. Park, E.J. & J.M. Pezzuto. 2002. Botanicals in cancer chemoprevention. *Cancer Metast. Rev.* **21:** 231–255.

30. Piotrowska, H., M. Kucinska & M. Murias. 2012. Biological activity of piceatannol: leaving the shadow of resveratrol. *Mutat. Res.* **750:** 60–82.

31. Pezzuto, J.M. 2006. Resveratrol as a cancer chemopreventive agent. In: *Resveratrol in Health and Disease.* B.B. Aggarwal & S. Shishodia, Eds.: 233–383. New York, New York: Marcel Dekker, Inc.

32. Khan, S.I., J. Zhao, A. Khan, *et al.* 2011. Potential utility of natural products as regulators of breast cancer-associated aromatase promoters. *Reprod. Biol. Endocrinol.* **9:** 91–101.

33. Strasser-Weippl, K. & P.E. Goss. 2005. Advances in adjuvant hormonal therapy for postmenopausal women. *J. Clin. Oncol.* **23:** 1751–1759.

34. Mukherjee, S., J.I. Dudley & D.K. Das. 2010. Dose-dependency of resveratrol in providing health benefits. *Dose–Response.* **8:** 478–500.

35. Bruckbauer, A., M.B. Zemel, T. Thorpe, *et al.* 2012. Synergistic effects of leucine and resveratrol on insulin sensitivity and fat metabolism in adipocytes and mice. *Nutrition & Metabolism.* **9:** 1–12.

36. Baur, J.A. & D.A. Sinclair. 2006. Therapeutic potential of resveratrol: the in vivo evidence. *Nat. Rev. Drug. Discov.* **5:** 493–506.

37. Bishayee, A. 2009. Cancer prevention and treatment with resveratrol: from rodent studies to clinical trials. *Cancer Prev. Res.* **2:** 409–418.

38. Kelloff, G.J. *et al.* 1999. Progress in cancer chemoprevention. *Ann. N.Y. Acad. Sci.* **889:** 1–13.

39. Fisher, B. *et al.* 2009. Tamoxifen for prevention of breast cancer: report of the National Surgical Adjuvant Breast and Bowel Project P-1 Study. *J. Natl. Cancer Inst.* **90:** 1371–1388.

40. Kelloff, G.J. *et al.* 1994. Surrogate endpoint biomarkers for Phase II cancer chemoprevention trials. *J. Cell. Biochem.* **19**(Suppl.): 1–9.

Ann. N.Y. Acad. Sci. ISSN 0077-8923

ANNALS OF THE NEW YORK ACADEMY OF SCIENCES

Issue: *Resveratrol and Health*

Resveratrol and its metabolites modulate cytokine-mediated induction of eotaxin-1 in human pulmonary artery endothelial cells

Joseph M. Wu, Tze-chen Hsieh, Ching-Jen Yang, and Susan C. Olson

Department of Biochemistry and Molecular Biology, New York Medical College, Valhalla, New York

Address for correspondence: Joseph M. Wu, Room 147, Department of Biochemistry and Molecular Biology, New York Medical College, Valhalla, NY 10595. Joseph_Wu@nymc.edu

Coronary heart disease (CHD) is a leading cause of death in many developed countries. Evidence has long implicated endothelial injury and inflammation as apical events in the pathogenesis of atherosclerosis, the primary cause of CHD. Numerous risk factors contribute to a damaged, inflamed endothelium. Conversely, cardioprotective agents targeting the dysfunctional endothelium have also been identified, notably from dietary sources. We have used cultured human pulmonary artery endothelial cells (HPAECs) to test the diet-mediated cardioprotective hypothesis. In this review, we summarize our recent findings on control of transcription and expression of inflammation biomarker eotaxin-1 in HPAECs exposed to single or combined proinflammatory cytokines interleukin-13 (IL-13) and tumor necrosis factor–α (TNF-α), and attenuation of the observed eotaxin-1 responses by prior or simultaneous treatment with resveratrol and its metabolites. Control of eotaxin-1 gene regulation may be considered an *in vitro* model to evaluate agents linking cardioprotection with endothelial cell damage and inflammation.

Keywords: resveratrol; cardioprotection; eotaxin-1

Atherosclerosis and coronary heart disease

Coronary heart disease (CHD) is the leading cause of death for men and women in the United States. Clinically, CHD presents as the narrowing of coronary arteries, restricting the blood supply to the peripheral tissues and organs.[1] The primary underlying cause of CHD is atherosclerosis (AS), the pathological thickening and loss of elasticity of arterial walls due to the formation of plaques.[1,2]

Atherosclerotic plaque formation is initiated by endothelial dysfunction and chronic inflammation, possibly resulting from repeated exposure to a variety of risk factors. Over time, the damaged endothelium transitions to a state marked by migration of smooth muscle cells into the intima, convergence of recruited monocytes, macrophages, and leukocytes, and release of cytokines and chemokines. These vasoactive and growth factors are released by both the injured/stressed endothelium and the cells recruited to its vicinity, whose interaction culminates in the formation of plaques and advanced, rupture-prone atherosclerotic lesions (Fig. 1). We have used cultured human pulmonary artery endothelial cells (HPAECs) to test the hypothesis that the grape-derived polyphenol resveratrol and its metabolites confer protection against CHD by suppressing inflammation gene expression. Our findings are summarized in this short review.

Inflammation and the dysfunctional endothelium

As proposed in the "response to injury" hypothesis, the coalescence of inflammation and a structurally/functionally compromised endothelium is an obligatory event in the pathogenesis of AS.[2,3] Experimental models of AS have shown that the vascular endothelium lining plays an important, active role in the egress of mononuclear leukocytes, as is evident from the recruitment and accumulation of monocytes, lymphocytes, and foam cells in the arterial intima. The capture/homing of leukocytes

doi: 10.1111/nyas.12151

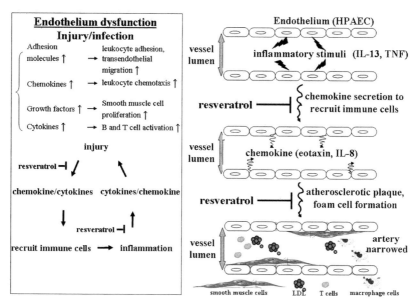

Figure 1. A scheme depicting AS as the clinical manifestation of multiple cellular dysfunctions, initiated by injury to the endothelium by a plethora of risk factors. The damaged endothelium loses its integrity, expresses adhesion molecules, for example, ICAM and VCAM, and recruits inflammatory cells, for example, monocytes, that become adherent to the endothelium. The oxidized LDL particles are taken by monocyte-derived macrophages to form fatty streaks that eventually transform into fibrous plaques, composed of a mixture of inflammatory and smooth muscle cells and debris. The rupture of fibrous plaques predisposes to formation of thrombi and severe complications of CHD. Cardioprotection by resveratrol may be attributed to its ability to act on the same multiple cellular targets adversely affected by extrinsic and intrinsic risk factors. These include inhibition of LDL oxidation, suppression of platelet aggregation, and inhibition of smooth muscle and endothelial cell proliferation and function, by resveratrol.

to the endothelial cells under conditions of blood flow is facilitated by the induction and expression of adhesion molecules, for example, VCAM-1 and ICAM-1, and cytokines and chemokines released by cells in the endothelial microenvironment.[4]

The relationship between inflammation and injured endothelium in AS and vascular pathology dates back before the turn of the 20th century to the time of Virchow, who theorized in the late 1880s that inflammation played an important role in disease processes.[5] Recently, Schwartz reported a positive correlation between inflammation in adventitia and the severity of AS.[6] Fabrican postulated that viral infection contributed to AS.[7] Minick *et al.* showed that AS occurred in rabbits infected by herpes virus.[8] Majno and Palade observed that histamine-type inflammation mediators caused endothelial cell separation in the postcapillary venules paralleled by the trapping of carbon particles in the basement membrane.[9,10] These and subsequent findings also showed that altered endothelial functions may be evaluated by activities/events emanating from dysfunctional endothelial cells and by

direct analysis of the compromised endothelium itself.

Red wine consumption confers protection against CHD

Population-based studies of an observation widely known as the French paradox show an inverse relationship between red wine drinkers and the risk for CHD.[1] *In vivo* studies have shown that red wine is more CHD-preventative compared to other alcoholic beverages; a 30–45% reduction in CHD risk occurs in individuals who consume a low to moderate amount of red wine as compared to those who drink excessively or those who abstain from the use of alcohol.[11] Animal and *in vitro* studies provide evidence that ethanol/red wine intake is beneficial to the cardiovascular system.[12] Nondrinkers fed a diet that included red wine showed a decrease in inflammation and oxidative stress-related biomarkers.[13]

The aforementioned studies showing that CHD prevention is associated with red wine consumption have led to the corollary notion that the ingestion of polyphenols in red wine, for example resveratrol,[14] may confer cardioprotection by targeting and suppressing key events in AS and CHD. This hypothesis has potential health implications, as it lends support to the notion that age-adjusted mortality and morbidity of CHD may be independently modulated by diet-based strategies and specific dietary ingredients.[15]

Cardioprotection by resveratrol targets the suppression of inflammation

Since inflammation is the initiating driver of AS and CHD, there is significant interest in the discovery and identification of novel CHD-relevant inflammation biomarkers. Possible leads might be found in the French paradox,[14,15] namely, that bioactive ingredients in red wine might prevent and offset the damaging effects of CHD through the suppression of chronic inflammation.[16,17] Testing this aspect of CHD prevention has been the recent interest of our laboratory. Our hypothesis is that suppression of inflammation gene regulation and expression in endothelial cells by the grape-derived polyphenol resveratrol and its metabolites can reduce atherosclerotic lesion formation and progression, thereby conferring protection against CHD. It is noteworthy that the anti-inflammation activity of resveratrol may be attributed to suppression of transcription factors, for example, NF-κB,[18] AP-1, and STAT3.[18] Resveratrol also inhibits TNF-α–induced phosphorylation of the NF-κB p65 subunit and prevents activation of IκB kinase (IKK) in coordination with the attenuation of NF-κB translocation to the nucleus.[18]

HPAECs as a model for identifying novel inflammation biomarkers and unraveling the cardioprotective potential of resveratrol

We have used a cultured HPAEC model to test our working hypothesis that grape chemicals, such as resveratrol, piceatannol, and resveratrol-4′-*O*-D-glucuronide, function to modulate inflammation[19] by inhibiting the transcription, synthesis, and, possibly, secretion of chemokine mediators in HPAECs exposed to proinflammatory cytokines IL-13 and TNF-α.

We have studied the induction of the chemokine eotaxin-1 in HPAECs exposed to IL-13 and TNF-α and modulation by resveratrol and its

metabolites. Chemokines are low molecular weight chemotactants best characterized in leucocyte trafficking and monocyte recruitment during the biogenesis and formation of atherosclerotic lesions.[20,21] Eotaxin is a chemokine discovered using the ovalbumin-sensitized guinea pig inflammation model.[22] Eotaxin is robustly expressed in the epithelium of asthmatic mice and plays a role in the recruitment of eosinophils to the site of inflammation through interaction with its cognate receptor CCR3.[23] In humans, eotaxin exists in multiple forms, as eotaxin-1/CCL11, eotaxin-2/CCL24, and eotaxin-3/CCL26.[24] They are synthesized and secreted by dermal fibroblast and bronchial epithelial cells[25,26] and seem to have integral roles in inflammation in these cells.[27,28] Studies on the mechanism of expression of eotaxin have identified participation by STAT6 and NF-κB;[29] binding sites for these transcription factors have been identified in the eotaxin gene promoter.[29] Exposure to cytokines IL-4 or IL-13 upregulates eotaxin expression in coordination with induced phosphorylation and nuclear translocation of STAT6.[29] TNF-α treatment induces eotaxin expression, in parallel with an increase in IκBα phosphorylation and degradation and accompanying nuclear translocation of NF-κB.[30]

Although earlier work had assigned a specific, restrictive role to eotaxin in eosinophil functioning, recent studies have shown that eotaxin is also secreted by HPAECs and seems to have a prominent presence in atherosclerotic lesions.[31,32] Contrary to ample knowledge concerning cytokine-mediated induction of eotaxin expression in fibroblasts and airway epithelial cells, little data are available on eotaxin regulation in control of cytokine-treated HPAECs. We therefore studied eotaxin gene regulation and expression in HPAECs exposed to proinflammatory cytokines IL-13 and TNF-α and modulation by resveratrol and its metabolites to gain insight into their respective contributions to inflammation and endothelial cells in the pathogenesis and protection of AS. A summary of our published findings appears below.

To test the effects of resveratrol and its metabolites, HPAECs were serum-starved overnight and then pretreated with resveratrol or its metabolites (resveratrol-4′-*O*-D-glucuronide, piceatannol, resveratrol-3-*O*-D-glucoside, resveratrol-3-*O*-D-glucuronide) for 1 h before the addition of

A

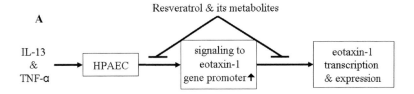

B

Assay	Fold changes in eotaxin-1 in response to treatment by IL-13 and TNF-α and modulation by pre-treatment with resveratrol		
		IL-13 (50 ng/ml) and TNF-α (10 ng/ml)	
	Control	– resveratrol	+ resveratrol (25 μM)
mRNA by RT-PCR [a]	1	58 ± 3	49 ± 5
eotaxin promoter analysis [b]	1	3.79 ± 0.4	1.5 ± 0.2
eotaxin promoter analysis [c]	1	6.7 ± 0.7	4.3 ± 1.0
Secreted eotaxin-1 [d]	1	53 ± 1.5	1.5 ± 0.2

Figure 2. (A) The HPAEC model showing control of eotaxin-1 expression and release by proinflammatory cytokines IL-13 and TNF-α and its modulation by resveratrol and its metabolites. (B) Summary of induction of eotaxin-1 by IL-13 and TNF-α and modulation by pre-treatment with resveratrol. (a) Total RNA was isolated from control and treated HPAECs at 3 h following stimulation, and eotaxin-1 mRNA was assayed by reverse transcription polymerase chain reaction (RT-PCR). The PCR products were separated on agarose gels according to size and visualized by ethidium bromide staining. Eotaxin-1 mRNA levels following treatments were quantified and presented as fold differences against control. Values were expressed as mean ± SEM for three experiments. (b,c) Effect of resveratrol and piceatannol on induction of eotaxin-1 gene promoter activity in response to treatment by IL-13/TNF-α. HPAECs were transfected using control plasmid (pGL3) or plasmids harboring the eotaxin-1 promoter–luciferase reporter (pEotx-1363 (b), pEotx-300 (c)). After transient transfection followed by an additional 48 h in culture, the cells were pretreated with resveratrol for 1 h and stimulated with IL-13 (50 ng/mL) and TNF-α (10 ng/mL) for 4 h. The luciferase activity was normalized to pRL-CMV activity and calculated as a fold against control. Values were expressed as mean ± SEM for three experiments. (d) Secreted eotaxin-1 levels in 24 and 48 h treated HPAEC culture media were determined by ELISA. Values were expressed as mean ± SEM for three experiments. Data in B are from Ref. 19.

IL-13 (50 ng/mL) or TNF-α (10 ng/mL), as a single agent in combination, for up to 48 h.[19] Changes in eotaxin-1 mRNA and transcription factors AP-1, STAT6, and NF-κB were assayed by molecular and biochemical methods. Similarly, mRNA and protein levels of signaling molecules ERK1/2, JNK, and JAK-1, known to affect the expression of the aforementioned eotaxin-1 gene transcription factors, were also determined. Secreted eotaxin-1 was monitored by ELISA. The study design and results are summarized in Figure 2.[19]

The eotaxin-1 mRNA level in HPAECs increased 58-fold in response to treatment by 50 ng/mL IL-13 and 10 ng/mL TNF-α, as assayed by RT-PCR.[19] To investigate transcriptional control of eotaxin by IL-13 and TNF-α in HPAECs, transfection experiments were performed using luciferase reporter plasmids under the control of different sized eotaxin promoters designated pEotx-1363 and pEotx300, respectively. These analyses showed that the combined IL-13 (50 ng/mL) and TNF-α (10 ng/mL)

elicited significant increases in reporter activity relative to activity of the control.[19] Pretreatment with 25 μM resveratrol significantly inhibited the up-regulation of eotaxin mRNA (from 58-fold to 49-fold).[19] Correspondingly, the 1363-bp eotaxin-1 gene promoter activity was decreased by >60% (from 3.8-fold to 1.5-fold), whereas the 300-bp eotaxin-1 gene promoter-driven luciferase reporter activity decreased by 35% (from 6.7-fold to 4.3-fold).[19]

Since STAT6 and NF-κB participate in transcriptional control of eotaxin-1 in cultured human fibroblasts and airway epithelial cells in response to proinflammatory cytokines,[30,33] we tested whether they also played a role in IL-13 and TNF-α–induced eotaxin-1 expression in HPAECs. Time-dependent changes on STAT6 and NF-κB protein expression were assayed by immunoblot analysis. Combined IL-13 and TNF-α elicited a 4- to 6-fold early increase (within minutes) in Y641-phosphorylated STAT6 that remained elevated to varying degrees over a longer duration (60 min).[19] In comparison, expression of total STAT6 and NF-κB was not changed, whereas the level of JAK1 operating upstream of STAT6 showed a steady decline.[19] Since the eotaxin-1 gene promoter spanning the upstream 1363 nucleotides also contains sequences targeted by AP-1 (which is under the control of ERK and JNK) immunoblot analysis was performed on changes in phosphorylated ERK and JNK. In HPAECs exposed to combined cytokines there were early (within minutes) increases in expression of both phosphorylated ERK and JNK, which continued for 20 min and then declined.[19] Treatment with resveratrol inhibited JAK1 expression, reduced phosphorylation of ERK, JNK, and STAT6, and decreased levels of the p65 subunit of NF-κB.[19]

A quantitative ELISA assay of released eotaxin-1 showed that secreted eotaxin-1 was barely detectable in the medium of unstimulated cells at both 24 and 48 h, and was amply elevated when stimulated with IL-13 or TNF-α and synergistically increased by their combination (Fig. 2).[19] The observed increase in eotaxin-1 in response to treatment by IL-13 and TNF-α was almost completely inhibited by resveratrol.[19] Taking the transcription and reporter gene results with the levels of secreted eotaxin-1, it may be suggested that in HPAECs the increase in eotaxin-1 mRNA levels by IL-13 and TNF-α occurred by transcriptional and posttranscriptional control mechanisms and was substantially modulated by resveratrol.

Whether resveratrol metabolites affected eotaxin-1 mRNA levels was also investigated. Piceatannol was similar to resveratrol in attenuating eotaxin-1 mRNA levels; the marked increase in eotaxin-1 mRNA levels induced by combined cytokines was inhibited by ∼20% by pretreatment with 25 μM piceatannol.[19] Reporter assay studies showed that induction of reporter plasmid activity by combined IL-13 (50 ng/mL) and TNF-α (10 ng/mL) was significantly inhibited in HPAECs pretreated with 25 μM piceatannol, and resulted in ∼75% and ∼15% decreases for the pEotx-1363 and pEotx-300 eotaxin-1 gene promoter constructs, respectively.[19] Moreover, pretreatment with piceatannol also almost completely inhibited secreted eotaxin-1 induced in response to 50 ng/mL IL-13 or 10 ng/mL TNF-α, alone or combined.[19] A ∼10% suppression of the IL-13 and TNF-α–elicited increase in eotaxin-1

mRNA expression was observed when HPAECs were first exposed to piceid or to either 3-*O*- or 4′-*O*-glucuronidated resveratrol.[19]

Implications and summary

Our findings indicate that the chemokine eotaxin-1 is induced in HPAECs in response to treatment by the cytokines TNF-α and IL-13. This is significant since eotaxin-1, in addition to its established role as an eosinophil-specific chemotactant, also plays a role in the cardiovascular system and in AS. Evidence supporting the involvement of eotaxin-1 in AS progression includes increases in eotaxin-1 levels and correlation with human atherosclerotic plaques and endothelial inflammation,[32] elevated circulating eotaxin-1 levels in patients with CHD,[28,34] associations between eotaxin-1 gene polymorphism and increased risk for myocardial infarction[35] as well as vascular smooth muscle cell proliferation and migration,[36] and increased expression of eotaxin-1 observed in vascular smooth muscle cells in human atheroma.[32]

Our studies also validate the hypothesis that cardioprotection conferred by resveratrol is in part mediated by modulation and attenuation of the inflammatory events involved in CHD initiation, as illustrated by suppression of eotaxin-1 expression. Moreover, attenuation of the upregulation of eotaxin-1 by proinflammatory cytokines in HPAECs can be replicated by the resveratrol metabolite piceatannol, and to a less significant degree by resveratrol glycosides (piceid)[37] and by glucuronidated and sulfated resveratrol. It is notable that both glucuronidated and sulfated resveratrol are metabolites that can be enzymatically generated from resveratrol, as previously demonstrated by studies using isolated rat intestine studies sections, and also in human feeding experiments.[38–40] To our knowledge, this is the first *in vitro* demonstration that a dietary agent and its metabolites with AS risk–reduction potential can significantly reduce the transcription and level of eotaxin-1.

In summary, the proinflammatory cytokines TNF-α and IL-13 induce eotaxin-1 mRNA expression and protein secretion in HPAECs. At the transcriptional level, control of eotaxin-1 is mediated by JAK1/STAT6 and NF-κB targeting the promoter activity of the eotaxin-1 gene, all of which are effectively suppressed by resveratrol, its hydroxylated metabolite piceatannol, and, to a lesser

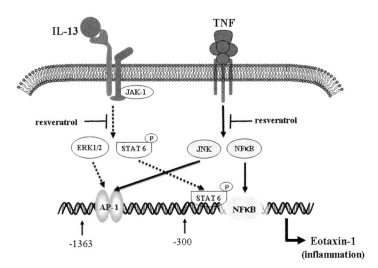

Figure 3. A proposed mechanism illustrating induction of eotaxin-1 gene transcription by IL-13 and TNF-α and modulation by resveratrol, adapted from our published studies[19] as a framework that links endothelial damage and inflammation with the synthesis and release of cytokines and chemokines relevant to AS and CHD. The proposed mechanism also shows cardioprotection by resveratrol (by extension, also piceatannol and resveratrol metabolites). Resveratrol suppresses the expression of eotaxin-1 induced by IL-13 and TNF-α by targeting the eotaxin-1 promoter activity and transcription, mediated in part by the ability of resveratrol to inhibit JAK-1/STAT6 and NF-κB p65 expression, as well as inhibition of JNK and ERK1/2 directed at AP-1.

extent, by a number of other resveratrol metabolites. It is noteworthy that the increase in eotaxin-1 secretion mediated by the cytokines IL-13 and TNF-α is almost completely inhibited by resveratrol (Fig. 2B), as well as by piceatannol.[19] This observation is novel in that it provides a readily quantifiable assay for testing the effects of resveratrol and, by extension, other cardioprotective agents on the production of secretory proteins with inflammation activities. The pronounced suppression of cytokine-elicited induction of secreted eotaxin-1 by resveratrol and its metabolites also suggests that posttranslational mechanisms may be affected to a significant degree. These results provide a mechanistic link between endothelial cell damage, inflammation via cytokine/chemokine mobilization—relevant to AS and CHD—and the evidence of cardioprotection by red wine polyphenols, resveratrol, piceatannol, and resveratrol metabolites (Fig. 3). Our results support the concept that bioactive components, such as those found in food and beverages consumed by the public, might provide cardioprotective benefits by regulating and modulating AS-relevant inflammatory genes such as eotaxin-1.

Acknowledgments

We thank Dr. Ole Vang, from the Department of Life Sciences and Chemistry, Roskilde University, Denmark, for the invitation to write this review. A portion of this review was presented by JMW as an invited speaker at the 2nd International Conference on Resveratrol and Health, held in Leicester, United Kingdom, December 5–7, 2012.

Our current studies on cardioprotection by resveratrol were supported in part by the Intramural Sponsored Research Program of New York Medical College to JMW.

Conflicts of interest

The authors declare no conflicts of interest.

References

1. Wu, J.M. *et al.* 2001. Mechanism of cardioprotection by resveratrol, a phenolic antioxidant present in red wine (review). *Int. J. Mol. Med.* **8:** 3–17.
2. Ross, R. 1999. Atherosclerosis—an inflammatory disease. *N. Engl. J. Med.* **340:** 115–126.
3. Ross, R. & J.A. Glomset. 1976. The pathogenesis of atherosclerosis (first of two parts). *N. Engl. J. Med.* **295:** 369–377.
4. Quehenberger, O. 2005. Thematic review series: the immune system and atherogenesis. Molecular mechanisms regulating monocyte recruitment in atherosclerosis. *J. Lipid Res.* **46:** 1582–1590.
5. Virchow, R. 1893. The Croonian lecture on the position of pathology among the biological studies: delivered before the Royal Society, March 16th, 1893. *Br. Med. J.* **1:** 561–565.

6. Schwartz, C.J. & J.R. Mitchell. 1962. Cellular infiltration of the human arterial adventitia associated with atheromatous plaques. *Circulation* **26:** 73–78.

7. Fabricant, C.G. *et al.* 1978. Virus-induced atherosclerosis. *J. Exp. Med.* **148:** 335–340.

8. Minick, C.R. *et al.* 1979. Atheroarteriosclerosis induced by infection with a herpesvirus. *Am. J. Pathol.* **96:** 673–706.

9. Majno, G. & G.E. Palade. 1961. Studies on inflammation. 1: the effect of histamine and serotonin on vascular permeability: an electron microscopic study. *J. Biophys. Biochem. Cytol.* **11:** 571–605.

10. Majno, G., S.M. Shea & M. Leventhal. 1969. Endothelial contraction induced by histamine-type mediators: an electron microscopic study. *J. Cell Biol.* **42:** 647–672.

11. Klatsky, A.L. 2010. Alcohol and cardiovascular health. *Physiol. Behav.* **100:** 76–81.

12. Lippi, G. *et al.* 2010. Moderate red wine consumption and cardiovascular disease risk: beyond the "French paradox". *Semin. Thromb. Hemost.* **36:** 59–70.

13. Hansen, A.S. *et al.* 2005. Effect of red wine and red grape extract on blood lipids, haemostatic factors, and other risk factors for cardiovascular disease. *Eur. J. Clin. Nutr.* **59:** 449–455.

14. Renaud, S. & M. de Lorgeril. 1992. Wine, alcohol, platelets, and the French paradox for coronary heart disease. *Lancet* **339:** 1523–1526.

15. Wu, J.M. & T.C. Hsieh. 2011. Resveratrol: a cardioprotective substance. *Ann. N.Y. Acad. Sci.* **1215:** 16–21.

16. Marier, J.F. *et al.* 2005. Production of *ex vivo* lipopolysaccharide-induced tumor necrosis factor-alpha, interleukin-1beta, and interleukin-6 is suppressed by trans-resveratrol in a concentration-dependent manner. *Can. J. Vet. Res.* **69:** 151–154.

17. Brown, L. *et al.* 2009. The biological responses to resveratrol and other polyphenols from alcoholic beverages. *Alcohol Clin. Exp. Res.* **33:** 1513–1523.

18. Manna, S.K., A. Mukhopadhyay & B.B. Aggarwal. 2000. Resveratrol suppresses TNF-induced activation of nuclear transcription factors NF-kappa B, activator protein-1, and apoptosis: potential role of reactive oxygen intermediates and lipid peroxidation. *J. Immunol.* **164:** 6509–6519.

19. Yang, C.J. *et al.* 2011. Control of eotaxin-1 expression and release by resveratrol and its metabolites in culture human pulmonary artery endothelial cells. *Am. J. Cardiovasc. Dis.* **1:** 16–30.

20. Mantovani, A. *et al.* The chemokine system in cancer biology and therapy. *Cytokine Growth Factor Rev.* **21:** 27–39.

21. Reape, T.J. & P.H. Groot. 1999. Chemokines and atherosclerosis. *Atherosclerosis* **147:** 213–225.

22. Jose, P.J. *et al.* 1994. Eotaxin: a potent eosinophil chemoattractant cytokine detected in a guinea pig model of allergic airways inflammation. *J. Exp. Med.* **179:** 881–887.

23. Pope, S.M. *et al.* 2005. The eotaxin chemokines and CCR3 are fundamental regulators of allergen-induced pulmonary eosinophilia. *J. Immunol.* **175:** 5341–5350.

24. Ponath, P.D. *et al.* 1996. Cloning of the human eosinophil chemoattractant, eotaxin. Expression, receptor binding, and functional properties suggest a mechanism for the selective recruitment of eosinophils. *J. Clin. Invest.* **97:** 604–612.

25. Watanabe, K., P.J. Jose & S.M. Rankin. 2002. Eotaxin-2 generation is differentially regulated by lipopolysaccharide and IL-4 in monocytes and macrophages. *J. Immunol.* **168:** 1911–1918.

26. Kobayashi, I. *et al.* 2004. Regulatory mechanisms of Th2 cytokine-induced eotaxin-3 production in bronchial epithelial cells: possible role of interleukin 4 receptor and nuclear factor-kappaB. *Ann. Allergy Asthma Immunol.* **93:** 390–397.

27. Komiya, A. *et al.* 2003. Concerted expression of eotaxin-1, eotaxin-2, and eotaxin-3 in human bronchial epithelial cells. *Cell Immunol.* **225:** 91–100.

28. Farahi, N. *et al.* 2007. Eotaxin-1/CC chemokine ligand 11: a novel eosinophil survival factor secreted by human pulmonary artery endothelial cells. *J. Immunol.* **179:** 1264–1273.

29. Matsukura, S. *et al.* 2001. Interleukin-13 upregulates eotaxin expression in airway epithelial cells by a STAT6-dependent mechanism. *Am. J. Respir. Cell Mol. Biol.* **24:** 755–761.

30. Hoeck, J. & M. Woisetschlager. 2001. STAT6 mediates eotaxin-1 expression in IL-4 or TNF-alpha-induced fibroblasts. *J. Immunol.* **166:** 4507–4515.

31. Abi-Younes, S. *et al.* 2000. The stromal cell-derived factor-1 chemokine is a potent platelet agonist highly expressed in atherosclerotic plaques. *Circ. Res.* **86:** 131–138.

32. Haley, K.J. *et al.* 2000. Overexpression of eotaxin and the CCR3 receptor in human atherosclerosis: using genomic technology to identify a potential novel pathway of vascular inflammation. *Circulation* **102:** 2185–2189.

33. Matsukura, S. *et al.* 1999. Activation of eotaxin gene transcription by NF-kappa B and STAT6 in human airway epithelial cells. *J. Immunol.* **163:** 6876–6883.

34. Economou, E. *et al.* 2001. Chemokines in patients with ischaemic heart disease and the effect of coronary angioplasty. *Int. J. Cardiol.* **80:** 55–60.

35. Zee, R.Y. *et al.* 2004. Threonine for alanine substitution in the eotaxin (CCL11) gene and the risk of incident myocardial infarction. *Atherosclerosis* **175:** 91–94.

36. Kodali, R.B. *et al.* 2004. CCL11 (Eotaxin) induces CCR3-dependent smooth muscle cell migration. *Arterioscler. Thromb. Vasc. Biol.* **24:** 1211–1216.

37. Romero-Perez, A.I. *et al.* 1999. Piceid, the major resveratrol derivative in grape juices. *J. Agric. Food Chem.* **47:** 1533–1536.

38. Patel, K.R. *et al.* Clinical pharmacology of resveratrol and its metabolites in colorectal cancer patients. *Cancer Res.* **70:** 7392–7399.

39. Walle, T. *et al.* 2004. High absorption but very low bioavailability of oral resveratrol in humans. *Drug Metab. Dispos.* **32:** 1377–1382.

40. Wenzel, E. & V. Somoza. 2005. Metabolism and bioavailability of trans-resveratrol. *Mol. Nutr. Food Res.* **49:** 472–481.

Ann. N.Y. Acad. Sci. ISSN 0077-8923

Resveratrol in primary and secondary prevention of cardiovascular disease: a dietary and clinical perspective

João Tomé-Carneiro,[1] Manuel Gonzálvez,[2] Mar Larrosa,[1] María J. Yáñez-Gascón,[1] Francisco J. García-Almagro,[2] José A. Ruiz-Ros,[2] Francisco A. Tomás-Barberán,[1] María T. García-Conesa,[1] and Juan Carlos Espín[1]

[1]Research Group on Quality, Safety and Bioactivity of Plant Foods, CEBAS-CSIC, Murcia, Spain. [2]Cardiology Service, Morales Meseguer University Hospital, Murcia, Spain

Address for correspondence: Juan Carlos Espín, Department of Food Science and Technology, Research Group of Quality, Safety and Bioactivity of Plant Foods, CEBAS-CSIC, 30100 Campus de Espinardo, Murcia, Spain. jcespin@cebas.csic.es

Primary prevention of cardiovascular disease (CVD) aims to avoid a first event in subjects that are at risk but have not yet been diagnosed with heart disease. Secondary prevention of CVD aims to avoid new events in patients with established heart disease. Both approaches involve clinical intervention and implementation of healthy lifestyles. The grape and wine polyphenol resveratrol (3,5,4′-trihydroxy-*trans*-stilbene) has shown cardioprotective benefits in humans. Most of these approaches deal with rather high doses and short follow-ups, and do not address the issue of long-term resveratrol consumption safety, especially in medicated individuals. Here, we review the trials conducted with resveratrol in patients at risk for or with established CVD, focusing on the two longest human clinical trials reported so far (1-year follow-up). We also discuss the expectations for resveratrol from a dietary and clinical perspective in relation to CVD. However, statistically significant changes in CVD-risk markers do not necessarily equal clinical significance in the daily care of patients.

Keywords: resveratrol; cardiovascular; grape; polyphenol; clinical trial; nutraceutical

Resveratrol as a dietary compound: myths and facts

Trans-resveratrol (3,5,4′-trihydroxy-*trans*-stilbene) is a nonflavonoid polyphenol belonging to the stilbenes group[1] whose bioactivity has been reported in many studies.[2] Resveratrol is a phytoalexin, i.e. a plant stress-inducible metabolite that is mainly induced in plants to face pathogen attacks as part of a number of defense mechanisms conceived to overcome unfavorable conditions. Occasionally, phytoalexins may be present in our diet when a fruit or vegetable has been previously exposed to a pathogen that induced the accumulation of the metabolite. There are a number of dietary phytoalexins, although they have negligible effects on health due to their extreme variability and very low concentration. As a phytoalexin, resveratrol can be found in grapes at very low quantities and can be induced under stress conditions.[3,4] Red wine resveratrol content can vary dramatically depending on the winemaking process, grape variety, geographical area, harvesting year, infections during growth, etc. The resveratrol content in red wine can range from undetectable to 14 mg/L, with a reported mean value of 1.9 ± 1.7 mg.[5] However, bearing in mind that this analysis was carried out using approximately 400 wine types and that the number of wine types worldwide is much higher (in Spain alone there are more than 20,000), this figure should be looked upon with caution. A more robust mean concentration value could be calculated if thousands of different types of wine from different countries and harvesting years were taken into consideration; but this huge task has not been done so far. In addition, the reproducibility of resveratrol content in different vintages of a particular type of wine has not yet been described. Other less significant sources of resveratrol are peanuts (0.02–1.8 mg/g),[6] some berries of the genera *Vaccinium*,[7] and pistachios.[8] Despite some suggestions that resveratrol is present in walnuts (on the internet and

doi: 10.1111/nyas.12150

even in some publications), to the best of our knowledge resveratrol content in walnuts has not been confirmed.

Thus, the presence of resveratrol in the human diet is probably almost negligible. Accordingly, the simple correlation of cardiovascular benefits of red wine and resveratrol is questionable, and a role for resveratrol in explaining the so-called French paradox,[9] associated with red wine consumption, has likely been overestimated.

The low bioavailability of resveratrol is a significant limitation. It is rapidly absorbed, metabolized, and excreted, with ABC transporters playing important roles in the whole process.[10–12] The limited concentration found in plasma has led to some skepticism regarding resveratrol's effects, but intervention studies looking to confirm said effects are still being carried out. However, in spite of its low bioavailability, evidence that beneficial activities occur in humans is beginning to emerge, and this phenomenon has been described as the "resveratrol paradox."[13] Bioavailability issues have provided the impetus for many investigations to assay very high resveratrol concentrations or to develop new formulations with enhanced bioavailability.[14,15] The use of high resveratrol concentrations or the increase of its absorption could raise safety concerns, and the risk/benefit balance of these approaches has not yet been established. The correlation between observed effects and the type or concentration of circulating resveratrol metabolites has not been unequivocally established.

The background: cardioprotection by resveratrol

Cardiovascular diseases (CVDs) are the major cause of premature death in Europe[16] and in the United States.[17] CVD-related deaths have declined over the past several years but the increasing deterioration of lifestyle, especially due to unbalanced diets and lack of physical activity, is strongly correlated with CVD, with the World Health Organization prediction of almost 24 million people dying from CVDs by 2030.

The causes of CVDs are multifactorial. Factors such as lifestyle (smoking, lack of physical activity, and poor dietary habits), elevated blood pressure, type 2 diabetes, and dyslipidemias are modifiable, whereas others, like age and gender, are not.

Atherosclerosis is the primary cause of CVD, and chronic inflammation plays a key role in its etiology and development.[18] Systemic low-grade chronic inflammation and fibrinolytic impairment are major risk factors underlying aging and age-related diseases such as atherosclerosis, arthritis, cancer, diabetes, dementia, obesity, metabolic syndrome, vascular diseases, and others.[19] The link between inflammation and the genesis, development, stability, and rupture of atherosclerotic plaques is well established.[20] In addition, since plaque rupture can precede thrombosis, the evolution of atherosclerotic events is closely related to thrombosis.[20]

Preclinical studies

Many preclinical studies (*in vitro* and animal models) have identified a number of mechanisms and targets by which resveratrol could exert benefits against CVDs.[2,21–23] These mechanisms are related to the improvement of vascular function, blood pressure, inflammatory state, cardiac injury, platelet aggregation, and oxidative stress, and to the regulation of metabolism and signaling pathways. Often, correlations between *in vitro* and animal data have been found. Although most studies have assayed very high resveratrol concentrations, some beneficial properties of resveratrol have been also observed at dietary doses.[2,21–33]

While the vast majority of *in vivo* studies with resveratrol have been carried out in rodents, strong evidence has been obtained from swine models, which present more physiological and anatomical similarities to humans, including the development of spontaneous atherosclerosis. On the other hand, animal models present substantial difficulties, such as animal maintenance and costs.[24,25] In a swine model of hypercholesterolemia and chronic myocardial ischemia, 100 mg/kg body weight/day resveratrol (a human equivalent dose (HED) of approximately 7 g for a 70 kg person) for seven weeks improved myocardial perfusion,[26] insulin sensitivity,[27] and regional left ventricular function and preserved perfusion to myocardium remote from an area of ischemia.[28]

The use of pathological animal models and specific cardiovascular damage and exposure to high doses of dietary compounds such as resveratrol for short times (weeks or a few months) are essential for exploring the possible therapeutic properties. However, such approaches are not representative of normal nutritional intake, as human beings regularly consume much lower doses of dietary compounds. In addition, long-term exposure to high resveratrol concentrations raises safety concerns, especially in subjects who take medications. Accordingly, direct extrapolation of conclusions drawn from certain types of animal pharmacological studies to humans can be questionable.

In regard to long-term conditions in swine models, Azorín-Ortuño *et al.*[29] reported that the daily intake of a grape extract containing low doses of resveratrol for 16 months (0.23 mg/kg/day; HED of 16 mg for a 70 kg person) prevented elastic fiber disruption, reduced the accumulation of fatty cells and superoxide anions (O_2^-), and diminished wall thickening in aortic arc tissue.[29] These effects seemed to be caused, at least in part, by a reduction in vascular oxidative stress and to the regulation of suppressors of cytokine signaling 1 and 3 (SOCS1 and 3) and fatty acid binding protein type 4 (FABP4) expression.[30] These studies showed cardiovascular benefits using a nutritional approach rather than a pharmacological one. However, it should be noted that dietary interventions in mild pathological models (early stages of atherosclerosis) can only exert moderate effects, which hampers their quantification and limits the determination of precise molecular mechanisms. Overall, despite the growing number of preclinical studies providing encouraging results concerning resveratrol's benefits against CVD, the objective of confirming the benefits and safety of resveratrol for human consumption is just now beginning.

Clinical trials dealing with resveratrol in patients with CVD

A role in cardiovascular protection has been the most acknowledged health benefit of resveratrol in patients with CVD. In this section, we briefly review the human clinical trials dealing with resveratrol in the CVD patient. Trials involving healthy people, where the quantification and interpretation of the possible benefits of resveratrol are less clear, are not covered here. Table 1 summarizes the published clinical trials involving resveratrol in patients undergoing either primary or secondary prevention of CVD.

To the best of our knowledge, the first trial involving CVD patients and resveratrol was reported by Brasnyo *et al.*[31] On a daily basis, type 2 diabetics consumed capsules containing either resveratrol (10 mg, $n = 10$) or placebo ($n = 9$) for one month in a randomized, double-blind, placebo-controlled trial. This trial reported improvement of insulin sensitivity, decreased blood glucose levels, and delayed glucose peaks after a test meal; these effects were correlated with the decrease of oxidative stress and the regulation of the Akt pathway, a well-known aspect of insulin signaling. Unfortunately, low sample size ($n = 19$), short follow-up (one month), and/or low resveratrol dose assayed (10 mg) limited the observation of effects in other CVD-risk markers. In addition, possible covariates, such as medication, were not taken into account in the statistical analyses; also, serobiochemical and hematological profiles of patients were not explored.

The effect of resveratrol on endothelial function in 34 metabolic syndrome patients was reported by Fujitaka *et al.*[32] In a randomized, crossover, unblinded, placebo-uncontrolled trial a group of patients ($n = 17$) consumed resveratrol (100 mg) for three months and then discontinued consumption for the same amount of time. The inverse pattern was followed by another group ($n = 17$). In both groups, endothelial function, measured as flow mediated dilation (FMD), increased approximately 4% to 9% and returned to baseline values after the discontinuation of resveratrol consumption. Blood pressure and inflammatory and atherogenic markers were not affected. But again, serobiochemical and hematological profiles were not monitored, patients' medication was not reported, and possible covariates were not taken into account in the statistical analyses.

Bhatt *et al.*[33] reported significant differences in several biological variables between type 2 diabetic subjects who consumed hypoglycemic drugs plus 250 mg resveratrol ($n = 28$) or only hypoglycemic drugs (control group, $n = 29$) daily for three months. These variables included fasting blood glucose, glycated hemoglobin HA_{1c}, systolic and diastolic blood pressures, total cholesterol, triglycerides, low-density lipoprotein cholesterol (LDLc), urea nitrogen, creatinine, and total protein levels. The trial was randomized, two-arm parallel, unblended, and placebo uncontrolled. No covariates were used in the statistical analysis and the female/male ratio was different between groups.

Magyar *et al.*[34] performed a randomized, two-arm parallel, placebo-controlled, double-blind trial

Table 1. Clinical trials dealing with RES in patients undergoing either primary or secondary prevention of CVD

Cohort (sample size)	Resveratrol dose and trial duration	Study outcome	Reference
Male subjects with type 2 diabetes mellitus (T2DM) (19)	Daily ingestion of 10 mg RES ($n = 10$) or placebo ($n = 9$) for 4 weeks. RES in capsules	Decrease of insulin resistance possibly due to a decrease of oxidative stress and improvement of insulin signaling via the Akt pathway	31
Patients with metabolic syndrome (34)	Total duration: 6 months. Effective RES consumption for 3 months: group A ($n = 17$) ingested 100 mg RES daily for 3 months and washed out for the following 3 months, and the inverse pattern for group B ($n = 17$). RES in capsules	In both groups, FMD increased approximately from 4% to 9% and returned to baseline values after discontinuation of RES treatment. No effects were observed on some inflammatory and atherogenic markers	32
Subjects with T2DM (62)	Three months daily ingestion of hypoglycemic drugs + 250 mg RES ($n = 28$) or only hypoglycemic drugs in control group ($n = 29$). Study products in capsules	RES improved systolic and diastolic blood pressures, HbAlc (–5%), total cholesterol and LDLc concentrations	33
Patients with stable CAD (40)	Three months daily ingestion of 10 mg RES in one of the groups. RES in capsules	RES decreased versus baseline LDLc (8%) and improved endothelial function (50%), left ventricular diastolic function (2%), and protected from unfavorable hemorheological changes. No effect on CRP and TNF-α	34
Overweight/obese and moderately insulin-resistant older adults (10)	RES capsules for 4 weeks in one of the three doses: 1, 1.5, and 2 g/day, taken in divided doses	Improved insulin sensitivity and post-meal plasma glucose. Results did not differ by dose. No drug interactions were observed during the study	35
Patients with stable angina pectoris (116)	Up to 60 days of oral supplementation with CF, RES, and RES + CF	Significant hsCRP decrease in all groups at the 30- and 60-day visits: 39.7% at 60 days for the CF group and 30.3% RES plus CF, at 60 days. The N-terminal prohormone of BNP was significantly lowered by RES (59.7% at 60 days), by CF (52.6% at 60 days), and by RES + CF (65.5% at 60 days). Slight changes from baseline in lipid markers (all groups)	36
Patients on statin treatment and at high risk of CVD (75)	Daily ingestion of 350 mg placebo ($n = 25$), resveratrol-containing grape extract (GE-RES, grape phenolics + 8 mg RES, $n = 25$) or conventional grape extract lacking RES (GE) for 6 months. Study products in capsules	GE-RES nutraceutical decreased ApoB (–9.8%) and LDLox (–20%) in patients beyond their treatment according to standard guidelines for primary prevention of CVD. No drug interactions were detected. No adverse affects on hematological profile, hepatic, thyroid, and renal functions	39

Continued

Table 1. *Continued*

Cohort (sample size)	Resveratrol dose and trial duration	Study outcome	Reference
Patients on statin treatment and at high risk of CVD (75). (Same cohort as in Ref. 39)	Daily ingestion of 350 mg placebo ($n = 25$), resveratrol-containing grape extract (GE-RES, grape phenolics + 8 mg RES, $n = 25$) or conventional grape extract lacking RES (GE, $n = 25$) for 6 months and the double dose for the following 6 months. Study products in capsules	GE-RES nutraceutical decreased hsCRP (−26%), TNF-α (−19.8%), PAI-1 (−16.8%) and IL-6/IL-10 ratio (−24%), and increased IL-10 (19.8%). No drug interactions were detected. No adverse affects on hematological profile, hepatic, thyroid, and renal functions	40
Patients with stable CAD (75)	Daily ingestion of 350 mg placebo ($n = 25$), resveratrol-containing grape extract (GE-RES, grape phenolics + 8 mg RES, $n = 25$) or conventional grape extract lacking RES (GE, $n = 25$) for 6 months and the double dose for the following 6 months. Study products in capsules	After 12 months: significant rise (23%) and decrease (57%) in adiponectin and PAI-1 levels, respectively, in GE-RES group vs. placebo. Non-HDL cholesterol decreased significantly in both GE and GE-RES groups (≈10%). No drug interactions or adverse effects were detected	41
Patients with stable CAD (35) (subpopulation of T2DM hypertensive male patients from cohort in Ref. 41)	Same as Ref. 41	In PBMCs isolated from GE-RES group patients: transcription downregulation of several important cytokines, and modulation of a network of microRNAs involved in the inflammatory response	75

ApoB, apolipoprotein B; BNP, brain natriuretic protein; CAD, coronary artery disease; CF, calcium fructoborate; CRP, C-reactive protein; CVD, cardiovascular disease; FMD, flow mediated dilation; GE, grape extract; GE-RES, resveratrol enriched grape extract; HbAlc, glycated hemoglobin; IL, interleukin; LDL-c, low-density lipoprotein cholesterol; LDLox, oxidized low-density lipoprotein; non-HDL, atherogenic load defined as the total cholesterol minus the high-density lipoprotein portion (total cholesterol-HDLc); PAI-1, plasminogen activator inhibitor type 1; PBMC, peripheral blood mononuclear cells; RES, resveratrol; T2DM, type 2 diabetes mellitus; TNF-α, tumor necrosis factor alpha.

involving 40 patients (26 men, 14 women) with stable coronary artery disease (CAD) who consumed either 10 mg resveratrol ($n = 20$) or placebo ($n = 20$) daily for three months. In comparison to baseline values, resveratrol intake decreased LDLc, improved endothelial function and left ventricular diastolic function, and provided protection against some unfavorable hemorheological changes. Inflammatory markers such as C-reactive protein (CRP) and tumor necrosis factor-α (TNF-α) increased approximately 50% in both placebo and resveratrol groups. No explanation was given for these results and no details were provided about the technique used to

measure these parameters. In spite of the medication received by these CAD patients, no safety parameters were evaluated and no covariates were used in the statistical analyses.

Crandall *et al.*[35] conducted a pilot trial on insulin sensitivity and glucose tolerance in overweight/obese and moderately insulin-resistant adults ($n = 7$ females and 3 males, 72 ± 3 years). Patients daily ingested 1, 1.5, or 2 g resveratrol (capsules) for one month. The study was open-labeled and uncontrolled. Some participants were under anti-hypertensive ($n = 4$) and statin ($n = 3$) treatments. The Matsuda index for insulin sensitivity improved and peak post-meal and 3-h glucose AUC decreased. No changes in hsCRP and serum lipid profile were observed versus baseline values. Notwithstanding the limitations regarding trial design, follow-up, and sample size, the improvement of insulin sensitivity upon resveratrol intake was clear. In addition, the specific search for possible drug interactions and the evaluation of some hepatic function–related enzymes was also included in this study. It is noteworthy that the previous study of Brasnyo *et al.*[31] also described an improvement in insulin sensitivity in diabetic patients upon intake of a 200-fold lower resveratrol dose (only 10 mg) during the same follow-up period (one month), which illustrates that higher resveratrol dosage (1–2 g) does not necessarily exert greater effects.

A more ambitious trial was conducted by Militaru *et al.*[36] in patients with stable angina pectoris who ingested calcium fructoborate (CF), resveratrol, or both for two months. The clinical trial was randomized, double-blinded, active-controlled, and had four arms. All groups received their usual medical care and treatment. One group of patients consumed a daily capsule (20 mg) of a powdered extract standardized to 50% resveratrol (10 mg); another group received the same resveratrol dose plus CF (112 mg/day); and a third group received only CF. One additional nonrandomized group served as control in which patients received only their usual medical care and treatment. Eighty-seven patients completed the 2-month trial and 29 followed in parallel their usual medical care and treatment. High-sensitivity CRP significantly decreased in all groups at the one- and two-month visits, especially in the CF group (39.7% at two months), followed by the resveratrol plus CF group (30.3% at two months); in addition, brain natriuretic peptide (BNP) was significantly lower in the resveratrol (59.7% at two months), CF (52.6% at two months), and resveratrol plus CF combination groups (65.5% at two months). Quality of life was improved in subjects who received both resveratrol and CF. No covariates were considered in the statistical analysis. Resveratrol seemed to be well tolerated, as no adverse effects were reported by the volunteers, although safety evaluation focusing on serobiochemical and hematological parameters was not carried out.

The above studies do not yet sufficiently fill the gaps regarding the cardioprotective role of resveratrol in a normal dietary context, as resveratrol is a minor compound in the total number of grape and wine phenolic compounds. In addition, there is a lack of long-term studies assessing resveratrol efficacy and safety in humans, especially in medicated patients with CVD. Thus, questions such as the following remain unanswered: How essential is resveratrol in comparison to the rest of grape phenolics? Is resveratrol effective at a dietary dose? and Is the long-term intake of resveratrol safe and effective, particularly in medicated subjects?

Grape resveratrol in primary prevention of cardiovascular disease

The phrase "primary prevention of CVD" denotes limiting or delaying a first event in subjects who may be at risk but have not yet been diagnosed with heart disease. Associations with ischemic vascular disease depend considerably on conventional risk factors and other markers of inflammation. In primary prevention, the main treatment goals deal with hypertension, diabetes, and blood lipid management, especially LDLc, which is feasible in massive routine hospital analyses and follow-up of these patients.[16] In this regard, the use of lipid-lowering statins is the first choice in primary care.[16,37,38] However, even in patients with gold-standard medication and achieved target risk markers, residual risk remains.[16] To complement the traditional risk factors, a number of nontraditional factors for CVD risk assessment are emerging, such as high-sensitivity C-reactive protein (hsCRP), plasminogen activator inhibitor type 1 (PAI-1), interleukin 6 (IL-6), TNF-α, serum amyloid A (SAA), oxidized fraction of LDL (oxLDL), soluble intercellular adhesion molecule type 1 (sICAM-1), lipoprotein-associated phospholipase A_2 (Lp-PLA2), apolipoprotein B (ApoB), and others. Although aging is a major risk factor for CVD—there is an important genetic basis in the onset of CVD—it is desirable to promote healthy lifestyles that prevent the appearance of risk factors, healthy lifestyles such as physical exercise, BMI < 25 kg/m^2, absence of smoking, and a plant-based diet with abundant fruits, vegetables, legumes, nuts, seeds, and low saturated fat intake.[16,17] The implementation of prevention guidelines is essential for patients undergoing primary prevention of CVD (diabetics, hypertensives, family history of CVD, familial dyslipidemia, etc.).[16] Guidelines include healthy lifestyles, dyslipidemia correction, blood

Ann. N.Y. Acad. Sci. 1290 (2013) 37–51 © 2013 New York Academy of Sciences.

pressure reduction, controlling diabetes, smoking cessation, antiplatelet therapy (aspirin and others), and the treatment of comorbidities that also raise CVD risk.

As stated in the previous section, there is a lack of long-term randomized clinical trials in patients despite an expectation owing to the preclinical benefits of resveratrol. To help address this, Tomé-Carneiro *et al.*[39,40] evaluated the dose-response impact of daily consumption of a resveratrol-enriched grape supplement for 12 months on atherogenic, inflammatory, and fibrinolysis-related markers in statin-treated patients undergoing primary prevention of CVD. The study design also aimed at ascertaining the role of the low resveratrol content in the grape extract compared to the rest of the polyphenolic fraction. In order to overcome the low and highly variable resveratrol content in grapes, Tomé-Carneiro *et al.*[39–41] used a patented procedure (WO 02/085137, ES 2177465; ES 2177465) to enhance the resveratrol concentration in the fruit. This procedure, based on the ultraviolet illumination of grapes,[4,42] uses specific controlled conditions to mimic a naturally occurring process. Grapes challenged by ultraviolet C (UVC) illumination produce resveratrol in response to this adverse condition. After UVC treatment, a resveratrol-containing grape extract (GE-RES) is obtained, thus offering the possibility of including resveratrol in the human diet within its natural edible matrix. In addition, the same grapes without UVC treatment are used to obtain a control grape extract (GE) that can be assayed in parallel with the GE-RES in order to evaluate the relevance of resveratrol against the rest of grape phenolics.

The products used in this clinical trial were provided by Actafarma S.L. (Pozuelo de Alarcón, Madrid, Spain).[39,40] Capsules contained 350 mg maltodextrin (placebo), 350 mg GE, or 350 mg GE-RES (Stilvid®). Both GE and GE-RES contained a similar polyphenolic content per capsule (151 ± 17 and 139 ± 18 mg, respectively), but the latter also contained 8.1 ± 0.5 mg resveratrol per capsule and other resveratrol derivatives (piceid and viniferins) in trace amounts (see supplementary material in Tomé-Carneiro *et al.*[39,40] for detailed qualitative and quantitative phenolic composition).

The study was a randomized, triple-blind, placebo-controlled trial with three parallel arms:

placebo, GE, and GE-RES (clinicaltrials.gov NCT01449110).[39,40] The primary endpoint was the change in either hsCRP or ApoB levels. Secondary outcomes were changes in PAI-1, IL-6, IL-10, adiponectin, IL-18, sICAM-1, TNF-α, total cholesterol, LDLc, high-density lipoprotein cholesterol (HDLc), oxLDL, triglycerides, and total atherogenic blood lipid load (measured as non-HDLc). Hematological and serobiochemical analyses were carried out at baseline, 6, and 12 months.

The inclusion and exclusion criteria defined for patient recruitment are indicated in Table 2A. Seventy-five eligible patients (34 males and 41 females) were randomly distributed into three groups (25 patients each) (Fig. 1A). All patients undergoing primary prevention for CVD were treated according to the European Society of Cardiology (ESC) guidelines and were on statin treatment. Detailed baseline characteristics of these patients (demographic, medication, and laboratory values) were reported,[39,40] and relevant covariates (gender, type of medication, age, smoking, etc.) were taken into consideration in the statistical analysis.[39,40]

Regarding atherogenic markers, the main outcome of this trial was a significant reduction of both ApoB and oxLDL, 9.8% and 20%, respectively, in the GE-RES group.[39] No significant effects were observed in the placebo and GE groups. It is known that elevated ApoB levels are correlated with smaller LDL particles, which are easily oxidized to yield oxLDL, thus increasing CVD risk.[43] Statins are effective in controlling LDL levels but their effects on ApoB and LDLox are not so relevant,[44] and this could be related, at least partially, to the residual risk that can persist in patients with optimized LDLc concentrations.[16] Consequently, it is important to control not only LDLc concentrations but also the atherogenicity of these particles through reduction of ApoB. In fact, the Canadian Cardiovascular Society proposed ApoB (values < 90 mg/dL) as a primary target therapy.[45,46] In the clinical study, the mean ApoB values of the GE-RES group moved from a risk phenotype (baseline mean value = 95 mg/dL) to a nonrisk phenotype (mean value = 85 mg/dL) at the end of the trial.[39] Although there is a debate regarding the usefulness of ApoB as a CVD risk–predicting marker,[16,47] therapy targeting ApoB could be of further benefit for statin-treated patients at high risk of CVD, like the ones included in the trial described above.[28] Hence,

Table 2. Inclusion and exclusion criteria in patients undergoing primary and secondary prevention of CVD[a]

(A) Primary prevention of CVD	(B) Secondary prevention of CVD
Main inclusion criteria	**Main inclusion criteria**

• Medical therapy, including statin treatment, according to the European Society of Cardiology (ESC) guidelines for more than 3 months before inclusion, and
• Age between 18 and 80 years, and
• Diabetes mellitus, or
• Hypercholesterolemia plus other cardiovascular risk factor:
    • Arterial hypertension, or
    • Active tobacco smoking, or
    • Overweight/obesity (BMI > 30 kg/m^2)
	• Stable angina or acute coronary syndrome at least 6 months before the inclusion in the study, and
	• Age between 18 and 80 years, and
	• Medical therapy according to the ESC guidelines for more than 3 months before inclusion, and
	• Left ventricular ejection fraction $\geq$ 45%, and
	• New York Heart Association (NYHA) functional class I–II

Main exclusion criteria:	**Main exclusion criteria:**
• Pregnancy, or • Age below 18 years or above 80 years, or • Habitual intake of food supplements (herbal preparations, antioxidant pills, etc.), or • Documented cardiovascular or cerebrovascular diseases (coronary acute syndrome, stroke, stable ischemic cardiopathy, arrhythmia, and others), or • Infectious disease, or • Neoplastic disease, or • Other known chronic pathology	• Pregnancy, or • Age below 18 years or above 80 years, or • Documented cardiovascular or cerebrovascular diseases (coronary acute syndrome, stroke, stable ischemic cardiopathy, arrhythmia, and others), or • Liver enzymes $\geq$ 3 over normal values, or • Renal failure (creatinine > 1.5 mg/dL), or • Steroid or anticoagulant treatment, or • Habitual intake of food supplements (herbal preparations, antioxidant pills, etc.), or • Infectious disease, or • Neoplastic disease, or • Other known chronic pathology

[a]Adapted from Tomé-Carneiro *et al.*[39–41]

in this set of patients GE-RES (a nutraceutical) exerted a beneficial effect, beyond the medication the patients were already taking.

Regarding inflammatory and fibrinolytic markers, no significant effects were observed in the placebo and conventional grape extract (GE) groups. In the GE-RES group, however, a dose-dependent decrease of hsCRP by 26% was observed after 12 months, which could also have clinical relevance. [The addition of CRP to risk charts has improved the ability to estimate 10-year cardiovascular risk;[48] thus, strategies targeting hsCRP in primary prevention could improve the prognosis for these patients.[49]] Other results included the decrease of TNF-α (−19.8%) and thrombogenic PAI-1 (−16.8%), which were well correlated with the decrease of hsCRP. Anti-inflammatory IL-10 levels increased (19.8%) and the proinflammatory IL-6/IL-10 ratio decreased (−24%). In addition, a clear trend toward the improvement of other markers, such as adiponectin, IL-18, and sICAM-1, was also observed.[40]

Neither resveratrol, its microbiota-derived metabolite dihydroresveratrol, nor their corresponding phase II metabolites (glucuronides, sulfates, and sulfoglucuronides) were detected in the plasma of these patients using state-of-the-art analytical techniques (HPLC-DAD-ESI-MS/MS, UHPLC-triple quadrupole (QqQ) MS detection, and HPLC-Q-TOF).[39,40] This could reflect the overnight fasting period prior to blood withdrawal and the low resveratrol amount consumed. The absence of detection of these compounds provides another example of the above-mentioned resveratrol paradox,[29] and highlights that the direct link between the effects observed and specific circulating metabolic resveratrol forms is an important topic of future research.

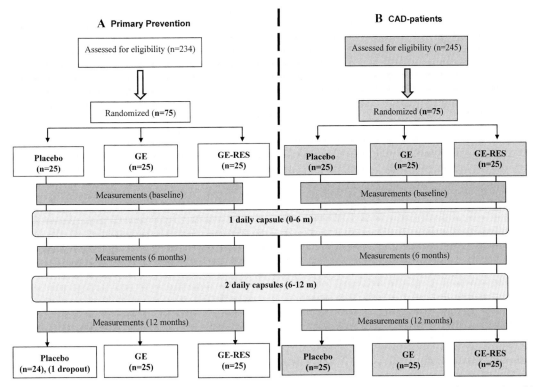

Figure 1. Design and flow of patients through the trials in primary (A) and secondary (B) prevention of CVD conducted by Tomé-Carneiro et al.[39–41]

Overall, the resveratrol-containing grape nutraceutical GE-RES exerted effects beyond those of the gold-standard medications in patients undergoing primary prevention of CVD. No cardiac events were recorded in the 1-year follow-up of this cohort ($n = 75$). Importantly, no drug interactions were found and no adverse effects were observed on the hematological profile or on the hepatic, thyroid, and renal functions of these patients after one year of follow-up. Although some positive effects were observed in the GE group, the presence of resveratrol in the grape extract seemed essential to exert the effects observed in the GE-RES group. A possible, though unconfirmed, synergistic action between statins and GE-RES was hypothesized.[39,40]

Grape resveratrol in secondary prevention of cardiovascular disease

Atherothrombosis results from complex interactions between modified lipoproteins, monocyte-derived macrophages, components of innate and adaptive immunity, and the normal cellular elements of the arterial wall. Inflammation plays a major role in all stages of atherothrombosis and participates in the local, myocardial, and systemic complications of atherosclerosis. Plaques cause clinical symptoms by producing flow-limiting stenoses (stable angina) or by provoking thrombi, with the consequent temporary (unstable angina) or permanent (myocardial infarction) interruption of blood flow. In addition, the activation of inflammatory pathways in atherothrombosis is not confined to coronary lesions but involves the participation of peripheral blood mononuclear cells (PBMCs), which are important players in atherosclerosis and in the acute manifestation of plaque destabilization.[50,51] In this regard, during the process of atherothrombosis some nuclear receptors respond to oxidative stress and inflammatory mechanisms by regulating the expression of genes involved in inflammation and lipid metabolism.[52,53]

Patients with established CAD are at very high risk of recurrent cardiovascular events.[54] Current guidelines in secondary prevention of CVD deal not only with clinical areas of intervention but also with the implementation of healthy lifestyles, including a healthy diet.[55] As mentioned in the previous section, resveratrol has been shown to provide cardiovascular benefits in CAD patients in a few short-term trials, and thus the evidence is still very limited.

Very recently, Tomé-Carneiro *et al.*[41] explored the effects of a GE-RES on patients with stable CAD, in a year-long dietary intervention. This is the longest follow-up period dealing with resveratrol in patients with CAD reported to date. Study products and trial design (Fig. 1B) were the same as described in the previous section for the clinical trial conducted in primary prevention patients of CVD.[39,40]

In this trial, patients with stable CAD were recruited according to the inclusion and exclusion criteria summarized in Table 2B (see Ref. 41 for detailed baseline characteristics of these patients such as type of CAD, demographic characteristics, laboratory values, medication). Here, the authors also used covariates (e.g., gender, type of medication, age, smoking) in the statistical analysis to discard confounding effects.[41] Inflammatory and fibrinolytic statuses were evaluated in these patients. The main outcome of the trial was a significant increase in adiponectin levels (23%), as well as a decrease in PAI-1 levels (57%) in the GE-RES group versus the placebo group. In addition, a noteworthy although non-statistically significant reduction in hsCRP values (−25% versus placebo) was observed.[41] The atherogenic blood lipid load, measured as non-HDLc, decreased significantly in both GE and GE-RES groups (10% and 13%, respectively). The authors highlighted the significance of the inverse relationship found between adiponectin and PAI-1, previously described in obese[56] and stable angina patients.[57] Whereas the increase of adiponectin has been suggested as a promising therapy for the prevention and treatment of CAD,[58] PAI-1 levels are higher in CAD patients[59] and can impair the fibrinolytic pathway, leading to acute myocardial infarction.[60] The combined improvement in circulating adiponectin, PAI-1, and hsCRP was in agreement with the previously described resveratrol-dependent upregulation of SIRT1/FOXO1 and PPAR-γ repression in relation to adipogenesis and vascular disease.[61,62]

CAD depends on interactions between the different pathways involved in inflammation and, increasingly, data suggest that integrated research work is needed to better understand the molecular basis of CAD.[63] In this regard, Tomé-Carneiro *et al.*

used isolated PBMCs from a subpopulation of the original cohort,[41,75] including only T2DM hypertensive male patients, to evaluate gene expression changes in these critical actors in atherosclerotic processes. A preliminary analysis using microarray chips showed a downregulation of proinflammatory gene expression in PBMCs isolated from GE-RES group patients.[41] Six inflammatory transcription factors were predicted to be significantly modulated, including Kruppel-like factor 2, NF-κB, activator protein-1, c-Jun, activating transcription factor 2, and CREB-binding protein. Twenty-seven genes that code for proteins present in the extracellular space were found to be downregulated. Functional analysis of this orchestrated downregulation revealed a significant inhibition of molecular pathways related to atherothrombotic signals, including inflammation, cell migration, and T cell interaction.[41] Validation by RT-PCR was then performed for a number of these genes and also for a group of inflammation-related microRNAs (miRs) found to be affected in the GE-RES group.[75] The results support the conclusion of a beneficial immunomodulatory effect for GE-RES, as the expression of the proinflammatory cytokines CCL3, IL-1β, and TNF-α was significantly reduced and that of the transcriptional repressor LRRFIP-1 increased in PBMCs from patients taking the GE-RES extract. Also, miR-21, miR-181b, miR-663, miR-30c2, miR-155, and miR-34a (involved in the regulation of the inflammatory response) were found to be highly correlated and modulated in the group consuming GE-RES for 12 months.[75]

Thirteen acute coronary syndromes (ACS) were recorded in this trial (no deaths or ST-elevation myocardial infarction events were recorded). In contrast to the five and six cardiac events that occurred in the placebo and GE groups, respectively, only two ACS were recorded in the GE-RES group. However, the authors acknowledged that a larger sample size and a longer follow-up are needed to confirm this positive trend.

As in the case of the primary prevention trial, no drug interactions or adverse effects were observed on the hematological profile or on the hepatic, thyroid, and renal functions of these patients.[41] Finally, the authors concluded that these overall results warrant further research on this nutraceutical as a possible safe coadjuvant food supplement in the follow-up of CAD patients.

Lessons from these trials: a dietary and clinical perspective

Resveratrol benefits have been reported in many *in vitro* and *in vivo* studies.[2,23] However, the evidence of cardioprotection in patients with CVD is still scarce (Table 1). Several questions arise when searching for confirmation regarding the efficacy and safety of resveratrol: How many trials are needed to confirm the effects observed? What are the most relevant markers or features to be evaluated in these patients? Which is the best rationale to establish the optimum sample size and follow-up? Are safety issues usually approached in the trials?

We have briefly reviewed here the clinical trials conducted by Tomé-Carneiro *et al.*[39–41] To date, these are the longest trials dealing with resveratrol both in patients at high risk of CVD and in patients with established heart disease (stable CAD). Whereas other clinical trials dealing with resveratrol had short-term follow-ups (up to three months), these were 1-year follow-up trials. In addition, the volunteers were patients treated according to accepted guidelines of CVD prevention, which was important in order to evaluate not only the possible additional benefits of a nutraceutical as a complement to the standard patients' medication, but also to assess possible drug interactions and adverse effects in these poly-medicated patients. Overall, results were quite promising and some novel interrogations were made. However, despite the improvement of the inflammatory, atherogenic, and fibrinolytic profile of these patients, and the absence of drug interactions or adverse effects, the authors highlighted that a much higher sample size and longer follow-up are required to evaluate a possible clinical effect. Thus, statistically significant results obtained from evaluating biomarkers related to CVD risk do not necessarily equal clinically significant results. The following question states the key point: Should one consider resveratrol to be a pharmaceutical drug or a dietary molecule (present in nutraceuticals) that can contribute to disease prevention or to the effectiveness of existing medical treatments for some diseases?

From a dietary point of view, the real challenge is to quantify the degree of prevention achieved, especially in healthy people. How should it be measured? Dietary molecules exert a relatively low bioactivity in comparison with standard drugs; thus it is reasonable to expect that possible effects of dietary compounds occur after low-quantity long-term intake (chronic exposure). These effects are expected to be low or moderate, which greatly hampers their quantification in terms of mechanisms and measurable (significant) changes. This is important because prevention is not necessarily associated with the decrease of so-called risk markers; for example, in CAD, risk markers such as hsCRP, TNF-α, LDLc, and many others are essential in the homeostasis of the organism and their levels are expected to be counter-balanced within normal ranges. For people in a normal, healthy state, the aim should be to prevent the disruption of physiological balance, and not simply to decrease risk marker levels, which may not necessarily be a good thing. It is only when biomarkers become severely altered (usually abnormally elevated) that it makes sense to bring their levels back to normal/controlled levels.

Recently, the lack of effects after resveratrol supplementation in healthy people has been reported in two short-term trials.[64,65] This idea is in agreement with the above-mentioned considerations in the sense that changes on the healthy (homeostatic) status of subjects should not be expected or targeted, since this could raise safety concerns. Another goal would be to maintain the homeostatic state or prevent its disruption, even though it seems obvious that assessing this preventive effect would require a very long follow-up.

From a clinical point of view, the future of resveratrol as a pharmaceutical drug is not clear. The multitarget activity of resveratrol could be another paradoxical drawback for this molecule—does it have effects in cancer, inflammation, oxidative stress, cardiovascular and neurodegenerative diseases, aging? In addition, current private funding (pharmaceutical industry) for conducting large, multicentric trials using resveratrol, as such, is lacking. Resveratrol is not a patent-protected molecule and possible clinical trials in patients funded by private companies are expected to be carried out with modified resveratrol analogs or with specific patented formulations.

It is essential to assess the resveratrol concentration *in vivo* required for beneficial benefits without side effects upon long-term exposure, especially in people taking medications. For example, high resveratrol doses, as frequently assayed in short-term trials, could affect the bioavailability of statins. It is known that the bioavailability of statins is affected by CYPs isoenzymes, including CYP3A4, together with uptake and efflux transporters that affect drug disposition.[66] High resveratrol doses can inhibit CYPs and interact with transporters,[67,68] which could modify the metabolism of statins, provoking serious adverse effects. Therefore, people (not only the ones with established disease but also those at risk or with mild disease) should be cautioned that the daily consumption of high doses of resveratrol (hundreds of milligrams to grams) for long periods of time might be harmful because of possible unknown interactions with medications.

There is an increasing recognition that despite the use of lipid-lowering therapies, some patients experience cardiovascular events. Recently, the AIM-HIGH trial (atherothrombosis intervention in metabolic syndrome with low HDL/high triglycerides: impact on global health outcomes) found no cardiovascular benefits from administering nicotinic acid (niacin) to statin-treated patients with established heart disease. In fact, although not statistically significant, there was a trend toward a greater risk of ischemic stroke.[69] Even though there is a debate regarding these results,[70,71] some niacin-based formulations used in primary and secondary prevention of CVD have been withdrawn from the market due to the above safety concerns. Also, fibrates, which are mainly indicated for patients with statin resistance or isolated hypertriglyceridemia or as an adjunct to other lipid-lowering therapies,[72] are not exempt from adverse effects like myopathy, increased serum creatinine, and cholelithiasis.[73] Taking into account all of the above, while statins remain the first line of clinical treatment to achieve blood lipid reduction, the search for complementary therapeutic/preventive strategies is essential.

The lack of strong clinical/scientific evidence prompted skepticism in many cardiologists regarding the cardioprotective effects of interventions with specific dietary molecules or food-derived concentrates. However, in a number of studies with large cohorts, cardiologists have begun to realize that the percentage of decrease in deaths from coronary heart disease attributed to risk factor changes through the implementation of healthy lifestyles, including the diet, can be higher than those attributed to specific treatments.[74]

To date, and according to the clinical trials conducted so far in CVD-prevention patients, resveratrol may exert cardioprotection by improving inflammatory, fibrinolytic, and atherogenic profiles, as well as improving glucose metabolism and endothelial function. However, the specific mechanisms related to these effects and the doses needed to achieve an optimum benefit/risk ratio have not been unequivocally established so far. In addition, the actual metabolite(s) responsible for the effects is not known.

In general, more long-term trials are needed to discard adverse effects or drug interactions when using higher resveratrol concentrations than those assayed by Tomé-Carneiro *et al.*,[39–41] with special attention to medicated people (either asymptomatic or with heart disease). Patients should not assume that natural products are inherently safe and ought to always ask their physicians for advice. Physicians, in turn, have to be aware that these natural products are consumed by millions of people (many under medication) without any type of control. The available evidence indicates that these products, including those containing resveratrol, could be helpful as medical treatment coadjuvants, in specific situations, for specific patients, and under specific conditions.

Acknowledgments

We thank Drs. Ole Vang and Karen Brown for the invitation to write this review. Part of this review was presented by JCE as an invited speaker at the 2nd International Conference on Resveratrol and Health, held in Leicester (UK), in December 5–7, 2012. The human clinical trials dealing with grape resveratrol, and described in the present review, were funded by the Projects CICYT BFU2007-60576 and ALG2011-22447 (Ministry of Economy and Competitiveness, MINECO, Spain), Fundación Séneca (grupo de excelencia GERM 06 04486, Murcia, Spain), and Consolider Ingenio 2010, CSD2007-00063 (Fun-*C*-Food, Spain). JTC was holder of a FPI-predoctoral grant (MINECO, Spain) and ML was holder of a JAE-Doc contract (CSIC, Spain).

Conflicts of interest

The authors declare no conflicts of interest.

References

1. Scalbert, A. & G. Williamson. 2000. Dietary intake and bioavailability of polyphenols. *J. Nutr.* **130:** 2073S–2085S.

2. Vang, O. *et al.* 2011. What is new for an old molecule? Systematic review and recommendations on the use of resveratrol. *PLoS One* **6:** e19881.

3. Langcake, P. & R.J. Pryce. 1976. The production of resveratrol by *Vitis vinifera* and other members of the *Vitaceae* as a response to infection or injury. *Physiol. Plant. Pathol.* **9:** 77–86.

4. Cantos, E., J.C. Espín & F.A. Tomás-Barberán. 2001. Postharvest induction modeling method using UV irradiation pulses for obtaining resveratrol-enriched table grapes: a new "functional" fruit? *J. Agric. Food Chem.* **49:** 5052–5058.

5. Stervbo, U., O. Vang & C. Bonnesen. 2007. A review of the content of the putative chemopreventive phytoalexin resveratrol in red wine. *Food Chem.* **101:** 449–457.

6. Sanders, M.A. & A.P. Majumdar. 2011. Colon cancer stem cells: implications in carcinogenesis. *Front. Biosci.* **16:** 1651–1662.

7. Rimando, A.M. *et al.* 2004. Resveratrol, pterostilbene, and piceatannol in Vaccinium berries. *J. Agric. Food Chem.* **57:** 4713–4719.

8. Tokusoglu, O., M.K. Unal & F. Yemis. 2005. Determination of the phytoalexin resveratrol (3,5,4′-trihydroxystilbene) in peanuts and pistachios by high-performance liquid chromatographic diode array (HPLC-DAD) and gas chromatography-mass Spectrometry (GC-MS). *J. Agric. Food Chem.* **53:** 5003–5009.

9. Renaud, S. & M. de Lorgeril. 1992. Wine, alcohol, platelets, and the French paradox for coronary heart disease. *Lancet* **339:** 1523–1526.

10. Alfaras, I. *et al.* 2010. Involvement of breast cancer resistance protein (BCRP1/ABCG2) in the bioavailability and tissue distribution of trans-resveratrol in knockout mice. *J. Agric. Food Chem.* **58:** 4523–4528.

11. van de Wetering, K. *et al.* 2009. Intestinal breast cancer resistance protein (BCRP)/Bcrp1 and multidrug resistance protein 3 (MRP3)/Mrp3 are involved in the pharmacokinetics of resveratrol. *Mol. Pharmacol.* **75:** 876–885.

12. Juan, M.E., E. González-Pons & J.M. Planas. 2010. Multidrug resistance proteins restrain the intestinal absorption of trans-resveratrol in rats. *J. Nutr.* **140:** 489–495.

13. Azorín-Ortuño M. *et al.* 2011. Metabolites and tissue distribution of resveratrol in the pig. *Mol. Nutr. Food Res.* **55:** 1154–1168.

14. Johnson, J.J. *et al.* 2011. Enhancing the bioavailability of resveratrol by combining it with piperine. *Mol. Nutr. Food Res.* **55:** 1169–1176.

15. Amiot, M.J. *et al.* 2013. Optimization of *trans*-Resveratrol bioavailability for human therapy. *Biochimie.* **95:** 1233–1238.

16. Graham, I. *et al.* 2007. European guidelines on cardiovascular disease prevention in clinical practice. fourth joint task force of the european society of cardiology and other societies on cardiovascular disease prevention in clinical practice (Constituted by representatives of nine societies and by invited experts). *Eur. Heart J.* **28:** 2375–2414.

17. Lloyd-Jones, D.M. *et al.* 2010. American Heart Association strategic planning task force and statistics committee. Defining and setting national goals for cardiovascular health promotion and disease reduction: The American Heart Association's strategic impact goal through 2020 and beyond. *Circulation* **121:** 586–613.

18. Ross, R. 1999. Atherosclerosis-an inflammatory disease. *N. Engl. J. Med.* **340:** 115–126.

19. Yu, P.B. & H.Y. Chung. 2006. The inflammatory process in ageing. *Rev. Clin. Gerontol.* **16:** 179–187.

20. Hansson, G.K. 2005. Inflammation, atherosclerosis, and coronary artery disease. *N. Engl. J. Med.* **352:** 1685–1695.

21. Wu, J.M. & T.C. Hsieh. 2011. Resveratrol: a cardioprotective substance. *Ann. N. Y. Acad. Sci.* **1215:** 16–21.

22. Wang, H. *et al.* 2012. Resveratrol in cardiovascular disease: what is known from current research? *Heart Fail Rev.* **17:** 437–448.

23. Tomé-Carneiro, J. *et al.* 2013. Resveratrol and clinical trials: the crossroad from in vitro studies to human evidence. *Curr. Pharm. Des.* In press.

24. Maxie, M.G. & W.F. Robinson. 2007. "Cardiovascular system." In *Jubb, Kennedy and Palmer's Pathology of Domestic Animals.* M.G. Maxie, Ed.: 1–103. Philadelphia: Elsevier Saunders.

25. Xiangdong, L. *et al.* 2011. Animal models for the atherosclerosis research: a review. *Protein Cell* **2:** 189–201.

26. Robich, M.P. *et al.* 2010. Resveratrol improves myocardial perfusion in a swine model of hypercholesterolemia and chronic myocardial ischemia. *Circulation* **122:** S142–S149.

27. Robich, M.P. *et al.* 2011. Resveratrol modifies risk factors for coronary artery disease in swine with metabolic syndrome and myocardial ischemia. *Eur. J. Pharmacol.* **664:** 45–53.

28. Robich, M.P. *et al.* 2012. Resveratrol preserves myocardial function and perfusion in remote nonischemic myocardium in a swine model of metabolic syndrome. *J. Am. Coll. Surg.* **215:** 681–689.

29. Azorín-Ortuño, M. *et al.* 2012. A dietary resveratrol-rich grape extract prevents the developing of atherosclerotic lesions in the aorta of pigs fed an atherogenic diet. *J. Agric. Food Chem.* **60:** 5609–5620.

30. Azorín-Ortuño, M. *et al.* 2012. Effects of long-term consumption of low doses of resveratrol on diet-induced mild hypercholesterolemia in pigs: a transcriptomic approach to disease prevention. *J. Nutr. Biochem.* **23:** 829–837.

31. Brasnyó, P. *et al.* 2011. Resveratrol improves insulin sensitivity, reduces oxidative stress and activates the Akt pathway in type 2 diabetic patients. *Br. J. Nutr.* **106:** 383–389.

32. Fujitaka, K. *et al.* 2011. Modified resveratrol Longevinex improves endothelial function in adults with metabolic syndrome receiving standard treatment. *Nutr. Res.* **31:** 842–847.

33. Bhatt, J.K., S. Thomas & M.J. Nanjan. 2012. Resveratrol supplementation improves glycemic control in type 2 diabetes mellitus. *Nutr. Res.* **32:** 537–541.

34. Magyar, K. *et al.* 2012. Cardioprotection by resveratrol: a human clinical trial in patients with stable coronary artery disease. *Clin. Hemorheol. Microcirc.* **50:** 179–187.

35. Crandall, J.P. *et al.* 2012. Pilot study of resveratrol in older adults with impaired glucose tolerance. *J. Gerontol. A. Biol. Sci. Med. Sci.* **67:** 1307–1312.

36. Militaru, C. *et al.* 2013. Oral resveratrol and calcium fructoborate supplementation in subjects with stable angina pectoris: effects on lipid profiles, inflammation markers, and quality of life. *Nutrition* **29:** 178–183.

37. Banegas, J.R. *et al.* 2011. Achievement of treatment goals for primary prevention of cardiovascular disease in clinical

practice across Europe: the EURIKA study. *Eur. Heart J.* **32:** 2143–2152.

38. Agewall, S. 2011. The large clinical statin trials. *Int. J. Cardiol.* **150:** 108–111.

39. Tomé-Carneiro, J. *et al.* 2012. Consumption of a grape extract supplement containing resveratrol decreases oxidized LDL and ApoB in patients undergoing primary prevention of cardiovascular disease: a triple-blind, 6-month follow-up, placebo-controlled, randomized trial. *Mol. Nutr. Food Res.* **56:** 810–821.

40. Tomé-Carneiro, J. *et al.* 2012. One-year consumption of a grape nutraceutical containing resveratrol improves the inflammatory and fibrinolytic status of patients in primary prevention of cardiovascular disease. *Am. J. Cardiol.* **110:** 356–363.

41. Tomé-Carneiro, J. *et al.* 2013. Grape resveratrol increases serum adiponectin and downregulates inflammatory genes in peripheral blood mononuclear cells: a triple-blind, placebo-controlled, one year clinical trial in patients with stable coronary artery disease. *Cardiovasc. Drugs Ther.* **27:** 37–48.

42. Cantos, E., J.C. Espín & F.A. Tomás-Barberán. 2002. Postharvest stilbene-enrichment of red and white table grape varieties using UV-C irradiation pulses. *J. Agric. Food Chem.* **50:** 6322–6329.

43. Ehara, S. *et al.* 2001. Elevated levels of oxidized low density lipoprotein show a positive relationship with the severity of acute coronary syndromes. *Circulation* **103:** 1955–1960.

44. Contois, J.H., G.R. Warnick & A.D. Sniderman. 2011. Reliability of low-density lipoprotein cholesterol, non-high-density lipoprotein cholesterol, and apolipoprotein B measurement. *J. Clin. Lipidol.* **5:** 264–272.

45. Grundy, S.M. 2002. Low-density lipoprotein, non-high-density lipoprotein, and apolipoprotein B as targets of lipid-lowering therapy. *Circulation* **106:** 2526–2529.

46. Genest, J. 2003. Recommendations for the management of dyslipidemias and the prevention of cardiovascular disease: summary of the 2003 update. *JAMC* **169:** 921–924.

47. Sniderman, A.D. *et al.* 2011. A meta-analysis of low-density lipoprotein cholesterol, non-high-density lipoprotein cholesterol, and apolipoprotein B as markers of cardiovascular risk. *Circ. Cardiovasc. Qual. Outcomes* **4:** 337–345.

48. Weil, B.R. *et al.* 2011. Relation of C-reactive protein to endothelial fibrinolytic function in healthy adults. *Am. J. Cardiol.* **108:** 1675–1679.

49. Reiner, Z. *et al.* 2011. European association for cardiovascular prevention and rehabilitation. ESC/EAS guidelines for the management of dyslipidaemias: the task force for the management of dyslipidaemias of the European Society of Cardiology (ESC) and the European Atherosclerosis Society (EAS). *Eur. Heart J.* **32:** 1769–1818.

50. Benagiano, M. *et al.* 2003. T helper type 1 lymphocytes drive inflammation in human atherosclerotic lesions. *Proc. Natl. Acad. Sci. USA* **100:** 6658–6663.

51. Lin, Z. *et al.* 2005. Kruppel-like factor 2 (KLF2) regulates endothelial thrombotic function. *Circ. Res.* **96:** e48–e57.

52. Libby, P. & F. Crea. 2010. Clinical implications of inflammation for cardiovascular primary prevention. *Eur. Heart J.* **31:** 777–783.

53. Smith, S.C., Jr *et al.* 2011. World heart federation and the preventive cardiovascular nurses association. AHA/ACCF secondary prevention and risk reduction therapy for patients with coronary and other atherosclerotic vascular disease: 2011 update: a guideline from the american heart association and american college of cardiology foundation endorsed by the world heart federation and the preventive cardiovascular nurses association. *J. Am. Coll. Cardiol.* **58:** 2432–2446.

54. World Health Organization. 2007. *Prevention of Cardiovascular Disease. Guidelines for Assessment and Management of Cardiovascular Risk.* Geneva: WHO Press.

55. Pauwels, E.K. 2011. The protective effect of the mediterranean diet: focus on cancer and cardiovascular risk. *Med. Princ. Pract.* **20:** 103–111.

56. Maruyoshi, H. *et al.* 2004. Adiponectin is inversely related to plasminogen activator inhibitor type 1 in patients with stable exertional angina. *Thromb. Haem.* **91:** 1026–1030.

57. Chan, K.C. *et al.* 2008. Atorvastatin administration after percutaneous coronary intervention in patients with coronary artery disease and normal lipid profiles: impact on plasma adiponectin level. *Clin. Cardiol.* **31:** 253–258.

58. Kohler, H.P. & P.J. Grant. 2000. Plasminogen-activator inhibitor type 1 and coronary artery disease. *N. Engl. J. Med.* **342:** 1792–1801.

59. Belalcazar, L.M. *et al.* 2011. Look Action for Health in Diabetes Research Group. Look action for health in diabetes research group. metabolic factors, adipose tissue, and plasminogen activator inhibitor-1 levels in type 2 diabetes: findings from the look ahead study. *Arterioscler. Thromb. Vasc. Biol.* **31:** 1689–1695.

60. Mertens, I. *et al.* 2005. Inverse relationship between plasminogen activator inhibitor-I activity and adiponectin in overweight and obese women. Interrelationship with visceral adipose tissue, insulin resistance, HDL-chol and inflammation. *Thromb. Haemost.* **94:** 1190–1195.

61. Picard, F. *et al.* 2004. Sirt1 promotes fat mobilization in white adipocytes by repressing PPAR-gamma. *Nature* **429:** 771–776.

62. Subauste, A.R. & C.F. Burant. 2007. Role of FoxO1 in FFA-induced oxidative stress in adipocytes. *Am. J. Physiol. Endocrinol. Metab.* **293:** E159–164.

63. Kazemian, P. *et al.* 2012. The use of Ω-3 poly-unsaturated fatty acids in heart failure: a preferential role in patients with diabetes. *Cardiovasc. Drugs Ther.* **26:** 311–320.

64. Yoshino, J. *et al.* 2012. Resveratrol supplementation does not improve metabolic function in nonobese women with normal glucose tolerance. *Cell Metab.* **16:** 658–664.

65. Poulsen, M.M. *et al.* 2012. High-dose resveratrol supplementation in obese men: an investigator-initiated, randomized, placebo-controlled clinical trial of substrate metabolism, insulin sensitivity, and body composition. *Diabetes.* **62:** 1186–1195.

66. Willrich, M.A., M.H. Hirata & R.D. Hirata. 2009. Statin regulation of CYP3A4 and CYP3A5 expression. *Pharmacogenomics* **10:** 1017–1024.

67. Chow, H.H. *et al.* 2010. Resveratrol modulates drug- and carcinogen-metabolizing enzymes in a healthy volunteer study. *Cancer Prev. Res. (Phila)* **3:** 1168–1175.

68. Planas, J.M. *et al.* 2012. The bioavailability and distribution of trans-resveratrol are constrained by ABC transporters. *Arch. Biochem. Biophys.* **527:** 67–73.

69. The AIM-HIGH Investigators. 2011. The role of niacin in raising HDL-C to reduce cardiovascular events in patients with atherosclerotic cardiovascular disease and optimally treated LDL-c AIM-HIGH: rationale and study design. *Am. Heart J.* **161:** 471–477.

70. Nicholls, S.J. 2012. The AIM-HIGH (Atherothrombosis intervention in metabolic syndrome with low HDL/High triglycerides: impact on global health outcomes) trial: to believe or not to believe? *J. Am. Coll. Cardiol.* **59:** 2065–2067.

71. Gouni-Berthold, I. & H.K. Berthold. 2013. The role of niacin in lipid-lowering treatment: are we aiming too high? *Curr. Pharm. Des.* **19:** 3094–3106.

72. Berglund, L. *et al.* 2012. Evaluation and treatment of hypertriglyceridemia: an Endocrine Society clinical practice guideline. *J. Clin. Endocrinol. Metab.* **97:** 2969–2989.

73. Chapman, M.J. *et al.* 2011. Triglyceride-rich lipoproteins and high-density lipoprotein cholesterol in patients at high risk of cardiovascular disease: evidence and guidance for management. *Eur. Heart J.* **32:** 1345–1361.

74. Di Chiara, A. & D. Vanuzzo. 2009. Does surveillance impact on cardiovascular prevention? *Eur. Heart J.* **30:** 1027–1029.

75. Tome-Carneiro, J. *et al.* 2013. One-year supplementation with a grape extract containing resveratrol modulates inflammatory-related microRNAs and cytokines expression in peripheral blood mononuclear cells of type 2 diabetes and hypertensive patients with coronary artery disease. *Pharmacol. Res.* doi:org/10.1016/j.phrs.2013.03.011.

Ann. N.Y. Acad. Sci. ISSN 0077-8923

ANNALS OF THE NEW YORK ACADEMY OF SCIENCES
Issue: *Resveratrol and Health*

Evidence for circulatory benefits of resveratrol in humans

Rachel H.X. Wong,[1] Alison M. Coates,[1] Jonathan D. Buckley,[1] and Peter R.C. Howe[1,2]

[1]Nutritional Physiology Research Centre, Sansom Institute for Health Research, University of South Australia, Adelaide, Australia. [2]Clinical Nutrition Research Centre, University of Newcastle, Callaghan, New South Wales, Australia

Address for correspondence: Peter R.C. Howe, Clinical Nutrition Research Centre, School of Biomedical Sciences & Pharmacy, University of Newcastle, Callaghan, NSW 2308, Australia. Peter.howe@newcastle.edu.au

Impairments of endothelial function, which can be assessed noninvasively by flow-mediated dilation (FMD) of the brachial artery, contribute to the development of cardiovascular disease. Associations between FMD and cognition suggest a vascular component in the loss of cognitive function. Certain vasoactive nutrients that have been shown to improve FMD may also have the potential to enhance cerebral perfusion and cognition. Preclinical studies show that *trans*-resveratrol can enhance nitric oxide bioavailability, thereby increasing endothelium-dependent vasodilation. We have now shown that acute administration of resveratrol elicits dose-dependent increases of FMD with greater potency than other vasoactive nutrients and that this benefit is sustained following regular consumption. We describe the potential implications of this vasodilator benefit of resveratrol and its role in enhancing cerebrovascular and cognitive functions.

Keywords: resveratrol; flow-mediated dilation; endothelial function; human; vasodilator responsiveness; *trans*-resveratrol

Overview

Poor circulatory function contributes to the pathogenesis of many lifestyle diseases including cardiovascular disease (CVD), inflammatory diseases, and dementia.[1] A healthy endothelium underpins a healthy circulation by regulating vasomotor, platelet, immune, and capillary transport functions and maintaining the structural integrity of blood vessels. Disruption of normal endothelial function, as occurs in hypertension or atherosclerosis, may reduce vasodilator responsiveness, promote abnormal and chronic vasoconstriction, and increase nonselective capillary permeability, platelet adhesion and aggregation, inflammation, and arterial remodeling. Certain vasoactive nutrients in foods, such as cocoa flavanols, have been found to improve the functionality of the endothelium,[2] which in turn may aid the prevention and/or management of CVD risk factors,[2] improve metabolic profiles,[3] and boost cognitive performance.[4] The latter may result from enhanced perfusion of brain tissue via improvement of cerebral circulatory function. Resveratrol, one of the numerous polyphenols in red wine and grapes,

has recently been identified as a vasoactive nutrient with the potential to enhance arterial health. Preclinical studies on resveratrol have consistently demonstrated its beneficial effects on arterial vasodilation, one of the numerous functions mediated by the vascular endothelium.[5] This short review will focus on the circulatory benefits of resveratrol in humans, as demonstrated in published clinical trials, and its potential to improve cerebrovascular perfusion and thereby enhance cognitive performance.

Importance of endothelial function

A healthy endothelium acts at the capillary level as a selectively permeable barrier between circulating blood and tissues, enabling nutrient and waste product exchange. At the arteriolar level, the endothelium controls vasomotor tone to regulate the flow of blood from large conduit arteries to the capillaries. It does so by secreting vasodilator substances, particularly nitric oxide (NO), which is produced by endothelial NO synthase (eNOS) to promote relaxation of the vascular smooth muscle cells (VSMC), or by secreting endothelin-1 to cause

doi: 10.1111/nyas.12155

vasoconstriction and promote VSMC proliferation. The release of endothelin-1, to some extent, also stimulates production of NO, which tends to counteract the constrictor response. As such, a normal healthy vasculature has a constant vasodilator tone, owing to the continuous release of NO in small amounts, and endothelial cells function as a "nonstick lining" that prevents cell adhesion and platelet aggregation and inhibits cell proliferation and thrombosis through the action of anticoagulants.[6] The endothelium also plays an important role in maintaining the structural integrity of blood vessels by inhibiting growth factors that promote hypertrophy and hyperplasia of VSMC, mainly via the action of NO working in concert with other vasoactive substances. The endothelium also plays a role in acute immune responses by expressing cell adhesion molecules on injured cell surfaces to attract leukocytes to initiate thrombosis and wound repair.[6]

Endothelial dysfunction

A shift in the profile of vasoactive mediators can cause a normal endothelium to become dysfunctional by upsetting the fine balance between vasodilators and vasoconstrictors, which impact both the structure and function of VSMC. In chronic inflammatory conditions, the endothelium produces a constant stream of proinflammatory cytokines promoting leukocyte adhesion to the endothelium. This hallmark characteristic marks the initial pathogenesis of atherosclerosis due to loss of eNOS-derived NO production or bioavailability, and manifests as impaired vasodilator responsiveness to vasodilator stimuli that eventually leads to the development of CVD.[7] Reduced NO bioavailability enhances proliferation of VSMC, leading to arterial remodeling and higher peripheral vascular resistance. Over time, this structural remodeling reduces permeability, increases blood flow resistance, and stiffens large conduit arteries. These effects occur throughout all blood vessels, including the brain, where a reduction in NO bioavailability in the cerebral endothelial cells plays a role in the impairment of cerebral vasodilator function[8] and is associated with an increased risk for stroke, transient ischemic attack,[9] and cognitive decline.[10] Moreover, as the cerebral capillary endothelium represents the blood–brain barrier, this critical component of cerebrovascular integrity is compromised by endothelial dysfunction, increasing the potential for accumulation of toxic substances in the highly vascularized basal ganglia, and thereby increasing the risk of neurodegenerative diseases.

Assessing endothelial vasodilator function

One endothelial function that can be readily measured noninvasively is arterial vasodilation. Endothelium-dependent vasodilation can be assessed by the technique of flow-mediated dilation (FMD) in the brachial artery, which uses a localized transient ischemia as a vasodilatory stimulus.[11] An acute increase in blood flow (reactive hyperemia) following forearm occlusion triggers upstream vasodilation in the brachial artery that is primarily mediated by eNOS-derived NO.[11] A reduced degree of dilation compared to a healthy artery may be attributed to the reduction in NO production or bioavailability, the loss of other functions, or even the absence of endothelial cells. Thus, if FMD is impaired, other endothelial functions are likely to be compromised. Aging,[12] hypertension,[13] obesity,[14] diabetes,[15] high cholesterol levels,[16] and smoking are all risk factors that have been shown to be associated with lower FMD values than in healthy controls. Thus, there is an inverse relationship between FMD and CVD. A recent meta-analysis demonstrated that FMD was at least as predictive as traditional risk factors (e.g., low-density lipoprotein (LDL) cholesterol, blood pressure) in predicting future cardiovascular events.[17] Meta-analyses have shown that in population groups with disease and in healthy populations, supplementing one's diet with vasoactive nutrients such as cocoa flavanols, tea catechins, or soy isoflavones with a single dose (acutely) and/or daily consumption over a period (chronically) may confer an improvement in FMD between 1.75% and 3.19% compared to placebo or control groups.[18–20] Therefore, early targeted vasoactive nutrient interventions that maintain or improve endothelial vasodilator function may be beneficial in reducing disease risks and for enhancing global circulation (i.e., to the brain and exercising muscles). In addition, poor systemic circulation can also affect cerebral perfusion, thereby resulting in brain atrophy, as evidenced by the correlation between FMD and whole brain volume ($r = 0.77$; measured by magnetic resonance imaging),[21] and loss of cognitive function. In fact, impaired FMD has been linked to poor cognitive performance in older adults with CVD risk factors.[22]

Evidence for circulatory benefits of resveratrol in humans

There are a growing number of publications describing the benefits of grape polyphenol consumption on human arterial function;[23–26] however, evidence for the efficacy of grape polyphenols on FMD in humans is limited, with mixed findings. Lekakis *et al.*[25] conducted a dietary intervention with polyphenols extracted from the leftover pomace from making red wine. They observed a significant improvement in absolute mean FMD (1.92% absolute increase, or 74% difference from placebo) 1 h after a single dose of 600 mg of red wine polyphenol extract in patients with coronary heart disease. FMD remained above baseline value (58% increase from baseline) 2 h postconsumption. In this extract, resveratrol was one of the many polyphenols present, but its content was low (0.54 mg) compared with other vasoactive polyphenols such as epicatechin (2.59 mg) and gallic acid (1.24 mg), which were therefore more likely to have mediated this improvement.[25] In a chronic supplementation trial with hypertensive adults who smoked and had hypercholesterolemia, Clifton[26] found a 1.10% absolute increase in FMD following four weeks of daily supplementation with 2000 mg of grape seed extract in which the main polyphenols present are proanthocyanidins, compared with a control group. A modest reduction in blood pressure has been reported in a meta-analysis of the effects of grape seed extract supplementation, but the effects on arterial function were attributed to the attenuation of intestinal cholesterol absorption and inhibition of LDL oxidation.[23] The exact mechanism by which grape seed extracts act to improve FMD is unclear. A more recent investigation observed no change in FMD or other cardiovascular biomarkers after supplementing coronary heart disease patients with 1300 mg of muscadine grape seed (encapsulated) daily for four weeks compared with the placebo group.[24]

Resveratrol was originally purported to be a nutrient for longevity, but experimental animal models have convincingly demonstrated the benefits of resveratrol for circulatory function and CVD risk factors.[5] However, human evidence attributing the benefit of resveratrol specifically to endothelial va-

sodilator function is fairly recent, and there is no evidence, as yet, of resultant improvement in clinical outcomes. Dietary supplements of resveratrol extracted from plant sources in varying doses and degrees of purity are available commercially, but evidence of the safety and efficacy of these products is scarce. Fujitaka *et al.*[27] recently observed a significant improvement in FMD (127% increase from baseline) after three months of daily supplementation with a combined administration of resveratrol (100 mg), vitamin D_3, quercetin, and rice bran phytate in adults with metabolic syndrome. No change was detected in cardiovascular and metabolic biomarkers. Although the evidence is promising, we need to better understand the relationship between individual polyphenol consumption and endothelial function. The first chronic resveratrol supplementation trial was published mid-2012 by a group in Hungary. They randomized patients with severe coronary heart disease to consume either 10 mg of resveratrol ($n = 20$) or placebo ($n = 20$) daily. The resveratrol used in the study was an extract derived from the root of the Japanese knotweed plant (*Polygonum cuspidatum*). After three months, FMD values increased twofold from baseline within the group that received resveratrol. The authors, however, failed to demonstrate a significant resveratrol-induced change in FMD compared to the placebo group, as the latter also improved after three months and the study was underpowered to detect a difference between groups.[28] Therefore, these studies have not provided definitive evidence that resveratrol itself is efficacious for improving endothelial vasodilator function.

We recently reported for the first time a dose-dependent effect of synthetic *trans*-resveratrol on endothelial function in humans.[29] Overweight/obese mildly hypertensive adults who had never been treated for hypertension were randomized in a double-blind crossover trial to take 0 (placebo), 30, 90, or 270 mg of encapsulated *trans*-resveratrol in a single dose, and an FMD assessment and venous blood samples were obtained 1 h after consumption to coincide with previously reported time-to-peak of resveratrol concentrations.[25] The protocol was repeated with the alternative doses at 1-week intervals. Acute resveratrol administration elicited a significant dose effect on plasma concentration ($P < 0.001$) and on FMD (up to 91% greater than the placebo FMD response,

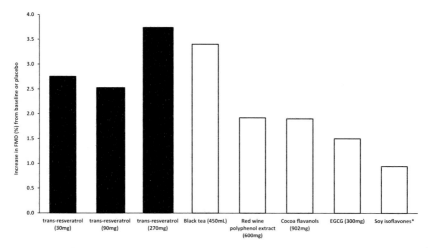

Figure 1. Acute increases of FMD from baseline FMD or placebo levels following single doses of *trans*-resveratrol[29] or other vasoactive nutrients: black tea,[30] red wine polyphenol extract,[25] cocoa flavanols,[2] epigallocatechin gallate (EGCG),[31] soy isoflavones.[18] *Results from meta-analysis.

$P < 0.01$). The mean absolute improvement in FMD compared to the placebo dose was between 2.50% and 3.67%,[29] and resveratrol appeared to be more potent than other vasoactive nutrients, for example, cocoa flavanols,[2] tea catechins,[30] epigallocatechin gallate (EGCG), and soy isoflavones,[18] all of which required higher doses to elicit similar acute improvements in FMD (Fig. 1). The higher relative potency of resveratrol may be attributable to its ability to work through multiple mechanisms such as SIRT1 upregulation, COX-1 inhibition, and stimulation of estrogen receptor activities to upregulate eNOS activity, thus increasing NO production/bioavailability and enhancing endothelial vasodilator function.[5]

In order to maintain healthy endothelial vasodilator function, the effects of vasoactive nutrients on FMD need to be sustainable following repeated administration. There is an emerging body of literature demonstrating acute increases of FMD with plant-derived supplements, but less evidence that such effects are sustainable following chronic consumption.[18] Cocoa flavanols are examples of vasoactive nutrients that have both acute and chronic effects on FMD.[2] The effect of a single dose of cocoa flavanols on FMD was more pronounced than the effect observed hours after ingesting cocoa flavanols following daily regular supplementation,[3] but nonetheless demonstrated that chronic consumption did not reduce the sensitivity of effect on FMD. The significance of the improvement in endothelial vasodilator function with cocoa flavanols has been recognized in a recently published scientific opinion on the substantiation of a nutrient health claim to the European Food Safety Authority.[32] This is the first official acknowledgment of the importance of FMD as an early indicator of arterial disease preceding the establishment of hypertension.[7]

Following our acute dose-response study of resveratrol,[29] we subsequently showed that the improvement in FMD persisted following daily resveratrol supplementation for six weeks (75 mg/day) in healthy obese adults.[33] Importantly, this latter study demonstrated that the improvement in FMD was not transient but a prolonged improvement (23% increase compared with placebo, $P = 0.021$, paired t-test) observed at least 18 h after participants had consumed their last dose of resveratrol. In addition, a single dose of resveratrol (75 mg) following chronic resveratrol supplementation resulted in a 35% greater acute FMD response than the equivalent placebo supplementation ($P = 0.002$). The magnitude of increase in FMD was inversely associated with baseline FMD ($r = -0.47$, $P = 0.01$), such that those with impaired vasodilator responsiveness showed greater improvement. This suggests that resveratrol supplementation may be most effective in those with impaired vasodilator function, and may therefore be most useful for assisting with the maintenance of normal vasodilator function in conditions that exhibit endothelial vasodilatory dysfunction. It has been estimated that a 1% absolute increase of FMD (10–20% relative improvement) would be clinically significant for primary CVD prevention,[11] reducing the risk of future cardiac events by 13%.[17] This magnitude of improvement following chronic resveratrol consumption exemplifies the potential for specific vasoactive nutrients to prevent future risk of CVD by maintaining normal circulatory function in a healthy population without overt disease. It is important to acknowledge that the efficacious 75 mg dose of pure *trans*-resveratrol that we administered cannot be achieved through regular intake from food sources. This would equate to drinking 3–27 L of red wine (depending on grape variety) or consuming 4.8 kg of red currants per day.[34] Doses used in both our acute and chronic studies were well tolerated by our participants.

Can circulatory effects of resveratrol mediate cognitive benefits?

The improvement in systemic vasodilator function with resveratrol or other vasoactive nutrients may be extended to the cerebral vasculature, and it is hypothesized that improved cerebral endothelial function may enhance cognitive performance.[35] Cocoa flavanols not only improve FMD[3] but have also been shown to increase cerebral perfusion during a cognitive task[36] and cognitive performance and mental fatigue following single dose consumption,[4] though these benefits were demonstrated in separate studies. Our recent trial of regular consumption of a polyphenol-rich extract from wild green oats[37] was the first demonstration that a vasoactive nutrient supplement could improve not only FMD but also cerebral vasodilator responsiveness. Considering that resveratrol has a greater potency than cocoa flavanols and may work via multiple mechanisms[5] to enhance vasodilator responsiveness, one may expect resveratrol to have similar or greater efficacy than the wild green oat extract for enhancing cerebral vascular and cognitive function. Using a crossover study design, Kennedy *et al.*[38] found that consumption of single doses (250 and 500 mg) of resveratrol by healthy young adults resulted in a dose-dependent overall increase in cerebral perfusion to active brain regions (measured by near-infrared spectroscopy) during a 9-min cognitive test battery. Although they found no

enhancement in cognitive performance following acute supplementation,[38] they recently reported a reduction in feelings of fatigue following chronic supplementation (500 mg/day for 28 days; data presented at the Resveratrol 2012 conference). The lack of improvement in cognitive performance noted by Kennedy *et al.*[38] may reflect the short duration of supplementation or the young age of the healthy participants (mean age 24.8 years), as endothelial vasodilator impairment is age-related. In a recent published intervention with cocoa flavanols,[39] elderly participants with mild cognitive impairment and several CVD risk factors performed significantly better on the trail-making test and verbal fluency tests following a high daily intake (990 mg) of cocoa flavanols for eight weeks. Therefore, the full potential of resveratrol for enhancing cerebral vascular function and cognitive performance warrants urgent evaluation in a population group with some degree of cognitive and vascular impairment. A direct and cost-effective alternative to functional magnetic resonance imaging in assessing the dependence of cognitive performance on cerebral perfusion is the use of functional transcranial Doppler ultrasound. This can be done noninvasively by measuring the increases in blood flow velocity in the middle cerebral artery resulting from downstream dilation of cerebral arterioles in response to cognitive stimuli.[40] Evaluating these variables simultaneously will provide a better understanding of the role of cerebral perfusion in cognitive performance.

Conclusion

There is increasing evidence from experimental and clinical studies for circulatory benefits of resveratrol. The benefits are in part attributable to the improvement of endothelial vasodilator function through increased NO production and/or bioavailability. Although the promising vasodilator benefits observed in clinical trials with varying levels of resveratrol supplementation (10 mg/day for 12 weeks,[28] 75 mg/day for 6 weeks,[33] 100 mg/day of resveratrol combination for 12 weeks[27]) are unlikely to be achieved through regular dietary intake, resveratrol is nonetheless more efficacious than other vasoactive nutrients tested. Therefore, more comprehensive dose-response trials of resveratrol supplements, particularly at lower doses, are warranted to further define long-term benefits in at-risk populations before recommendations can be made for its use in disease prevention. A lower intake of resveratrol that may be obtainable from food sources may prove equally efficacious in a longer term study, particularly in individuals with impaired FMD. For now, resveratrol is available as a supplement and approval is being sought to incorporate it as a novel ingredient in functional foods. Considering that resveratrol has multiple mechanistic actions,[5] it will be important to establish whether, in enhancing FMD, resveratrol is acting on the endothelium to increase NO bioavailability or directly on the smooth muscle to modulate vasodilator responsiveness. In view of the acute[29] and chronic[27,28,33] effects of resveratrol on systemic vascular function and on cerebral blood flow,[38] it will be of interest to see whether resveratrol consumption can also improve cerebral circulatory function and whether this correlates with changes in cognitive performance and stroke risk. Such evidence will be pivotal for our understanding of the role of resveratrol in primary prevention.

Acknowledgment

The authors would like to thank Dr. Iris Kunz, DSM Nutritional Products, for providing feedback on the review.

Conflicts of interest

The authors have no conflicts of interest.

References

1. Ruitenberg, A., T. den Heijer, S.L.M. Bakker, *et al.* 2005. Cerebral hypoperfusion and clinical onset of dementia: the Rotterdam study. *Ann. Neurol.* **57:** 789–794.
2. Davison, K., A.M. Coates, J.D. Buckley & P.R. Howe. 2008. Effect of cocoa flavanols and exercise on cardiometabolic risk factors in overweight and obese subjects. *Int. J. Obes. (Lond).* **32:** 1289–1296.
3. Hooper, L., K. Colin, A. Asmaa, *et al.* 2012. Effects of chocolate, cocoa, and flavan-3-ols on cardiovascular health: a systematic review and meta-analysis of randomized trials. *Am. J. Clin. Nutr.* **95:** 740–751.
4. Scholey, A.B, S.J. French, P.J. Morris, *et al.* 2009. Consumption of cocoa flavanols results in acute improvements in mood and cognitive performance during sustained mental effort. *J. Psychopharmacol.* **24:** 1505–1514.
5. Li, H., N. Xia & U. Förstermann. 2012. Cardiovascular effects and molecular targets of resveratrol. *Nitric Oxide* **26:** 102–110.
6. Félétou, M. 2011. The endothelium, part I: multiple functions of the endothelial cells—focus on endothelium-derived vasoactive mediators. D.N. Granger & J.P. Granger, Eds. San Rafael, CA: Morgan & Claypool Life Sciences.
7. Celermajer, D.S., K.E. Sorensen, C. Bull, *et al.* 1994. Endothelium-dependent dilation in the systemic arteries of asymptomatic subjects related to coronary risk

factors and their interaction. *J. Am. Coll. Cardiol.* **24:** 1468–1474.
8. Zimmermann, C. & R.L. Haberl. 2003. L-arginine improves diminished cerebral CO2 reactivity in patients. *Stroke* **34:** 643–647.
9. Markus, H. & M. Cullinane. 2001. Severely impaired cerebrovascular reactivity predicts stroke and TIA risk in patients with carotid artery stenosis and occlusion. *Brain* **124:** 457–467.
10. Silvestrini, M., P. Pasqualetti, R. Baruffaldi, *et al.* 2006. Cerebrovascular reactivity and cognitive decline in patients with Alzheimer disease. *Stroke* **37:** 1010–1015.
11. Thijssen, D.H.J., M.A. Black, K.E. Pyke, *et al.* 2011. Assessment of flow-mediated dilation in humans: a methodological and physiological guideline. *Am. J. Physiol Heart Circ. Physiol.* **300:** H2–H12.
12. Yavuz, B.B., B. Yavuz, D.D. Sener, *et al.* 2008. Advanced age is associated with endothelial dysfunction in healthy elderly subjects. *Gerontology* **54:** 153–156.
13. Palmieri, V., C. Russo, S. Pezzullo, *et al.* 2011. Relation of flow-mediated dilation to global arterial load: impact of hypertension and additional cardiovascular risk factors. *Int. J. Cardiol.* **152:** 225–230.
14. Davison, K., S. Bircher, A. Hill, *et al.* 2010. Relationships between obesity, cardiorespiratory fitness, and cardiovascular function. *J. Obes.* **2010:** Article ID 191253, 7 pp.
15. Henry, R.M.A., I. Ferreira, P.J. Kostense, *et al.* 2004. Type 2 diabetes is associated with impaired endothelium-dependent, flow-mediated dilation, but impaired glucose metabolism is not: the Hoorn Study. *Atherosclerosis* **174:** 49–56.
16. Vladimirova-Kitova, L., T. Deneva, E. Angelova, *et al.* 2008. Relationship of asymmetric dimethylarginine with flow-mediated dilatation in subjects with newly detected severe hypercholesterolemia. *Clin. Physiol. Funct. Imaging* **28:** 417–425.
17. Inaba, Y., J.A. Chen & S.R. Bergmann. 2010. Prediction of future cardiovascular outcomes by flow-mediated vasodilatation of brachial artery: a meta-analysis. *Int. J. Cardiovasc. Imaging* **26:** 631–640.
18. Hooper, L., P.A. Kroon, E.B. Rimm, *et al.* 2008. Flavonoids, flavonoid-rich foods, and cardiovascular risk: a meta-analysis of randomized controlled trials. *Am. J. Clin. Nutr.* **88:** 38–50.
19. Ras, R.T., P.L. Zock & R. Draijer. 2011. Tea consumption enhances endothelial-dependent vasodilation; a meta-analysis. *PLoS One* **6:** e16974.
20. Li, S.H, X. Liu, Y.Y. Bai, *et al.* 2010. Effect of oral isoflavone supplementation on vascular endothelial function in postmenopausal women: a meta-analysis of randomized placebo-controlled trials. *Am. J. Clin. Nutr.* **91:** 480–486.
21. Cohen, R.A., A. Poppas, D.E. Forman, *et al.* 2009. Vascular and cognitive functions associated with cardiovascular disease in the elderly. *J. Clin. Exp. Neuropsychol.* **31:** 96–110.
22. Forman, D.E., R.A. Cohen, K.F. Hoth, *et al.* 2008. Vascular health and cognitive function in older adults with cardiovascular disease. *Artery Res.* **2:** 35–43.
23. Feringa, H.H.H., D.A. Laskey, J.E. Dickson & C.I. Coleman. 2011. The effect of grape seed extract on cardiovascular risk markers: a meta-analysis of randomized controlled trials. *J. Am. Diet Assoc.* **111:** 1173–1181.

24. Mellen, P.B., K.R. Daniel, K.B. Brosnihan, *et al.* 2010. Effect of muscadine grape seed supplementation on vascular function in subjects with or at risk for cardiovascular disease: a randomized crossover trial. *J. Am. Coll. Nutr.* **29:** 469–475.

25. Lekakis, J., L.S. Rallidis, I. Andreadou, *et al.* 2005. Polyphenolic compounds from red grapes acutely improve endothelial function in patients with coronary heart disease. *Eur. J. Cardiovasc. Prev. Rehabil.* **12:** 596–600.

26. Clifton, P.M. 2004. Effect of grape seed extract and quercetin on cardiovascular and endothelial parameters in high-risk subjects. *J. Biomed. Biotechnol.* **5:** 272–278.

27. Fujitaka, K., H. Otani, F. Jo, *et al.* 2011. Modified resveratrol Longevinex improves endothelial function in adults with metabolic syndrome receiving standard treatment. *Nutr. Res.* **31:** 842–847.

28. Magyar, K., R. Halmosi, A. Palfi, *et al.* 2012. Cardioprotection by resveratrol: a human clinical trial in patients with stable coronary artery disease. *Clin. Hemorheol. Microcirc.* **50:** 179–187.

29. Wong, R.H.X., P.R.C. Howe, J.D. Buckley, *et al.* 2011. Acute resveratrol supplementation improves flow-mediated dilatation in overweight/obese individuals with mildly elevated blood pressure. *Nutr. Metab. Cardiovasc. Dis.* **21:** 851–856.

30. Widlansky, M.E., S.J. Duffy, N.M. Hamburg, *et al.* 2005. Effects of black tea consumption on plasma catechins and markers of oxidative stress and inflammation in patients with coronary artery disease. *Free Radic. Biol. Med.* **38:** 499–506.

31. Widlansky, M.E., N.M. Hamburg, E. Anter, *et al.* 2007. Acute EGCG supplementation reverses endothelial dysfunction in patients with coronary artery disease. *J. Am. Coll. Nutr.* **26:** 95–102.

32. EFSA. 2012. Scientific opinion on the substantiation of a health claim related to cocoa flavanols and maintenance of normal endothelium-dependent vasodilation pursuant to Article 13(5) of Regulation (EC) No 1924/2006. *EFSA Journal* **10:** 2809.

33. Wong, R.H.X., N.M. Berry, A.M. Coates, *et al.* 2012. Sustained improvement of vasodilator function by resveratrol in obese adults. *J. Hypertens.* **30:** e70.

34. Chachay, V.S., C.M. Kirkpatrick, I.J. Hickman, *et al.* 2011. Resveratrol—pills to replace a healthy diet? *Br. J. Clin. Pharmacol.* **72:** 27–38.

35. Sinn, N. & P.R.C. Howe. 2008. Mental health benefits of omega-3 fatty acids may be mediated by improvements in cerebral vascular function. *Biosci. Hypotheses* **1:** 103–108.

36. Francis, S.T., K. Head, P.G. Morris & I.A. Macdonald. 2006. The effect of flavanol-rich cocoa on the fMRI response to a cognitive task in healthy young people. *J. Cardiovasc. Pharmacol.* **47:** S215–S220.

37. Wong, R.H., P.R. Howe, A.M. Coates, *et al.* 2013. Chronic consumption of a wild green oat extract (Neuravena) improves brachial flow-mediated dilatation and cerebrovascular responsiveness in older adults. *J. Hypertens.* **31:** 192–200.

38. Kennedy, D.O., E.L. Wightman, J.L. Reay, *et al.* 2010. Effects of resveratrol on cerebral blood flow variables and cognitive performance in humans: a double-blind, placebo-controlled, crossover investigation. *Am. J. Clin. Nutr.* **91:** 1590–1597.

39. Desideri, G., C. Kwik-Uribe, D. Grassi, *et al.* 2012. Benefits in cognitive function, blood pressure, and insulin resistance through cocoa flavanol consumption in elderly subjects with mild cognitive impairment: the Cocoa, Cognition, and Aging (CoCoA) study. *Hypertension* **60:** 794–801.

40. Badcock, N.A., G. Holt, A. Holden & D.V.M. Bishop. 2012. dopOSCCI: a functional transcranial Doppler ultrasonography summary suite for the assessment of cerebral lateralization of cognitive function. *J. Neurosci. Meth.* **204:** 383–388.

Ann. N.Y. Acad. Sci. ISSN 0077-8923

ANNALS OF THE NEW YORK ACADEMY OF SCIENCES

Issue: *Resveratrol and Health*

Osteogenic effects of resveratrol *in vitro*: potential for the prevention and treatment of osteoporosis

Ali Mobasheri[1,2] and Mehdi Shakibaei[3]

[1]Medical Research Council-Arthritis Research UK Centre for Musculoskeletal Ageing Research, Arthritis Research UK Pain Centre, Arthritis Research UK Centre for Sport, Exercise, and Osteoarthritis, Faculty of Medicine and Health Sciences, The University of Nottingham, United Kingdom. [2]Center of Excellence in Genomic Medicine Research (CEGMR), King Fahad Medical Research Center, King Abdulaziz University, Jeddah, Kingdom of Saudi Arabia. [3]Institute of Anatomy, Ludwig Maximilian University Munich, Germany

Address for correspondence: Mehdi Shakibaei, Institute of Anatomy, Musculoskeletal Research Group, Ludwig-Maximilian-University Munich, Pettenkoferstrasse 11, D-80336 Munich, Germany. mehdi.shakibaei@med.uni-muenchen.de

There are a number of pharmacological agents for the treatment of bone mineral loss and osteoporosis. Hormone replacement therapy (HRT) with estrogen is an established treatment, but it has several adverse side effects and can increase the risk of cancer, heart disease, and stroke. There is increasing interest in nutritional factors and naturally occurring phytochemical compounds with the potential for preventing age-related and postmenopausal bone loss. Resveratrol (3,5,4′-trihydroxy-*trans*-stilbene) is a polyphenolic phytoestrogen with osteogenic and osteoinductive properties. It can modify the metabolism of bone cells and has the capacity to modulate bone turnover. This paper provides an overview of current research on resveratrol and its effects on bone cells *in vitro*, highlighting the challenges and opportunities facing this area of research, especially in the context of providing nutritional support for postmenopausal women who may not benefit from HRT and older patients with various forms of arthritis, metabolic bone disease, and osteoporosis.

Keywords: resveratrol; phytoestrogen; osteogenesis; osteoporosis; menopause

Introduction

Despite being calcified, bone is a living and dynamic tissue that constantly turns over and renews itself. The osteon in cortical bone is the micromechanical unit that responds to the biomechanical, endocrine, and nutritional stimuli that are responsible for the physiological maintenance of bone extracellular matrix (ECM).[1] Old bone is degraded by bone-resorbing osteoclasts and is replaced with new bone produced by bone-synthesizing osteoblasts.[2] However, the delicate balance between bone synthesis and bone degradation is lost with aging, resulting in low bone density and osteoporosis. Osteoporosis is a metabolic disease of bones that causes them to become more porous, gradually making them weaker, more brittle, more fragile, and more likely to fracture. The increased porosity is the result of an imbalance in the bone remodeling process, whereby bone resorption, mediated by osteoclasts, outpaces bone formation, mediated by osteoblasts. Consequently, osteoporosis reduces bone mineral density and mass, making long bones significantly more prone to fractures. Osteoporosis-induced bone fractures commonly occur in the spine, wrist, and hips, but can affect other bones such as the arm or the pelvis. Reduced bone mineral density can be a feature of bone remodeling in arthritis; subchondral bone sclerosis is also associated with age-related joint degeneration.[4]

Nonhormonal treatments for osteoporosis: bisphosphonates

Significant progress has been made over the past five decades in the nonhormonal treatment of osteoporosis.[5] Bisphosphonates (BPs) are a class of drugs that are used to treat osteoporosis and related bone diseases by preventing the loss of bone mass.

doi: 10.1111/nyas.12145

These drugs were developed in the early 1960s as potential treatments for bone diseases. Five decades later, BPs are the most frequently prescribed drugs for the treatment of osteoporosis and other diseases characterized by increased bone resorption. In patients with postmenopausal osteoporosis, BPs reduce osteoclast activity back to healthy, premenopausal levels, thereby decreasing the rate of bone loss. BP drugs increase bone mass, strengthen bones, and reduce the incidence of fractures, including severe fractures of the hip and spine. BPs approved for the treatment and/or prevention of osteoporosis include alendronate (Fosamax, Fosamax Plus D; Merck, Whitehouse Station, New Jersey, USA), ibandronate (Boniva; Genentech, South San Francisco, California, USA), zoledronic acid (Reclast; Novartis, Basel, Switzerland), and risedronate (Actonel, Actonel with Calcium, and Atelvia; Warner Chilcott, Dublin, Ireland). Other BPs include etidronate, raloxifene, and teriparatide, for the secondary prevention of osteoporotic fragility fractures in postmenopausal women. In addition to osteoporosis, BPs are also used to lower calcium levels in the blood and to treat Paget's disease of bone (which causes bones to become weak and deformed) and bone-related cancers, alleviating pain and weakness. In addition, BPs are also used following other forms of cancer treatment, such as chemotherapy and hormone therapies, both of which can weaken bones. They can also prevent some cancers from spreading to bone. Therefore, BPs are an enormously important class of drugs in modern medicine, and in addition to their therapeutic potential for osteoporosis and related bone diseases, they are potential therapeutic agents for disease modification in osteoarthritis.[6] Discussion of the side effects of BPs is beyond the scope of this review. We refer the readers to the NIH website for further information (http://nihseniorhealth.gov/osteoporosis/treatmentandresearch/01.html). However, bone is also highly responsive to sex hormones, particularly estrogen, and its turnover can be regulated by estrogen-like compounds.

Hormonal treatments for osteoporosis: estrogen

Estrogen plays a fundamental role in skeletal growth and bone homeostasis in both men and women.[7] Although the term *estrogen* actually refers to a large number of steroidal and nonsteroidal molecules ca-pable of inducing estrus, in the context of this article, *estrogen* refers to a pharmacological agent in hormone replacement therapy (HRT) to prevent postmenopausal bone loss in older women.[8] Taking estrogen orally in various formulations or as an adhesive skin patch increases circulating levels of this hormone and compensates for its loss after menopause, thus relieving the symptoms of menopause. It is especially recommended after menopause to prevent osteoporosis in women. It slows down the loss of bone minerals and increases bone thickness. Estrogen has been shown to prevent bone loss and lower the risk of hip fractures in postmenopausal women. Estrogen deficiency can also affect young women, and oral estrogen is prescribed to young women with hormonal imbalances.[9]

Estrogen deficiency is also linked to disturbances in the redox state. The acute loss of estrogens has been shown to increase the levels of reactive oxygen species (ROS), activate nuclear factor κB (NF-κB), and stimulate the production of proinflammatory cytokines such as interleukin 1β (IL-1β) and tumor necrosis factor α (TNF-α).[10] The production of proinflammatory cytokines is a common feature of many different types of inflammatory bone and joint disorders. Interestingly, proinflammatory cytokine production and release is attenuated by HRT.[10] Therefore, for long-term preservation of bone mineral density, women are advised to take estrogen for at least seven years after menopause.[8] This strategy is thought to reduce the risk of developing osteoarthritis and osteoporosis. However, this duration of therapy may have little effect on bone density in women over 75, who have the highest risk of developing fractures.[8] Studies also suggest that age-related bone loss may be the result of estrogen deficiency in men as well as postmenopausal women.[11] These studies highlight the fact that estrogen is important for the maintenance of bone mineral density in both men and women.

However, estrogen use is associated with a number of undesired side effects that include headache, fluid retention, weight gain, and swollen breasts. In addition to these minor side effects, there are reports that suggest an increased risk of breast or uterine cancer, heart failure, or stroke in some women. Therefore, it may not be recommended for women who have a family or personal history of heart disease, stroke, blood clots, or breast cancer. The Women's Health Initiative (WHI) study linked the

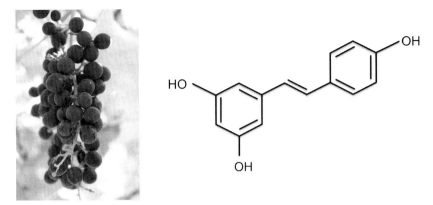

Figure 1. Resveratrol, also known as *trans*-resveratrol, 3,5,4′-trihydroxy-*trans*-stilbene, is produced by grape vines in response to fungal infections. It is induced by stress, injury, or ultraviolet irradiation. Resveratrol is also found in *Polygonum cuspidatum* and several other plant species. Resveratrol has anti-inflammatory, anticarcinogenic, antimutagenic, antineoplastic, and antioxidant properties.

use of HRT to an increase in a woman's risk of depression and cardiovascular sequelae including stroke.[12] Many experts recommend that long-term estrogen replacement therapy only be considered for women with a significant risk for osteoporosis that outweighs the risks of taking HRT. Like other drugs and hormone treatments, estrogen has side effects and should be taken at the lowest dose and for the shortest possible duration. Women who experience side effects from taking estrogen are advised to seek help from their medical practitioner.

Phytoestrogens and resveratrol

The side effects of estrogen therapy highlight a medical need for safer treatments for bone mineral loss and associated bone and joint disorders. As suggested earlier, the term *estrogen* refers to a large number of steroidal and nonsteroidal molecules, many of which naturally exist in our food and the environment. Phytoestrogens are plant-derived compounds found in a wide variety of foods. They are capable of substituting for estrogens[13] and may be implicated in lowering the risk of osteoporosis, heart disease, breast cancer, and menopausal symptoms.[14] Phytoestrogens possess estrogenic and antiestrogenic effects, and some of them are considered to be endocrine disruptors with the potential to cause adverse health effects.[14] Some phytoestrogens can enhance bone formation, increase bone mineral density, and increase the expression of bone markers including alkaline phosphatase, osteocalcin, osteopontin, and type I collagen.[15] Resvera-

trol, also known as 3,5,4′-trihydroxy-*trans*-stilbene, is a polyphenolic phytoestrogen and phytoalexin present in plants such as grapes, berries, and peanuts (Fig. 1). It has a variety of potentially beneficial health effects and has been reported to possess anti-inflammatory, immunomodulatory, and antioxidative capabilities.[16] The subsequent sections highlight selected research articles on the effects of resveratrol on bone.

In vitro and *in vivo* effects of resveratrol on bone

Resveratrol has been shown to stimulate bone cell proliferation and differentiation. One of the first studies of resveratrol action on bone cells was carried out using osteoblastic MC3T3-E1 cells. This study demonstrated the ability of resveratrol to directly stimulate the proliferation and differentiation of osteoblasts.[17] Resveratrol dose dependently increased DNA synthesis and alkaline phosphatase (ALP) and prolyl hydroxylase activities in MC3T3-E1 cells. The effects of resveratrol were antagonized by the antiestrogen drug tamoxifen. Turner *et al.* carried out an *in vivo* study published in 1999 to determine if resveratrol can act as an estrogen agonist in growing rats.[18] Their 6-day study in weanling rats aimed to determine the dose response of orally administered resveratrol on estrogen target tissues. They used resveratrol concentrations including 1, 4, 10, 40, and 100 μg/day. Using 10% ethanol as a solvent had no significant effect on any of the measurements. They found that resveratrol had no effect on body weight, uterine wet weight, uterine epithelial cell height, cortical bone histomorphometry, or serum cholesterol. Based on the *in vivo* data obtained, they proposed that resveratrol has little or no estrogen agonism on reproductive and nonreproductive estrogen target tissues and may be an estrogen antagonist. Similar work carried out by Durbin *et al.* has shown that resveratrol supplementation of 6-month-old Brown Norway male rats had no bone protective effects and may even have detrimental bone effects.[16] In contrast, work by Liu *et al.* has shown that resveratrol from *Polygonum cuspidatum* increases bone mineral density in the epiphysis of the ovariectomized female rat model.[19] This model is much more relevant to hormone-dependent osteoporosis and provides more tangible evidence for using resveratrol for protecting against bone loss induced by estrogen deficiency.

These studies highlight the fact that *in vitro* and *in vivo* data are not always directly comparable. Also, data from animal models, especially rodents, are often conflicting and the outcomes depend on the type of model that was employed. Although rodent data may not always be directly translatable to humans, the ovariectomized female rat is probably the most suitable animal model for research on drugs and natural compounds for treating osteoporosis.

More recent data from our own work suggest that resveratrol affects sirtuin 1 (Sirt1). The *Sirt1* gene encodes a member of the sirtuin family of proteins, homologs to the yeast Sir2 protein, which are known to regulate epigenetic gene silencing. Members of the sirtuin family are histone deacetylases characterized by a sirtuin core domain. Sirt1 is a NAD^+-dependent histone deacetylase. Sirtuins are believed to function as intracellular regulatory proteins with mono-ADP–ribosyltransferase activity. The effects of resveratrol on Sirt1 influence its interactions with receptor activator of NF-κB ligand (RANKL) and the bone-specific transcription factor Runx2, in bone-derived cells and mesenchymal stem cells (MSCs), respectively.[20,21]

The RANKL/RANK/osteoprotegerin (OPG) system plays an important role in the regulation of bone resorption.[22] RANKL is a cytokine and a member of the TNF superfamily. It stimulates osteoclast differentiation and augments bone loss. We recently used high-density bone cultures to investigate the effects of resveratrol on RANKL during bone morphogenesis *in vitro*.[20] We observed that RANKL induced

formation of tartrate-resistant acid phosphatase–positive multinucleated cells that exhibited morphological features of osteoclasts. RANKL also induced NF-κB activation. RANKL upregulated the expression of p300 (a histone acetyltransferase), which, in turn, promoted acetylation of NF-κB. However, in cultures pretreated with resveratrol, this activation was inhibited. Resveratrol also suppressed the activation of IκBα kinase and the phosphorylation and degradation of IκBα. Resveratrol inhibited RANKL-induced acetylation and nuclear translocation of NF-κB in a time- and concentration-dependent manner. In addition, activation of Sirt1 by resveratrol induced Sirt1–p300 association in both bone-derived and preosteoblastic cells, leading to deacetylation of RANKL-induced NF-κB, inhibition of NF-κB transcriptional activation, and osteoclastogenesis. Cotreatment with resveratrol activated the bone transcription factor Cbfa1 and Sirt1 and induced the formation of Sirt1–Cbfa1 complexes. This *in vitro* study demonstrated that resveratrol-activated Sirt1 plays important roles in regulating the balance between bone resorption and bone production. This was the first study that highlighted the mechanisms underlying the therapeutic potential of resveratrol for treating osteoporosis and arthritis-related bone loss.[20]

In a more recent study, we examined whether activation of Sirt1 by resveratrol affects osteogenic differentiation. We employed monolayer and high-density cultures of MSCs and preosteoblastic cells and treated them with an osteogenic induction medium with or without the Sirt1 inhibitor nicotinamide and/or resveratrol in a concentration-dependent manner. MSCs and preosteoblastic cells differentiated into osteoblasts when exposed to osteogenic induction medium. Osteogenesis was blocked by nicotinamide, resulting in adipogenic differentiation and expression of the adipose transcription regulator PPARγ (peroxisome proliferator–activated receptor). However, in nicotinamide-treated cultures, pretreatment with resveratrol significantly enhanced osteogenesis by increasing expression of Runx2 (a transcription factor that encodes a nuclear protein with a Runt DNA-binding domain), and decreased the expression of PPARγ. Activation of Sirt1 by resveratrol in MSCs increased its binding to PPARγ and repressed PPARγ activity by involving its cofactor nuclear receptor corepressor (NCoR). The modulatory effects of resveratrol on nicotinamide-induced expression of PPARγ and its cofactor NCoR were found to be partly mediated by the association between Sirt1 and Runx2 and by the deacetylation of Runx2. Knockdown of Sirt1 protein expression by antisense oligonucleotides abolished the inhibitory effects of resveratrol, namely, nicotinamide-induced Sirt1 suppression and Runx2 acetylation, suggesting that the acetylation of Runx2 is related to down-regulated Sirt1 expression. This study suggests that Runx2 acetylation/deacetylation is important during osteogenic differentiation in MSCs.[21]

Synergistic actions of resveratrol and curcumin

Combinations of phytochemicals and phytoestrogens are thought to exert synergistic effects *in vitro* and *in vivo*. Recently, we have critically reviewed the scientific evidence and rationale for the development of phytochemicals such as curcumin and resveratrol as nutraceuticals for joint health.[23] Curcumin and resveratrol have the capacity to target NF-κB signaling and inflammation in osteoarthritis. Recent studies from our laboratories have focused on the synergistic anti-inflammatory effects of curcumin and resveratrol on cartilage cells (chondrocytes), when these agents are used in combination. *In vitro*, resveratrol and curcumin have been shown to inhibit IL-1β–induced apoptosis in chondrocytes, by inhibition of caspase 3 and downregulation of the NF-κB pathway.[24–27] Resveratrol and curcumin have also been shown to suppress NF-κB–dependent proinflammatory mediators such as PGE$_2$, leukotriene B$_4$ (LTB$_4$), COX2, MMP-1, MMP-3, and MMP-13. These studies highlight the fact that combinations of these phytochemicals may be more effective than the individual compounds by themselves. Treatment with curcumin and resveratrol suppresses the expression of NF-κB–regulated gene products involved in inflammation (e.g., COX2, MMP-3, MMP-9, and vascular endothelial growth factor [VEGF]).[25] Combinations of curcumin and resveratrol inhibit apoptosis and prevent activation of caspase 3.[25] Closer examination of the signaling pathway has shown that IL-1β–induced NF-κB activation can be suppressed directly by mixtures of curcumin and resveratrol through inhibition of IKK and proteasome activation, inhibition of IκBα phosphorylation and degradation, and inhibition of nuclear transloca-

tion of NF-κB. Combining curcumin and resveratrol also activates MEK/Erk signaling. The mitogen-activated protein kinase (MAPK) pathway is stimulated in differentiated chondrocytes and is an important signaling cascade for the maintenance of the chondrocyte phenotype. Activation of this pathway is thought to be required for the maintenance of chondrocyte differentiation and survival. These observations support the enhanced potential of combination therapy, with both anti-inflammatory and antiapoptotic capabilities mediated by inhibition of multiple components of the NF-κB pathway, to treat osteoarthritis and osteoporosis.

Recent work suggests that resveratrol has osteogenic effects on MSCs.[13] For example, resveratrol promotes osteogenesis of human MSCs by upregulating Runx2 gene expression by activating the Sirt1–FOXO3a axis.[28] Resveratrol enhances the canonical Wnt signaling pathway, thus promoting osteoblastic differentiation of MSCs.[28] Resveratrol also enhances osteoblastic differentiation in MSCs via Erk1/2 activation.[29]

In addition, *in vitro* combinations of resveratrol and curcumin have the synergistic potential to promote chondrogenic and osteogenic differentiation of MSCs by targeting NF-κB. For example, treating MSC cultures with curcumin has been shown to suppress NF-κB, thus establishing a microenvironment in which the effects of proinflammatory cytokines are antagonized.[30] This facilitates the chondrogenesis of MSC-like progenitor cells co-cultured with primary chondrocytes.[30] The use of this strategy *in vitro* may support the regeneration of articular cartilage in cell-based cartilage repair techniques, such as autologous chondrocyte implantation (ACI), since cell-based repair of lesions in articular cartilage will be compromised in already inflamed joints. Resveratrol-mediated modulation of Sirt1 and Runx2 promotes osteogenic differentiation of MSCs.[21] Our work also suggests that acetylation and deacetylation of Runx2 are critical for osteogenic differentiation.[21]

Based on these results, we (and others) have proposed that combining these natural compounds may potentially be a more useful strategy for supporting cartilage and bone health than using each individual compound alone. The data available suggest that combinations of phytochemicals work well in culture, but further research is required in animal models and human subjects.

Resveratrol, sirtuins, and mitochondrial function

The identification of naturally occurring compounds capable of altering mitochondrial function could complement strategies to reduce cartilage degradation in osteoarthritis.[31] Similar approaches may support bone turnover in osteoporosis. Regulating cartilage and bone metabolism, autophagy, and apoptosis may be achieved naturally, through pharmacological and physiological modulation of sirtuins. As described earlier, sirtuins are a family of seven NAD^+-dependent deacetylases that may be activated by NAD^+ and the antioxidant phytochemical resveratrol.[32] Resveratrol has been shown to protect chondrocytes against oxidant injury and apoptosis through its effects on mitochondrial repolarization and ATP production.[33] The authors have recently reviewed the potential benefits of resveratrol for enhancing chondrocyte function.[23,34] Dietary supplementation with resveratrol and related antioxidant phytoestrogens may be another important nutritional preventive strategy for osteoarthritis and osteoporosis, especially in people with compromised antioxidant systems. Indeed, it has been reported that resveratrol, as a natural polyphenolic compound, can protect various tissues against oxidative damage: its chemical structure contains electron donors that can prevent hydroxyl radical and superoxide anion formation, thereby suppressing lipid peroxidation, protein oxidation, and DNA damage.[35,36]

Conclusions

The aim of this article was to review the effects of resveratrol on bone cells *in vitro* and highlight the osteogenic and osteoinductive effects of this compound in studies of bone cells in culture. Dietary resveratrol may have potential benefits for modulating bone resorption in age-related, hormone-dependent, and postmenopausal osteoporosis. Cross-sectional studies have demonstrated a positive association between higher fruit intake and higher bone mineral density.[37,38] Therefore, there is considerable interest in finding natural alternatives in foods and combining them with vitamins for further synergistic action on bone.[39] This highlights the potential of natural osteoinductive phytoestrogens such as resveratrol for the nutritional

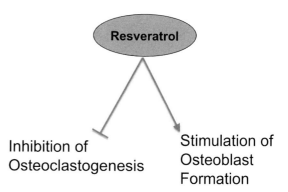

Figure 2. The effects of resveratrol on osteoclastogenesis and osteoblast formation.

support of bone. The schematics in Figures 2 and 3 summarize the key effects of resveratrol on bone cells (osteoblasts and osteoclasts) and MSCs. The currently available *in vitro* data support the role for resveratrol in bone health in general. However, it is important to note that the potential for using resveratrol in the treatment of osteoporosis is currently underdeveloped and requires further investigation and extensive clinical trials. The major challenges facing this area of research are the safety and bioavailability of resveratrol.

According to the data available on TOXNET (http://toxnet.nlm.nih.gov/), safety issues related to the consumption of natural forms of resveratrol are relatively minor. Pregnant women and nursing mothers are advised to avoid the use of resveratrol-containing supplements; they should also avoid the use of wine as a primary source of resveratrol. There are no reported safety concerns for older women. However, closer examination of the evidence available suggests that the issue of the safety of resveratrol (and its analogues) is controversial. In 2010, the pharmaceutical company GlaxoSmithKline (GSK) suspended a clinical trial of SRT501 (http://www.clinicaltrials.gov/show/NCT00920556), a proprietary form of resveratrol, due to safety concerns, and terminated the study. The pharmacokinetics, bioavailability, and safety profile of *trans*-resveratrol have recently been studied in healthy human volunteers.[40] The study was a double-blind, randomized, placebo-controlled investigation of increasing concentrations of *trans*-resveratrol (25, 50, 100, or 150 mg), given orally, six times a day, for a maximum of 13 doses. Peak plasma concentrations of

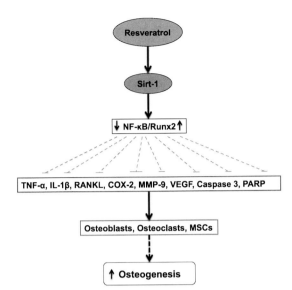

Figure 3. Proposed signaling pathway summarizing the molecular targets of resveratrol in bone and its effects on osteogenesis.

trans-resveratrol were reached at 0.8–1.5 h after oral ingestion, and these were higher after morning administration. Although repeated oral administration of high doses with short dosing intervals was well tolerated, this approach produced relatively low plasma concentrations of *trans*-resveratrol; 150 mg of *trans*-resveratrol resulted in a peak plasma concentration (C_{max}) of 63.8 ng/mL.

Another underdeveloped area relating to research on resveratrol is the paucity of clinical trials. No convincing randomized clinical trials have been conducted to test the *in vivo* efficacy and safety of resveratrol thus far. The poor bioavailability of resveratrol is a major problem affecting the design of clinical trials of various oral formulations. Once this issue has been satisfactorily addressed, large-scale clinical trials will be needed to determine whether resveratrol supplementation will prove beneficial for bone health in estrogen-deficient young patients and cohorts of elderly men and women over 75 years of age. Finally, resveratrol analogues act as antagonists of osteoclast activity and promoters of osteoblast function.[41] Despite the suspension of the clinical trial of SRT501, there are opportunities for the pharmaceutical industry for developing resveratrol analogues with enhanced gastrointestinal absorption and bioavailability for modulating bone remodeling. Future work will need to evaluate the risk–benefit ratio of resveratrol supplementation and to consider the cost of supplements. We and other investigators will be evaluating the emerging evidence for the potential beneficial effects of resveratrol on bone health (as we have recently done for glucosamine[42]) and will propose new strategies for the design of clinical trials aimed at identifying beneficial physiological effects on bone.

Acknowledgments

A.M. is the co-ordinator of the D-BOARD Consortium funded by European Commission Framework 7 program (EUFP7; HEALTH.2012.2.4.5–2, project number 305815, Novel Diagnostics and Biomarkers for Early Identification of Chronic Inflammatory Joint Diseases). A.M. also wishes to acknowledge the support of Arthritis Research U.K. and the Medical Research Council. The authors wish to apologize to all those scientists whose work could not be cited due to space limitations.

Conflicts of interest

The authors declare no conflicts of interest.

References

1. Ascenzi, M.G. & A.K. Roe. 2012. The osteon: the micromechanical unit of compact bone. *Front Biosci.* **17:** 1551–1581.
2. Del Fattore, A., A. Teti & N. Rucci. 2012. Bone cells and the mechanisms of bone remodelling. *Front Biosci.* **4:** 2302–2321.
3. Rosen, C.J. 2000. Pathogenesis of osteoporosis. *Baillieres Best Pract. Res. Clin. Endocrinol. Metab.* **14:** 181–193.
4. Burr, D.B. & M.A. Gallant. 2012. Bone remodelling in osteoarthritis. *Nat. Rev. Rheumatol.* **8:** 665–673.
5. Rizzoli, R. 2007. Osteoporosis: non-hormonal treatment. *Climacteric* **10:** 74–78.
6. Spector, T.D. 2003. Bisphosphonates: potential therapeutic agents for disease modification in osteoarthritis. *Aging Clin. Exp. Res.* **15:** 413–418.
7. Weitzmann, M.N. & R. Pacifici. 2006. Estrogen deficiency and bone loss: an inflammatory tale. *J. Clin. Invest.* **116:** 1186–1194.
8. Felson, D.T., Y. Zhang, M.T. Hannan, *et al.* 1993. The effect of postmenopausal estrogen therapy on bone density in elderly women. *N. Engl. J. Med.* **329:** 1141–1146.
9. Popat, V.B., K.A. Calis, V.H. Vanderhoof, *et al.* 2009. Bone mineral density in estrogen-deficient young women. *J. Clin. Endocrinol. Metab.* **94:** 2277–2283.
10. Martin-Millan, M. & S. Castaneda. 2013. Estrogens, osteoarthritis and inflammation. *Joint Bone Spine.* doi: 10.1016/j.jbspin.2012.11.008.
11. Khosla, S., L.J. Melton, 3rd, E.J. Atkinson, *et al.* 1998. Relationship of serum sex steroid levels and bone turnover

markers with bone mineral density in men and women: a key role for bioavailable estrogen. *J. Clin. Endocrinol. Metab.* **83:** 2266–2274.

12. Wassertheil-Smoller, S. *et al.* 2004. Depression and cardiovascular sequelae in postmenopausal women. The Women's Health Initiative (WHI). *Arch. Intern. Med.* **164:** 289–298.

13. Schilling, T. *et al.* 2012. Effects of phytoestrogens and other plant-derived compounds on mesenchymal stem cells, bone maintenance and regeneration. *J. Steroid Biochem. Mol. Biol.* doi: 10.1016/j.jsbmb.2012.12.006.

14. Patisaul, H.B. & W. Jefferson. 2010. The pros and cons of phytoestrogens. *Front Neuroendocrinol.* **31:** 400–419.

15. Chiang, S.S. & T.M. Pan. 2013. Beneficial effects of phytoestrogens and their metabolites produced by intestinal microflora on bone health. *Appl. Microbiol. Biotechnol.* **97:** 1489–1500.

16. Csiszar, A. 2011. Anti-inflammatory effects of resveratrol: possible role in prevention of age-related cardiovascular disease. *Ann. N.Y. Acad. Sci.* **1215:** 117–122.

17. Mizutani, K. *et al.* 1998. Resveratrol stimulates the proliferation and differentiation of osteoblastic MC3T3-E1 cells. *Biochem. Biophys. Res. Commun.* **253:** 859–863.

18. Turner, R.T. *et al.* 1999. Is resveratrol an estrogen agonist in growing rats? *Endocrinology* **140:** 50–54.

19. Liu, Z.P. *et al.* 2005. Effects of trans-resveratrol from *Polygonum cuspidatum* on bone loss using the ovariectomized rat model. *J. Med. Food* **8:** 14–19.

20. Shakibaei, M., C. Buhrmann & A. Mobasheri. 2011. Resveratrol-mediated SIRT-1 interactions with p300 modulate receptor activator of NF-kappaB ligand (RANKL) activation of NF-kappaB signaling and inhibit osteoclastogenesis in bone-derived cells. *J. Biol. Chem.* **286:** 11492–11505.

21. Shakibaei, M. *et al.* 2012. Resveratrol mediated modulation of Sirt-1/Runx2 promotes osteogenic differentiation of mesenchymal stem cells: potential role of Runx2 deacetylation. *PLoS One* **7:** e35712.

22. Boyce, B.F. & L. Xing. 2007. Biology of RANK, RANKL, and osteoprotegerin. *Arthritis Res. Ther.* **9:** S1.

23. Mobasheri, A. *et al.* 2012. Scientific evidence and rationale for the development of curcumin and resveratrol as nutraceutricals for joint health. *Int. J. Mol. Sci.* **13:** 4202–4232.

24. Csaki, C. *et al.* 2008. Regulation of inflammation signalling by resveratrol in human chondrocytes *in vitro*. *Biochem. Pharmacol.* **75:** 677–687.

25. Csaki, C., A. Mobasheri & M. Shakibaei. 2009. Synergistic chondroprotective effects of curcumin and resveratrol in human articular chondrocytes: inhibition of IL-1beta-induced NF-kappaB-mediated inflammation and apoptosis. *Arthritis Res. Ther.* **11:** R165.

26. Shakibaei, M. *et al.* 2008. Resveratrol suppresses interleukin-1beta-induced inflammatory signaling and apoptosis in human articular chondrocytes: potential for use as a novel nutraceutical for the treatment of osteoarthritis. *Biochem. Pharmacol.* **76:** 1426–1439.

27. Shakibaei, M. *et al.* 2007. Resveratrol inhibits IL-1 beta-induced stimulation of caspase-3 and cleavage of PARP in human articular chondrocytes *in vitro*. *Ann. N.Y. Acad. Sci.* **1095:** 554–563.

28. Tseng, P.C. *et al.* 2011. Resveratrol promotes osteogenesis of human mesenchymal stem cells by upregulating RUNX2 gene expression via the SIRT1/FOXO3A axis. *J. Bone Miner. Res.* **26:** 2552–2563.

29. Dai, Z. *et al.* 2007. Resveratrol enhances proliferation and osteoblastic differentiation in human mesenchymal stem cells via ER-dependent ERK1/2 activation. *Phytomedicine* **14:** 806–814.

30. Buhrmann, C. *et al.* 2010. Curcumin mediated suppression of nuclear factor-kappaB promotes chondrogenic differentiation of mesenchymal stem cells in a high-density co-culture microenvironment. *Arthritis Res. Ther.* **12:** R127.

31. Kim, J. *et al.* 2010. Mitochondrial DNA damage is involved in apoptosis caused by pro-inflammatory cytokines in human OA chondrocytes. *Osteoarthritis Cartilage* **18:** 424–432.

32. Morris, B.J. 2013. Seven sirtuins for seven deadly diseases of aging. *Free Radic. Biol. Med.* **56:** 133–171.

33. Dave, M. *et al.* 2008. The antioxidant resveratrol protects against chondrocyte apoptosis via effects on mitochondrial polarization and ATP production. *Arthritis Rheum.* **58:** 2786–2797.

34. Mobasheri, A. 2012. Intersection of inflammation and herbal medicine in the treatment of osteoarthritis. *Curr. Rheumatol. Rep.* **14:** 604–616.

35. Sinha, K., G. Chaudhary & Y.K. Gupta. 2002. Protective effect of resveratrol against oxidative stress in middle cerebral artery occlusion model of stroke in rats. *Life Sci.* **71:** 655–665.

36. Lopez-Velez, M., F. Martinez-Martinez & C. Del Valle-Ribes. 2003. The study of phenolic compounds as natural antioxidants in wine. *Crit. Rev. Food Sci. Nutr.* **43:** 233–244.

37. Shen, C.L. *et al.* 2012. Fruits and dietary phytochemicals in bone protection. *Nutr. Res.* **32:** 897–910.

38. Sacco, S.M., M.N. Horcajada & E. Offord. 2013. Phytonutrients for bone health during ageing. *Br. J. Clin. Pharmacol.* **75:** 697–707.

39. Lai, C.Y. *et al.* 2011. Preventing bone loss and weight gain with combinations of vitamin D and phytochemicals. *J. Med. Food* **14:** 1352–1362.

40. Almeida, L. *et al.* 2009. Pharmacokinetic and safety profile of trans-resveratrol in a rising multiple-dose study in healthy volunteers. *Mol. Nutr. Food Res.* **53:** S7–S15.

41. Kupisiewicz, K. *et al.* 2010. Potential of resveratrol analogues as antagonists of osteoclasts and promoters of osteoblasts. *Calcif. Tissue Int.* **87:** 437–449.

42. Henrotin, Y. *et al.* 2013. Physiological effects of oral glucosamine on joint health: current status and consensus on future research priorities. *BMC Res. Notes* **6:** 115.

Ann. N.Y. Acad. Sci. ISSN 0077-8923

ANNALS OF THE NEW YORK ACADEMY OF SCIENCES

Issue: *Resveratrol and Health*

Resveratrol in mammals: effects on aging biomarkers, age-related diseases, and life span

Julia Marchal, Fabien Pifferi, and Fabienne Aujard

UMR 7179 Centre National de la Recherche Scientifique, Muséum National d'Histoire Naturelle, Brunoy, France

Address for correspondence: Fabienne Aujard, UMR 7179 Centre National de la Recherche Scientifique, Muséum National d'Histoire Naturelle, 1 avenue du Petit Château, 91800 Brunoy, France. aujard@mnhn.fr

Through its antioxidant, anticarcinogenic, and anti-inflammatory properties, resveratrol has become a candidate for drug development in the context of aging studies. Scientific evidence has highlighted its potential as a therapeutic agent for cardiovascular diseases and some cancers but also as an antiaging molecule. Resveratrol is thought to mimic the beneficial effects of chronic and moderate calorie restriction. Nevertheless, no study has demonstrated the prolongation of life span in healthy nonobese mammal models. This review summarizes recent findings on the effects of resveratrol on aging and life span in mammals. In our opinion, more studies should be performed to assess the effects of a chronic dietary intake of resveratrol in long-lived species close to humans, such as nonhuman primates. This will certainly generate more evidence about the ability of resveratrol to achieve the physiological benefits that have been observed in small mammal laboratory models and feature the eventual unwanted secondary effects that may occur under high levels of resveratrol.

Keywords: resveratrol; nutrition; antiaging strategy; life span; mimetic effect

Over the past 20 years, interest in the benefits of natural polyphenolic compounds has increased: several epidemiological studies have suggested that there is a relationship between the consumption of foods rich in polyphenols and the prevention of certain diseases.[1] The polyphenolic compound resveratrol is a molecule synthesized in many plants, such as peanuts, blueberries, pine nuts, and grapes, which protects them against fungal infection and ultraviolet irradiation.[2] Since the early 1990s, scientists have suggested that it could be the molecule responsible for the French paradox. Indeed, in the southwestern population of France, the low occurrence of coronary heart diseases and cardiovascular diseases—despite the consumption of a high saturated fat diet—was correlated to some extent with the regular consumption of red wine, which contains high levels of resveratrol.[3,4] The growing interest in the use of such a molecule in scientific research is also due to its pleiotropic action. Resveratrol exerts its various biological actions on a variety of targets, including the cell surface and some intracellular receptors, the molecules of signal transduction, metabolism,

and DNA repair proteins and transcription factors.[5] Some studies have shown that these actions were flexible depending on the dose, cell type studied, genetic variation within a population, and species[6] (Table 1).

Many studies have reported the beneficial virtues of resveratrol,[7] especially with regard to the development of metabolic disorders, such as metabolic syndrome or type 2 diabetes, and to the development of certain age-related diseases. While biogerontologists have relied on its high antioxidant properties to slow the aging rate and delay the onset of age-related diseases, several reports have indicated that resveratrol could be the most promising candidate to mimic the beneficial effects induced by a chronic calorie restriction (CR) without malnutrition.[8] Since resveratrol may follow the identical metabolic pathway to CR, notably through the activation of sirtuins, a class of NAD-dependent proteins that possess antiaging activity by regulating transcription, apoptosis, and stress resistance, as well as energy regulation efficiency,[9] it has been suggested that it could prolong life span as well. However, the description

doi: 10.1111/nyas.12214

Table 1. Current models used in studies on resveratrol

Models	Size (weight)	Life span	Experimental advantages
Invertebrates			
Yeast (Saccharomycotina)	6–50 μm	30–40 cell divisions	Short life span, known
Nematode (Rhabditidae)	1 mm	3 weeks	genome, rapid
Fly (Drosophilidae)	2–4 mm	1 month	replication
Vertebrates			
Fish (Nothobranchiidae)	5–6 cm	3–6 months	Short-lived mammals, genetic lineage, rapid reproduction
Mice (Muridae)	7–10 cm (20–50 g)	2–3 years	
Rats (Muridae)	35–50 cm (200–600 g)	2–4 years	
Swine (Suidae)	(1–1.3 m)	22–27 years	Medium-lived mammals, physiology and systems close to humans
Nonhuman primate (prosimian, Cheirogaleidae)	25–30 cm (80–100 g)	6–8 years	Medium-lived primates, phylogenetically close to humans
Nonhuman primate (simian, Cercopithecidae)	50–60 cm (3–6 kg)	30–35 years	Medium-lived primates, phylogenetically close to humans
Humans	150–190 cm (50–100 kg)	70–90 years	Random clinical trials

of such mimetic effects remains somehow indecisive and scarce, particularly in long-lived species, including humans. Even though data are promising in invertebrate models, the evidence is still poor in vertebrates, especially mammals. Besides, longitudinal studies in relevant animal models would be of great help in understanding the mechanisms by which this compound can naturally play its antiaging action, whether or not it mimics the effects of CR. Selected surrogate aging biomarkers that assess energy balance, endocrine function, and cognitive and motor abilities may be used to evaluate the individual phenotype associated with advancing age as well as the health status in animals subjected to antiaging strategies, and such profiles may better correlate with biological age than with chronological age. This review aims to focus and report the effect of acute or chronic intake of resveratrol in mammals, on aging markers, and on the onset of diseases associated with age and longevity. Such results are of major importance in the validation and in the long-term implementation of the use of resveratrol supplementation in humans, especially in the therapeutic context of aging studies.

Resveratrol's effects on aging biomarkers

There is compelling evidence from animal and human studies supporting the hypothesis that aging is a plastic process.[10] It was assumed that aging is not a frozen event but could rather be modulated by environmental factors such as dietary habits. Numerous studies have shown that resveratrol has exhibited many beneficial effects on overall health, corroborating the beneficial effects found in CR studies.[11,12]

Resveratrol seems to be promising as an antidiabetic molecule, as it modulates insulin secretion, preserves pancreatic β cells, promotes the consumption of glucose by muscle cells, and improves insulin sensitivity in peripheral tissues as shown in rodent *in vitro* studies,[13] nonhuman primates,[14] and humans, *in vivo*[15] and *in vitro*.[16] However, recently

Poulsen *et al.* demonstrated no significant variations on either glucoregulatory functions or insulin sensitivity in obese men treated with high doses of resveratrol.[17] Importantly, the effects of resveratrol on insulin secretion and induced insulin sensitivity seem to be modulated *in vitro* by the activation of SIRT1[18] and AMPK.[19]

It has been demonstrated that resveratrol intake exerts favorable metabolic adaptation similar to the one observed during a CR diet, in several mammals including in humans.[20,21] These energy-balance regulations include reduction in sleeping metabolic rate and resting metabolic rate (RMR), but a 30-day resveratrol intake failed to decrease energy expenditure in obese humans as with CR.[22] Another 15-week follow-up study demonstrated that low or high doses of resveratrol did not increase energy intake in obese mice submitted to a high-fat diet; neither did they induce changes in metabolism (body weight and adiposity).[23] Resveratrol is also known to promote mitochondrial biogenesis, especially in muscle cells,[24] suggesting that the increase in RMR may be due to a rise in quantity and quality of mitochondria.

Some effects of resveratrol on biomarkers of aging have been proven to be relatively consistent. Resveratrol prevents cellular damage caused by reactive oxygen species and also plays an important role in inflammatory processes and inhibits aggregation of arterial thrombotic plaques.[25] In healthy subjects, resveratrol protects neurons from apoptosis induced by oxidative stress and by inflammation *in vivo*[26] and *in vitro*.[27] In models of induced Alzheimer's-like disease, resveratrol inhibits the aggregation of β-amyloid peptide, thereby causing a reduction in the formation of senile plaques.[28]

Nevertheless, recent studies have shown inconsistent effects of resveratrol on some specific biomarkers of aging. For example, a daily dose of resveratrol (0.0062 or 0.04 mg) enhances IGF-1 production in the specific brain region in adult mice, which has been linked to improved cognitive performances.[29] In contrast, high doses (2.5 g/day) of resveratrol taken for one month in adult (20–70 years old) healthy humans decreases circulating IGF-1 after ingestion, a reduction that is thought to explain the chemopreventive activity of resveratrol by limiting cellular growth and proliferation through the regulation of IGF-1 concentration.[30] Finally, after one year of treatment in adult nonhuman primates (3–4 years old, *Microcebus murinus*) receiving 200 mg/kg of body weight once a day, no difference was found in total IGF-1 plasma levels between resveratrol-supplemented and control animals.[31]

Some theories of aging state that minimizing the reproductive functions, which results in limited energy expenditure, could potentially lead to a lengthening of life span as seen under CR.[32] Previous research demonstrated the beneficial impact of resveratrol on sexual hormone and sperm quality in rats,[33] but there was no effect after one year of treatment in nonhuman primates.[31]

Although resveratrol, and natural polyphenolic extracts in general, are increasingly used in human studies, notably concerning the *in vitro* study of their antioxidant and neuroprotective properties in therapy against neurodegenerative diseases,[34] little evidence is available regarding a potential beneficial effect of resveratrol on cognitive skills. The study by Kennedy *et al.* in 2010 showed that an acute *trans*-resveratrol intake of 250 or 500 mg did not change cognitive performance in healthy young adult (25-year-old) humans, although 45 min after ingestion, resveratrol induced an increase in cerebral blood flow and blood oxygenation.[35] In adult (3–6 months) and in aged (22–24 months) rodents, doses of 1–50 mg/kg of resveratrol seem to have no effect on working[36,37] and spatial reference memories.[38] Very few studies have investigated the effect of resveratrol on spontaneous age-related memory deficits. Abraham and Johnson observed no effect of a 4-week resveratrol supplementation on spatial working memory in old mice (22–24 months).[36] Conversely, 12-week supplementation of a resveratrol analog improved spatial working memory without any effect on spatial reference memory in old rats.[39] In adult nonhuman primates (3–4 years old), 2 years of a 200 mg/kg/day resveratrol treatment revealed higher cognitive performances in treated animals when compared to control animals during the test of spontaneous alternation (working memory), and resveratrol enhanced the spatial memory skills tested in a Barnes-like maze.[40]

Numerous current studies on resveratrol highlight a number of positive effects on biomarker evolution during aging, particularly with regard to markers of energy balance and metabolism. Nonetheless, further studies are required, particularly in healthy subjects during normal aging.

Resveratrol's effects on age-related disease onset

Nutrition plays a critical role in the prevention and in the development of age-related diseases. In humans, few data are available regarding the effectiveness of resveratrol as a preventive or curative treatment against some chronic metabolic diseases, including type 2 diabetes and obesity. Clinical trials hold promise for the use of resveratrol to improve the overall health and prevention of chronic diseases associated with aging. However, further research is necessary and justified in order to understand the particular relationships between bioavailability in the whole organism and in target organs.

Resveratrol positively affects many mechanisms responsible for the development of cardiovascular diseases. As a strong antioxidant molecule, it prevents lipid peroxidation.[41] The antioxidant power of resveratrol results from the activation of specific antioxidant enzymes including superoxide dismutase or peroxidase. These enzymes are themselves key players in the cellular protection against reactive oxygen species. It was also shown that a treatment of 12.5 mg/kg of resveratrol limits the malondialdehyde levels in healthy rat brains.[42] Additionally, resveratrol prohibits, in a dose-dependent manner, the entry of oxidized low-density lipoprotein (LDL) into the vascular system wall. It also exerts beneficial counteracting effects on the adverse effects of a fat-rich diet in adult rodents by decreasing body mass, blood pressure, and the occurrence of cardiovascular diseases.[43] In the literature, *in vivo* and *in vitro* studies suggest the involvement of SIRT1 in cardiovascular diseases and in cardioprotection by resveratrol.[44] However, most of these studies are based on the pharmacological modulation of SIRT1 through various molecules such as resveratrol.

While at low doses (5–20 μM), resveratrol protects against type 2 diabetes, and cardiovascular and neurodegenerative diseases, high concentrations of resveratrol (10–40 mM) exert chemotherapeutic effects inducing cell cycle arrest and causing cancer cell apoptosis.[6] It is perhaps in the area of chemoprevention that resveratrol offers the most promising results. There are an increasing number of studies on this subject, increasing the knowledge about this polyphenol that is able to delay or completely stop the various stages of development of certain kinds of cancers. Another study discovered that cells convert resveratrol into an anticancer agent that can target and prevent cancer cells from developing and proliferating.[45] More specifically, it was shown that the enzyme cytochrome P450, found in various tumors, is capable of metabolizing resveratrol into a phytoestrogen, the piceatannol, endowed with anticancer properties.[46] In addition to its antioxidant quality, several studies have revealed that resveratrol protects the brain from free radical damage by acting as a shield against free radicals and cellular oxidative stress. Similarly, the effect of resveratrol in neurodegenerative diseases has been attributed to its ability to protect neuronal cells against various attacks *in vitro*, including those caused by oxidative stress.[26,47]

In brief, resveratrol is a very promising agent in the area of chemoprevention, as it mediates many cellular targets involved in cancer signaling pathways. But overall, great care must be taken regarding other diseases associated with aging, such as coronary heart disease and diabetes, indicating the need for longitudinal animal studies and human clinical trials.

Resveratrol's effects on life span

A longer life span may be achieved through two mechanisms. The first is by slowing down the aging rate from adulthood. A chronic resveratrol supplementation started into adulthood could therefore delay the onset of metabolic diseases associated with aging, as well as the general decline in body functions found with age, and thus extend life span. The second is that life span can be sustained if the tolerance to aging is increased, that is, when the capacity to survive during age-related adverse events is improved or made more efficient. Resveratrol may be effective in both preventing senescence-related dysfunctions and in delaying the onset of certain age-associated diseases or even treating chronic metabolic disorders. However, all these effects, as beneficial as they are, are not necessarily translated into greater—median or maximal—survival in treated individuals.

Resveratrol has been reported to significantly extend life span in yeast[48] and short-lived invertebrates, such as flies and nematodes,[49] and in a recent vertebrate model for aging studies, the turquoise killifish (*Nothobranchius furzeri*).[50] Meta-analytic techniques were recently used by Hector *et al.* from published data to characterize the effect of resveratrol on invertebrate and fish life span.[51] While the life span of the turquoise killifish was positively affected by the resveratrol treatment, results are less clear for flies and nematodes, as there was an important variability between the studies.[51] Moreover, resveratrol was able to restore the median life span in obese mice given a high fat diet in comparison with the control fed mice.[11] To date, no evidence exists concerning the efficiency of resveratrol in increasing life span in nonobese mammals, whether the treatment starts during the early stages of life or during adulthood.[52–54]

It is thought that resveratrol can increase life span because of its CR-mimicking effects and because of the highlighted similar cellular pathway activation. Nevertheless, CR induced an 80% increase in the life span of unicellular organisms and some invertebrates, and a 20–40% increase in small mammals.[55] It should, however, be remembered that the two CR studies in nonhuman primates (rhesus macaques), conducted by the National Institute on Aging and in the Wisconsin National Primate Research Center, gave divergent results for a beneficial effect on longevity, despite positive effects on health span.[56,57] Additionally, CR has proven to be detrimental or ineffective in some rodent lines.[58,59] The processes of aging and life expectancy are certainly not only determined by the regulation of one pathway, that is SIRT1.[60,61] Several laboratory studies have shown a minimum life span–prolonging effect of sirtuins.[62,63] Another analysis showed no direct effect of resveratrol on sirtuin activation but rather an increase in cAMP-phosphodiesterase IV inhibitors, resulting in the regulation of SIRT1 and PGC1-α.[22,64]

In conclusion, the present review reported the beneficial effects of resveratrol in different mammalian species, including humans, and generally reflected the effects observed during chronic caloric restriction without malnutrition. Although most of these effects have been observed in individuals without age-associated pathology but who are overweight or obese, they indicate the role of resveratrol in metabolic regulation and the antiaging efficacy of this intervention. One explanation is the positive and rapid changes induced by resveratrol, which lead to adaptive metabolic response associated with an energy balance regulation and maintenance of overall health. In addition, data on the effects of this molecule on longevity in healthy but nonobese mammals are rare, and we recommend that longitudinal studies on experimental models close to humans, such as nonhuman primates, multiply. Indeed, there are several advantages to the use of nonhuman primates versus clinical trials in humans: the availability of large cohorts of primates, the cost of breeding and animal care compared to the cost of clinical studies, the most rigorous experimental design with direct control of food intake or drug use in captive primates, and finally the possibility of *ex vivo* studies after a variable period of treatment. Data and results of such studies could also address the long-term undesirable side effects, particularly under high-dose protocols, and the long-term dose-dependent effects, to consolidate the fact that resveratrol may be used with caution in humans.

Conflicts of interest

The authors declare no conflicts of interest.

References

1. Gollücke, A.P. & D.A. Ribeiro. 2012. Use of grape polyphenols for promoting human health: a review of patents. *Recent Pat Food Nutr. Agric.* **4:** 26–30.
2. Bavaresco, L. 2003. Role of viticultural factors on stilbene concentrations of grapes and wine. *Drugs Exp. Clin. Res.* **29:** 181–187.
3. Renaud, S. & M. de Lorgeril. 1992. Wine, alcohol, platelets, and the French paradox for coronary heart disease. *Lancet* **339:** 1523–1526.
4. Wu, J.M. *et al.* Mechanism of cardioprotection by resveratrol, a phenolic antioxidant present in red wine (review). *Int. J. Mol. Med.* **8:** 3–17.
5. Pervaiz, S. & A.L. Holme. 2009. Resveratrol: its biologic targets and functional activity. *Antioxid Redox Signal* **11:** 2851–2897.
6. Aggarwal, B.B. *et al.* 2004. Role of resveratrol in prevention and therapy of cancer: preclinical and clinical studies. *Anticancer Res.* **24:** 2783–2840.
7. Chachay, V.S. *et al.* 2011. Resveratrol—pills to replace a healthy diet? *Br. J. Clin. Pharmacol.* **72:** 27–38.
8. Wood, J.G. *et al.* 2004. Sirtuin activators mimic caloric restriction and delay ageing in metazoans. *Nature* **430:** 686–689.
9. Yamamoto, H. *et al.* 2007. Sirtuin functions in health and disease. *Mol. Endocrinol.* **21:** 1745–1755.
10. Kirkwood, T.B. 2008. Gerontology: healthy old age. *Nature* **455:** 739–740.
11. Baur, J.A. *et al.* 2006. Resveratrol improves health and survival of mice on a high-calorie diet. *Nature* **444:** 337–342.
12. Baur, J.A. *et al.* 2010. Dietary restriction: standing up for sirtuins. *Science* **329:** 1012–1013.

13. Szkudelski, T. & K. Szkudelska. 2011. Anti-diabetic effects of resveratrol. *Ann. N.Y. Acad. Sci.* **1215:** 34–39.

14. Marchal, J. *et al.* 2012. Effects of chronic calorie restriction or dietary resveratrol supplementation on insulin sensitivity markers in a primate, *Microcebus murinus.* *PLoS One* **7:** e34289.

15. Elliott, P.J. *et al.* 2009. Resveratrol/SRT501. Sirtuin SIRT1 activator, treatment of type 2 diabetes. *Drugs Fut.* **34:** 291–295.

16. Vetterli, L. *et al.* 2011. Resveratrol potentiates glucose-stimulated insulin secretion in INS-1E beta-cells and human islets through a SIRT1-dependent mechanism. *J. Biol. Chem.* **286:** 6049–6060.

17. Poulsen, M.M. *et al.* 2013. High-dose resveratrol supplementation in obese men: an investigator-initiated, randomized, placebo-controlled clinical trial of substrate metabolism, insulin sensitivity, and body composition. *Diabetes* **62:** 1186–1195.

18. Sun, C. *et al.* 2007. SIRT1 improves insulin sensitivity under insulin-resistant conditions by repressing PTP1B. *Cell Metab.* **6:** 307–319.

19. Um, J.H. *et al.* 2010. AMP-activated protein kinase-deficient mice are resistant to the metabolic effects of resveratrol. *Diabetes* **59:** 554–563.

20. Heilbronn, L.K. *et al.* 2006. Effect of 6-month calorie restriction on biomarkers of longevity, metabolic adaptation, and oxidative stress in overweight individuals: a randomized controlled trial. *JAMA* **295:** 1539–1548.

21. Civitarese, A.E. *et al.* 2007. Diet, energy metabolism and mitochondrial biogenesis. *Curr. Opin. Clin. Nutr. Metab. Care* **10:** 679–687.

22. Timmers, S. *et al.* 2011. Calorie restriction-like effects of 30 days of resveratrol supplementation on energy metabolism and metabolic profile in obese humans. *Cell Metab.* **14:** 612–622.

23. Tauriainen, E. *et al.* 2011. Distinct effects of calorie restriction and resveratrol on diet-induced obesity and fatty liver formation. *J. Nutr. Metab.* **2011:** 525094.

24. Zheng, Y.Y. *et al.* 2012. Dietary agents in cancer prevention: an immunological perspective. *Photochem. Photobiol.* **88:** 1083–1098.

25. Ramprasath, V.R. & P.J. Jones. 2010. Anti-atherogenic effects of resveratrol. *Eur. J. Clin. Nutr.* **64:** 660–668.

26. Sharma, M. & Y.K. Gupta. 2002. Chronic treatment with trans-resveratrol prevents intracerebroventricular streptozotocin induced cognitive impairment and oxidative stress in rats. *Life Sci.* **71:** 2489–2498.

27. Candelario-Jalil, E. *et al.* 2007. Resveratrol potently reduces prostaglandin E2 production and free radical formation in lipopolysaccharide-activated primary rat microglia. *J. Neuroinflam.* **10:**25.

28. Albani, D. *et al.* 2010. Neuroprotective properties of resveratrol in different neurodegenerative disorders. *Biofactors* **36:** 370–376.

29. Harada, N. *et al.* 2011. Resveratrol improves cognitive function in mice by increasing production of insulin-like growth factor-I in the hippocampus. *J. Nutr. Biochem.* **22:** 1150–1159.

30. Brown, V.A. *et al.* 2010. Repeat dose study of the cancer chemopreventive agent resveratrol in healthy volunteers: safety, pharmacokinetics, and effect on the insulin-like growth factor axis. *Cancer Res.* **70:** 9003–9011.

31. Dal-Pan, A. *et al.* 2011. Caloric restriction or resveratrol supplementation and ageing in a non-human primate: first-year outcome of the RESTRIKAL study in *Microcebus murinus.* *Age* **33:** 15–31.

32. Holliday, R. 2006. Food, fertility and longevity. *Biogerontology* **7:** 139–141.

33. Juan, M.E. *et al.* 2005. Trans-resveratrol, a natural antioxidant from grapes, increases sperm output in healthy rats. *J. Nutr.* **135:** 757–760.

34. Cuzzola, V.F. *et al.* 2012. Pharmacogenomic update on multiple sclerosis: a focus on actual and new therapeutic strategies. *Pharmacogen. J.* **12:** 453–461.

35. Kennedy, D.O. *et al.* 2010. Effects of resveratrol on cerebral blood flow variables and cognitive performance in humans: a double-blind, placebo-controlled, crossover investigation. *Am. J. Clin. Nutr.* **91:** 1590–1597.

36. Abraham, J. & R.W. Johnson. 2009. Consuming a diet supplemented with resveratrol reduced infection-related neuroinflammation and deficits in working memory in aged mice. *Rejuvenation Res.* **12:** 445–453.

37. Girbovan, C. *et al.* 2012. Repeated resveratrol administration confers lasting protection against neuronal damage but induces dose-related alterations of behavioral impairments after global ischemia. *Behav. Pharmacol.* **23:** 1–13.

38. Gacar, N. *et al.* 2011. Beneficial effects of resveratrol on scopolamine but not mecamylamine induced memory impairment in the passive avoidance and Morris water maze tests in rats. *Pharmacol. Biochem. Behav.* **99:** 316–323.

39. Joseph, J.A. *et al.* 2008. Cellular and behavioral effects of stilbene resveratrol analogues: implications for reducing the deleterious effects of aging. *J. Agric. Food Chem.* **56:** 10544–10551.

40. Dal-Pan, A. *et al.* 2011. Cognitive performances are selectively enhanced during chronic caloric restriction or resveratrol supplementation in a primate. *PLoS One* **6:** e16581.

41. Kasdallah-Grissa, A. *et al.* 2006. Resveratrol, a red wine polyphenol, attenuates ethanol-induced oxidative stress in rat liver. *Life Sci.* **80:** 1033–1039.

42. Mokni, M. *et al.* 2007. Effect of resveratrol on antioxidant enzyme activities in the brain of healthy rats. *Neurochem. Res.* **32:** 981–987.

43. Baur, J.A. & D.A. Sinclair. 2006. Therapeutic potential of resveratrol: the *in vivo* evidence. *Nat. Rev. Drug Discov.* **5:** 493–506.

44. Csiszar, A. *et al.* 2008. Vasoprotective effects of resveratrol and SIRT1: attenuation of cigarette smoke-induced oxidative stress and proinflammatory phenotypic alterations. *Am. J. Physiol. Heart Circ. Physiol.* **294:** H2721–H2735.

45. Delmas, D. *et al.* 2011. Resveratrol, a phytochemical inducer of multiple cell death pathways: apoptosis, autophagy and mitotic catastrophe. *Curr. Med. Chem.* **18:** 1100–1121.

46. Piotrowska, H. *et al.* 2011. Biological activity of piceatannol: leaving the shadow of resveratrol. *Mutat. Res.* **750:** 60–82.

47. Alvira, D. *et al.* 2007. Comparative analysis of the effects of resveratrol in two apoptotic models: inhibition of complex

I and potassium deprivation in cerebellar neurons. *Neuroscience* **147:** 746–756.

48. Howitz, K.T. *et al.* 2003. Small molecule activators of sirtuins extend *Saccharomyces cerevisiae* lifespan. *Nature* **425:** 191–196.

49. Bass, T.M. *et al.* 2007. Effects of resveratrol on lifespan in *Drosophila melanogaster* and *Caenorhabditis elegans*. *Mech. Ageing Dev.* **128:** 546–552.

50. Terzibasi, E. *et al.* 2006. The short-lived fish Nothobranchius furzeri as a new model system for aging studies. *Exp. Gerontol.* **42:** 81–89.

51. Hector, K.L. *et al.* 2012. The effect of resveratrol on longevity across species: a meta-analysis. *Biol. Lett.* **8:** 790–793.

52. Pearson, K.J. *et al.* 2008. Resveratrol delays age-related deterioration and mimics transcriptional aspects of dietary restriction without extending life span. *Cell Metab.* **8:** 157–168.

53. Miller, R.A. *et al.* 2011. Rapamycin, but not resveratrol or simvastatin, extends life span of genetically heterogeneous mice. *J. Gerontol. A. Biol. Sci. Med. Sci.* **66:** 191–201.

54. Strong, R. *et al.* 2012. Evaluation of resveratrol, green tea extract, curcumin, oxaloacetic acid, and medium-chain triglyceride oil on life span of genetically heterogeneous mice. *J. Gerontol. A. Biol. Sci. Med. Sci.* **68:** 6–16.

55. Smith, D.L. *et al.* 2010. Calorie restriction: what recent results suggest for the future of ageing research. *Eur J Clin Invest.* **40:** 440–450.

56. Colman, R.J. *et al.* 2009. Caloric restriction delays disease onset and mortality in rhesus monkeys. *Science* **325:** 201–204.

57. Mattison, J.A. *et al.* 2012. Impact of caloric restriction on health and survival in rhesus monkeys from the NIA study. *Nature* **489:** 318–321.

58. Ferguson, M. *et al.* 2008. Comparison of metabolic rate and oxidative stress between two different strains of mice with varying response to caloric restriction. *Exp. Gerontol.* **43:** 757–763.

59. Liao, C.Y. *et al.* 2010. Genetic variation in the murine lifespan response to dietary restriction: from life extension to life shortening. *Aging Cell.* **9:** 92–95.

60. Hu, Y. *et al.* 2011. The controversial links among calorie restriction, SIRT1, and resveratrol. *Free Radic. Biol. Med.* **15; 51:** 250–256.

61. Houtkooper R.H. *et al.* 2012. Sirtuins as regulators of metabolism and healthspan. *Nat. Rev. Mol. Cell. Biol* **13:** 225–238.

62. Burnett, C. *et al.* 2011. Absence of effects of Sir2 overexpression on lifespan in *C. elegans* and *Drosophila*. *Nature* **477:** 482–485.

63. Viswanathan, M. & L. Guarente. 2011. Regulation of *Caenorhabditis elegans* lifespan by sir-2.1 transgenes. *Nature* **477:** E1–E2.

64. Park, S.J. *et al.* 2012. Resveratrol ameliorates aging-related metabolic phenotypes by inhibiting cAMP phosphodiesterases. *Cell* **148:** 421–433.

Ann. N.Y. Acad. Sci. ISSN 0077-8923

ANNALS OF THE NEW YORK ACADEMY OF SCIENCES
Issue: *Resveratrol and Health*

Resveratrol in metabolic health: an overview of the current evidence and perspectives

Morten Møller Poulsen, Jens Otto Lunde Jørgensen, Niels Jessen, Bjørn Richelsen, and Steen Bønløkke Pedersen

Department of Endocrinology and Internal Medicine, MEA, Aarhus University Hospital and Institute of Clinical Medicine, Aarhus University, Denmark

Address for correspondence: Morten Møller Poulsen, M.D., Department of Endocrinology and Internal Medicine, MEA, Aarhus University Hospital, Tage Hansens Gade 2, 8000 Aarhus, Denmark. mmp@ki.au.dk

In the search for novel preventive and therapeutic modalities in the management of metabolic diseases and obesity, resveratrol has attracted great attention over the past decades. Preclinical trials suggest that resveratrol mimics the metabolic effects of calorie restriction (CR) via activation of silent mating type information regulation 2 homolog 1 (SIRT1). In experimental animals, this potential translates into prevention or improvement of glucose metabolism, anti-inflammation, cancer, and nonalcoholic fatty liver disease. Moreover, and in accordance with CR, supplementation with resveratrol promotes longevity in several primitive species and protects against diet-induced metabolic abnormalities in rodents. Despite the substantial preclinical evidence, human clinical data are very scarce, and even though the compound is widely distributed as an over-the-counter human nutritional supplement, its therapeutic rationale has not been well characterized. In this review, we provide a brief overview of the field and discuss the future scientific directions of resveratrol research.

Keywords: resveratrol; metabolism; *in vitro*; *in vivo*; clinical trials

The obesity paradigm

Throughout the world, obesity is a rapidly increasing problem gradually approaching epidemic levels, and associated comorbidities such as type 2 diabetes are projected to rise steadily during the years to come. Even though the steadily increasing obesity incidence has recently been reported to have leveled off in some places, the prevalence clearly indicates a serious public health concern, as obesity predisposes to increased overall morbidity and mortality.

Through conventional weight loss regimens, considerable weight losses may be achieved, but irrespective of the chosen regimen, weight maintenance at a lower set point often fails. As the conventional preventive and therapeutic options therefore seem inadequate, physicians are instead obliged to resort to medical treatment of the obesity-associated conditions and complications, often at advanced stages of the diseases. This approach is by all means suboptimal, but serves as the best alternative, leaving room for novel preventive and therapeutic modalities.

Calorie restriction

It has been known for nearly a century that calorie restriction (CR) induces health-promoting effects. Reducing calorie intake to 20–40% below the *ad libitum* intake without compromising nutritional demands preserves various aspects of metabolic health and furthermore promotes longevity in various organisms. For this reason, CR has been widely used as a preclinical investigational tool in describing the processes of aging. Since the first observations in the 1930s by McCay *et al.*,[1] the potential has correspondingly been demonstrated in diverse primitive organisms and animal species.

Sirtuins

The molecular basis underlying the favorable effects of CR remains subject to scientific debate. Despite these controversies, one common denominator recurs, namely, the silent mating type information regulator 2 homolog 1 (SIRT1). SIRT1 is

doi: 10.1111/nyas.12141

Ann. N.Y. Acad. Sci. 1290 (2013) 74–82 © 2013 New York Academy of Sciences.

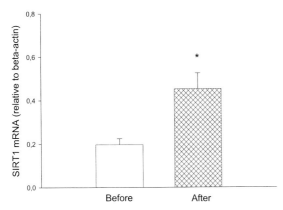

Figure 1. Metabolic control of SIRT1 in human adipose tissue. SIRT1 mRNA expression was evaluated by RT-PCR in isolated subcutaneous abdominal adipocytes obtained by biopsy before (white box) and after (hatched box) 6 days of total fasting in nine obese women. Results presented as means ± SEM. Statistical comparison was performed by student's paired *t*-test. *$P < 0.02$. From Ref. 3, with permission.

part of a family of highly conserved proteins capable of modifying various proteins posttranslationally. As the name implies, SIRT1 is the mammalian homolog to the *Saccharomyces cerevisiae* Sir2 (silent information regulator 2) protein. The sirtuins have a stoichiometric requirement for the cofactor nicotinamide adenine dinucleotide (NAD^+) to biochemically modify their substrates.[2] By means of posttranslational modifications, the sirtuins affect numerous and various transcription factors that ultimately translate into physiological alterations, many of which involve highly conserved metabolic pathways potentially interfering with aging processes and the development of lifestyle-related diseases. Recently, we have shown that SIRT1 is also metabolically regulated in human adipose tissue as we found a twofold increase in SIRT1 expression in subcutaneous adipose tissue from human volunteers in response to CR for one week (Fig. 1).[3]

Because long-term fasting is not a realistic possibility in humans, the search for chemical sirtuin activators has increased during the past decade. Among these so-called sirtuin-activating compounds (STACs) with purported potential to mimic the cellular response to caloric restriction, the small polyphenolic molecule resveratrol is one of the first to be identified and is probably the best characterized.

Resveratrol

Resveratrol was initially identified and described as an isolate of the poisonous but medicinal white hellebore (*Veratrum album*, L. var. *grandiflorum* Maxim. Ex Baker) in a Japanese paper in 1939.[4] Today it is known to be widely distributed in nature and synthesized by various plants in response to external stressors and infections. Resveratrol (3,5,4′-trihydroxy-*trans*-stilbene) is a small polyphenolic compound chemically belonging to the stilbenoid class, and in the lay press, resveratrol is probably best known as a constituent of grapes and wine, albeit in minute amounts.

The awareness of this compound was accelerated by a publication from Jang *et al.* in 1997 in which resveratrol displayed chemopreventive properties both *in vitro* and *in vivo*.[5] The next milestone came in 2003 in a paper by the Sinclair group in which resveratrol was established to stimulate SIRT1, thereby increasing yeast lifespan by 70%.[6] One year later, the same group succeeded in reproducing the life-extending potential of resveratrol in worms and flies.[7] In 2006, the Sinclair group demonstrated a resveratrol-mediated shift in the physiology of middle-aged mice kept on a high-calorie diet toward that of mice fed a standard diet, thereby significantly increasing their survival.[8] Even though data in human subjects are very scarce, the compound is widely distributed as an over-the-counter nutritional supplement with an array of alleged salutary effects in relation to human health. In fact, resveratrol is one of the most prevalent substances among individuals in the United States who routinely consume multiple nutritional supplements.[9]

Experimental dosing

At the cellular level, the most commonly applied resveratrol concentration is 50 μM[10,11] ($\approx$11,400 ng/mL), and the generally accepted range of *in vitro* activity is 5–100 μM.[12] These *in vitro* concentrations are distinctly above the plasma concentrations achieved *in vivo* after conventional ingestion and absorption. In a phase I dose-escalation study, a single dose of 5.0 g generated a C_{max} of only 2.4 μM ($\approx$ 500 ng/mL).[13] In another study assessing resveratrol pharmacokinetics following repeated dosing of 0.5–5.0 g daily for 28 days, both average ($C_{average}$) and maximum (C_{max}) values of parent resveratrol increased with the dose, but still ranged from only

0.04–0.55 µM and 0.19–4.24 µM, respectively.[14] On this basis, the likelihood of benefiting from resveratrol as a result of ordinary dietary intake appears dubious, since a conventional diet at best provides a few milligrams of resveratrol daily. Furthermore, resveratrol is rapidly metabolized by hepatic glucoronidation and sulfonidation processes, and these metabolites are present in higher circulating amounts than the native compound. On this basis, it has been speculated that the resveratrol metabolites might have biological effects.

Biological targets

Multiple downstream targets of resveratrol action have been reported. Among these, PGC1α[11] appears rather reproducible, and deacetylation of PGC1α is commonly used as a proxy of SIRT1 activity. Other frequently reported targets include PPARγ, NF-κB, TNF-α, SREBP1, CIDEA, FOXO, ROS, and eNOS.[15] Recently, Park *et al.* proposed another pathway in which resveratrol at high concentrations acts as a competitive inhibitor of cAMP-degrading phosphodiesterases, leading to elevated cAMP levels and indirect SIRT1 activation.[16]

Preclinical evidence

At the preclinical level, resveratrol has demonstrated reproducible effects in modifying various aspects of metabolic health. This finding is consistent overall with the suggestion that resveratrol acts as a CR mimetic. In terms of cellular experiments, various aspects of resveratrol action have been investigated. Resveratrol seems to be a strong anti-inflammatory compound in cell culture as well as in animal models. In numerous rodent models, resveratrol has reduced the levels of well-known proinflammatory biomarkers, such as TNF-α, NF-κB, IL-6, IL-10, and IL-1β.[17] In line with the anti-inflammatory effects, isolated antioxidative effects have also been repeatedly reported.[18]

We have demonstrated that resveratrol also exhibits very strong anti-inflammatory effects in human adipose tissue explants.[10] This observation could be of great clinical importance, as the low-grade inflammation associated with obesity may be the underlying mechanism coupling obesity and its metabolic consequences (Fig. 2).

Another prominent effect of resveratrol is the improvement of glucose homeostasis, which has been demonstrated in diverse animal models.[8,19] Due to the close association between diabetes and obesity, a range of obesity-related measures have also been explored, but only very few studies have been able to demonstrate an antiobesity potential for resveratrol.[11]

In addition to improved glucose homeostasis, it has been suggested that resveratrol prevents ectopic lipid accumulation, particularly in the liver.[8,11] In fact, the capacity of preventing hepatic steatosis due to high-fat feeding is one of the most robust and reproducible findings at the preclinical level, and multiple mechanisms have been proposed to account for this effect. Based on our own rodent model, we demonstrate that resveratrol prevents nonalcoholic fatty liver disease induced by high-fat diet, independently of the generally accepted anti-inflammatory potential. Mechanistically, an increased number of hepatic mitochondria seem to be involved, and on the basis of gene expression patterns, we suggest that UCP2 might be causatively linked to the observed effect (Fig. 3).[20]

Furthermore, resveratrol has demonstrated chemopreventive potential in relation to diverse cancer types, including mammary[21] and colonic cancer.[22] Resveratrol has been shown to provide neuroprotection,[23] and in cardiovascular health, resveratrol has demonstrated cardioprotective potential, partly due to antihypertensive[24] and lipid-lowering[25] properties. Additionally, recent studies have demonstrated that resveratrol modifies the biological pathways of bone metabolism; resveratrol promotes osteoblastogenesis and antagonizes osteoclasts *in vitro*,[26] and these initial findings have been substantiated by animal studies of osteoporosis, in which resveratrol demonstrates beneficial properties.[27]

Besides the life-extending effect in yeast mentioned above,[6] similar potential has been shown in primitive animal species, including worms and flies.[7] Considering rodents, two independent studies have demonstrated that the transcriptional response to resveratrol supplementation resembles the alterations induced by CR.[19,28] Despite these similarities, resveratrol supplementation has not extended lifespan in metabolically healthy rodents.[28] However, the compound has significantly restored the life span of mice suffering from metabolic abnormalities due to obesity induced by high-fat diet.[8]

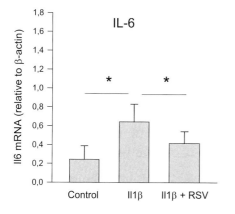
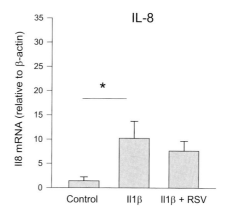
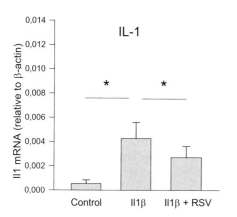
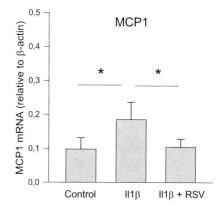
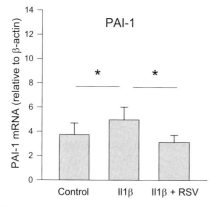
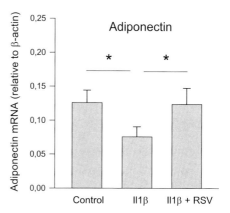

Figure 2. Anti-inflammatory potential of resveratrol in adipose tissue explants: effect of resveratrol (RSV) treatment on IL-1β–induced adipokine mRNA expression in human adipose tissue. Human adipose tissue fragments were incubated with IL-1β (2 ng/mL) either alone or concomitant with RSV (50 μM) for 24 h. Total RNA was extracted for measuring the mRNA expression levels of IL-6, IL-8, IL-1, MCP-1, PAI-1, and adiponectin by quantitative RT-PCR. The results are expressed relative to controls (*N* = 8) and the bars indicate means ± SEM. Differences between group means were determined using one-way analysis of variance with Bonferroni *post hoc* test. *$P < 0.05$. From Ref. 10, with permission.

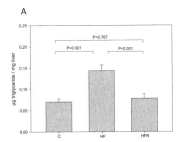 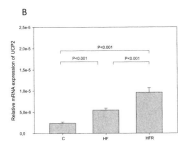 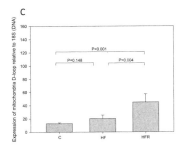

Figure 3. Prevention of nonalcoholic fatty liver disease. Male Wistar rats were fed for 8 weeks, after which they were sacrificed and relevant tissues were collected for subsequent analysis; C, rats fed a control diet ($n = 12$); HF, rats fed a high-fat diet ($n = 12$); HFR, rats fed a high-fat diet supplemented with resveratrol ($n = 12$). (A) Liver triglyceride content was determined by ethanolic KOH saponification followed by assay for glycerol. (B) Liver UCP2 mRNA expression relative to 18S mRNA evaluated by RT-PCR. (C) Liver mitochondria count quantified as relative expression of mitochondrial DNA, D-loop, relative to nonmitochondrial 18S DNA. Values are group means with vertical bars indicating SEM. Individual group comparisons evaluated by Student's *t*-test. From Ref. 20, with permission.

Clinical evidence

Although the vast majority of the 5,000+ published studies on resveratrol have been performed *in vitro* or in animal models, sporadic clinical trials on efficacy outcomes are by now reported. The three most methodologically robust intervention studies were published in December 2011 by Timmers *et al.*,[29] in October 2012 by Yoshino *et al.*,[30] and our own contribution published in December 2012.[31] In the study by Timmers *et al.*, 11 obese but otherwise healthy male participants received a daily dose of 150 mg resveratrol or placebo for 30 days in a double-blind crossover design with an intervening washout phase of four weeks. Metabolic examinations were carried out before and after entering both intervention periods. Significant albeit moderate improvements were recorded in various metabolic markers, including improvement of insulin sensitivity assessed by HOMA-IR, decrease of systolic and mean arterial blood pressure with no changes in diastolic blood pressure, lowering of sleeping metabolic rate suggesting improved metabolic efficiency, and diminished intrahepatic lipid content. Furthermore, this study demonstrated metabolically favorable alterations in pertinent biomarkers including triglycerides, liver transaminases (ALT), leptin, and TNF-α. Finally, microarray analysis revealed that gene sets related to mitochondrial oxidative phosphorylation were significantly increased, whereas genes related to cytokine signaling were significantly decreased, and specific western blotting analysis of skeletal muscle indicated resveratrol-induced AMPK acti-

vation and increased protein levels of SIRT1 and PGC1α. In the work by Yoshino *et al.*, 29 nonobese (BMI < 30 mg/m^2) postmenopausal women with normal glucose tolerance were randomized to a daily dose of 75 mg resveratrol ($N = 15$) or placebo ($N = 14$) for 12 weeks. Before and after the intervention period, the participants underwent exhaustive metabolic examination, including hyperinsulinemic euglycemic clamp, indirect calorimetry, MR spectroscopy, and muscle and adipose tissue biopsies. Resveratrol supplementation failed to affect any physiological parameters or putative molecular targets.

This is consistent with the findings in our own human clinical trial:[31] in an investigator-initiated, randomized, double-blinded, placebo-controlled, parallel-group design, 24 male volunteers were randomly assigned treatment for four weeks with tablets containing 500 mg trans-resveratrol three times daily or matched placebo tablets. Participants were 18–68 years of age and obese (BMI > 30 kg/m^2) but otherwise healthy. Extensive metabolic examinations including assessment of glucose turnover, insulin sensitivity (hyperinsulinemic euglycemic clamp), resting energy expenditure, assessment of ectopic and visceral fat (NMR spectroscopy), and 24 h ambulatory blood pressure were performed before and after the treatment. Insulin sensitivity was similar in both groups, and endogenous glucose production and the turnover and oxidation rates of glucose remained unchanged. Resveratrol supplementation also had no effect on blood pressure, resting energy expenditure, and oxidation

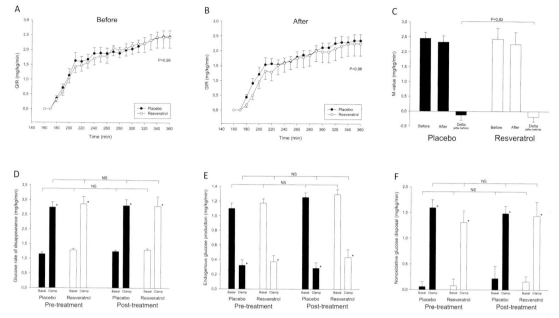

Figure 4. Insulin sensitivity and glucose metabolism. Glucose metabolism was examined before and after 4 weeks of resveratrol or placebo supplementation; 500 mg thrice daily. Throughout the figure, filled bars and dots indicate placebo group ($N = 12$) and open bars and dots indicate resveratrol group ($N = 12$). Results are presented as group means ± SEM. Insulin sensitivity was assessed by a hyperinsulinemic euglycemic clamp. The participants were clamped at a blood glucose level of ~5 mmol/L with an insulin infusion of 0.5 mU/kg/min. (A) and (B) The glucose infusion rate (GIR) before and after intervention, respectively. *P*-values reflect between-group differences assessed by two-way repeated measures ANOVA. (C) The corresponding whole body insulin sensitivity, the M-value, defined as the mean GIR during the last 30 min of the clamp. *P*-value reflects potential treatment effect analyzed by two-way repeated measures ANOVA. (D) Glucose rate of disappearance (R_d). (E) Endogenous glucose production (EGP). (F) Nonoxidative glucose disposal (NOGD). In (D)–(F), * indicates a statistical significant within-group effect of the insulin stimulation evaluated by a paired *t*-test. Overall comparisons of potential treatment effects were performed by two-way repeated measures ANOVA in basal and clamp situation, respectively. NS, nonsignificant. From Ref. 31, with permission.

rates of lipid, ectopic, and visceral fat content, or inflammatory and metabolic biomarkers (Fig. 4).

In addition to these three studies described above, a few other small studies have been performed. Briefly, Brasnyo *et al.* reported that administration of 5 mg resveratrol ingested twice daily for four weeks significantly decreased oxidative stress and improved HOMA-IR in type 2 diabetic men compared to controls ($N = 10$ in the active group and $N = 9$ in the control group).[32] In accordance with this finding, Bhatt *et al.* demonstrated improvements of HbA1c, total cholesterol, and systolic blood pressure due to three months of resveratrol supplementation (250 mg daily; both groups cotreated with conventional antidiabetic agents; $N = 31 + 31$) in type 2 diabetic subjects.[33] In an open-label study, Crandall *et al.* described improvement of postprandial glycemia (decline of post-meal glucose AUC) in elderly participants with impaired glucose tolerance

(1.0, 1.5, or 2.0 g daily for four weeks, $N = 10$).[34] In contrast, Ghanim *et al.* failed to detect any effect on glucose metabolism in healthy individuals receiving 40 mg resveratrol daily for six weeks ($N = 10 + 10$); however, significant reductions were found in ROS, TNF-α, IL-6, and CRP.[35] Anti-inflammatory potential was also described by Tome-Carneiro *et al.*; 75 participants at high risk of cardiovascular disease (CVD) were assigned to placebo, low-, or high-dose (8 mg daily) resveratrol groups for one year. In comparison with placebo and low-dose groups, resveratrol supplementation in the high-dose group significantly decreased hs-CRP, TNF-α, PAI1, and IL-6/IL-10 ratio.[36] Regarding cardiovascular effects, Magyar *et al.* suggest that 10 mg resveratrol daily for three months improved left ventricular diastolic function and decreased low density lipo-proteins (LDL) in postmyocardial patients ($N = 20 + 20$).[37] Wong *et al.* investigated the acute effect of resveratrol on flow-mediated dilatation of the brachial artery in obese subjects and found a dose-dependent effect of 30, 90, and 270 mg resveratrol assessed 1 h after ingestion ($N = 19$).[38] Finally, Kennedy *et al.* explored acute effects on cognitive functions in healthy subjects, but found no effects upon assessment 45 min after ingestion of 250 or 500 mg resveratrol. However, a significant and dose-dependent increase in cerebral blood flow was demonstrated.[39]

In terms of human safety and pharmacokinetic properties, the available data are fairly solid, and both acute exposure to high doses of resveratrol (5 g daily for 28 days)[14] as well as more chronic exposure to lower doses (8 mg daily for one year)[36] have not induced any observable adverse events.

Discussion and perspectives

Sirtuins make up an exclusive class of highly evolutionarily conserved proteins. Given their involvement in mediating ubiquitous metabolic processes, they have attracted attention as therapeutic targets. As illustrated throughout this paper, the scientific field of sirtuin biology, including the potential role of resveratrol in mediating the proposed SIRT1-mediated metabolic effects, is a highly complex field of great scientific interest.

Based on our own rodent study, resveratrol convincingly prevented NAFLD in our designated DIO rats, which is in accordance with existing data. Moreover, our rodent data provide a novel mechanism whereby resveratrol may prevent hepatic steatosis. However, in contrast to a similar human clinical trial, resveratrol failed to demonstrate any metabolic effect under the given circumstances. The conflicting human data remain remarkable, but our negative findings are supported by another well-designed clinical study in nonobese women. Several metabolic studies are in the pipeline investigating varying doses, time schedules, and clinical potential in relation to baseline morbidity. Time will tell whether or not our negative outcome may be tied to methodological limitations or to the fact that our volunteers were too healthy to demonstrate any effect of resveratrol.

Future studies should particularly focus on dose-response relationships and preferably also compare the effects of treatment duration and various premorbid states, as these may be prerequisites for clinical effect. Besides, the primary objective of this paper relates primarily to metabolic parameters, leaving open the possibility for human effects in other diverse areas, including neurodegeneration, cardiovascular diseases, and cancer. Furthermore, the pharmacodynamic properties of the compound need to be definitively established. Reviewing the literature, and based on our human clinical trial, the compound is well-tolerated at the applied dose and unit of time. Nonetheless, potential untoward effects have to be borne in mind when conducting future clinical investigations. Until long-term clinical trials, now in progress, have been conducted, chronic intake of resveratrol in doses above the concentration contained in natural food sources should be considered experimental.

Taken as a whole, this paper—and research on resveratrol in general—serves as an illustrative example of the major challenges associated with translating basic research into human clinical practice.[40] Moreover, there are numerous examples in modern medicine of major discordance between treatment effects obtained in animal and human studies.[41]

Regardless of our own negative clinical findings, the research into human effects of resveratrol is in its infancy, and we need additional RCTs to ultimately define the role of resveratrol in metabolic health. Irrespective of the direction of future human clinical data published in the years to come, the scientific field of sirtuin biology remains an area of great interest.

Acknowledgments

This work was supported by grants from the Danish Agency for Science Technology and Innovation (Grant 09-072323), The Novo Nordisk Foundation, Karen Elise Jensens Foundation, The Toyota Foundation, Elvira and Rasmus Riisfort Foundation, Ejnar Danielsens Foundation, and the AP Møller Maersk Foundation. The work is part of the research program LIRMOI Research Center (www.LIRMOI.com), which is supported by the Danish Council for Strategic Research (Grant 10-093499).

Conflicts of interest

The authors have no conflicts of interest.

References

1. McCay, C.M., M.F. Crowell & L.A. Maynard. 1989. The effect of retarded growth upon the length of life span and upon the ultimate body size. *Nutrition* **5:** 155–171.

2. Villalba, J.M. & F.J. Alcain. 2012. Sirtuin activators and inhibitors. *Biofactors* **38**: 349–359.

3. Pedersen, S.B., J. Olholm, S.K. Paulsen, *et al.* 2008. Low Sirt1 expression, which is upregulated by fasting, in human adipose tissue from obese women. *Int. J. Obes.* **32**: 1250–1255.

4. Takaoka, M.J. 1939. Of the phenolic substances of white hellebore (*Veratrum grandiflorum*). *J. Faculty Sci. Hokkaido Imperial Univ.* **3**: 1–16.

5. Jang, M., L. Cai, G.O. Udeani, *et al.* 1997. Cancer chemopreventive activity of resveratrol, a natural product derived from grapes. *Science* **275**: 218–220.

6. Howitz, K.T., K.J. Bitterman, H.Y. Cohen, *et al.* 2003. Small molecule activators of sirtuins extend Saccharomyces cerevisiae lifespan. *Nature* **425**: 191–196.

7. Wood, J.G., B. Rogina, S. Lavu, *et al.* 2004. Sirtuin activators mimic caloric restriction and delay ageing in metazoans. *Nature* **430**: 686–689.

8. Baur, J.A., K.J. Pearson, N.L. Price, *et al.* 2006. Resveratrol improves health and survival of mice on a high-calorie diet. *Nature* **444**: 337–342.

9. Block, G., C.D. Jensen, E.P. Norkus, *et al.* 2007. Usage patterns, health, and nutritional status of long-term multiple dietary supplement users: a cross-sectional study. *Nutr. J.* **6**: 30.

10. Olholm, J., S.K. Paulsen, K.B. Cullberg, *et al.* 2010. Anti-inflammatory effect of resveratrol on adipokine expression and secretion in human adipose tissue explants. *Int. J. Obes.* **34**: 1546–1553.

11. Lagouge, M., C. Argmann, Z. Gerhart-Hines, *et al.* 2006. Resveratrol improves mitochondrial function and protects against metabolic disease by activating SIRT1 and PGC-1alpha. *Cell* **127**: 1109–1122.

12. Goldberg, D.M., J. Yan & G.J. Soleas. 2003. Absorption of three wine-related polyphenols in three different matrices by healthy subjects. *Clin. Biochem.* **36**: 79–87.

13. Boocock, D.J., G.E. Faust, K.R. Patel, *et al.* 2007. Phase I dose escalation pharmacokinetic study in healthy volunteers of resveratrol, a potential cancer chemopreventive agent. *Cancer Epidemiol. Biomarkers Prev.* **16**: 1246–1252.

14. Brown, V.A., K.R. Patel, M. Viskaduraki, *et al.* 2010. Repeat dose study of the cancer chemopreventive agent resveratrol in healthy volunteers: safety, pharmacokinetics, and effect on the insulin-like growth factor axis. *Cancer Res.* **70**: 9003–9011.

15. Baur, J.A., Z. Ungvari, R.K. Minor & D.G. Le Couteur. 2012. Are sirtuins viable targets for improving healthspan and lifespan? *Nat. Rev. Drug Discov.* **11**: 443–461.

16. Park, S.J., F. Ahmad, A. Philp, *et al.* 2012. Resveratrol ameliorates aging-related metabolic phenotypes by inhibiting cAMP phosphodiesterases. *Cell* **148**: 421–433.

17. Bujanda, L., E. Hijona, M. Larzabal, *et al.* 2008. Resveratrol inhibits nonalcoholic fatty liver disease in rats. *BMC Gastroenterol.* **8**: 40.

18. Gomez-Zorita, S., A. Fernandez-Quintela, M.T. Macarulla, *et al.* 2011. Resveratrol attenuates steatosis in obese Zucker rats by decreasing fatty acid availability and reducing oxidative stress. *Br. J. Nutr.* **107**: 202–210.

19. Barger, J.L., T. Kayo, J.M. Vann, *et al.* 2008. A low dose of dietary resveratrol partially mimics caloric restriction and retards aging parameters in mice. *PLoS One* **3**: e2264.

20. Poulsen, M.M., J.O. Larsen, S. Hamilton-Dutoit, *et al.* 2012. Resveratrol up-regulates hepatic uncoupling protein 2 and prevents development of nonalcoholic fatty liver disease in rats fed a high-fat diet. *Nutr. Res.* **32**: 701–708.

21. Provinciali, M., F. Re, A. Donnini, *et al.* 2005. Effect of resveratrol on the development of spontaneous mammary tumors in HER-2/neu transgenic mice. *Int. J. Cancer* **115**: 36–45.

22. Sengottuvelan, M. & N. Nalini. 2006. Dietary supplementation of resveratrol suppresses colonic tumour incidence in 1,2-dimethylhydrazine-treated rats by modulating biotransforming enzymes and aberrant crypt foci development. *Br. J. Nutr.* **96**: 145–153.

23. Jeon, B.T., E.A. Jeong, H.J. Shin, *et al.* 2012. Resveratrol attenuates obesity-associated peripheral and central inflammation and improves memory deficit in mice fed a high-fat diet. *Diabetes* **61**: 1444–1454.

24. Rivera, L., R. Moron, A. Zarzuelo & M. Galisteo. 2009. Long-term resveratrol administration reduces metabolic disturbances and lowers blood pressure in obese Zucker rats. *Biochem. Pharmacol.* **77**: 1053–1063.

25. Cho, S.J., U.J. Jung & M.S. Choi. 2012. Differential effects of low-dose resveratrol on adiposity and hepatic steatosis in diet-induced obese mice. *Br. J. Nutr.* **108**: 2166–2175.

26. Boissy, P., T.L. Andersen, B.M. Abdallah, *et al.* 2005. Resveratrol inhibits myeloma cell growth, prevents osteoclast formation, and promotes osteoblast differentiation. *Cancer Res.* **65**: 9943–9952.

27. Habold, C., I. Momken, A. Ouadi, *et al.* 2011. Effect of prior treatment with resveratrol on density and structure of rat long bones under tail-suspension. *J. Bone Miner. Metab.* **29**: 15–22.

28. Pearson, K.J., J.A. Baur, K.N. Lewis, *et al.* 2008. Resveratrol delays age-related deterioration and mimics transcriptional aspects of dietary restriction without extending life span. *Cell Metab.* **8**: 157–168.

29. Timmers, S., E. Konings, L. Bilet, *et al.* 2011. Calorie restriction-like effects of 30 days of resveratrol supplementation on energy metabolism and metabolic profile in obese humans. *Cell Metab.* **14**: 612–622.

30. Yoshino, J., C. Conte, L. Fontana, *et al.* 2012. Resveratrol supplementation does not improve metabolic function in nonobese women with normal glucose tolerance. *Cell Metab.* **16**: 658–664.

31. Poulsen, M.M., P.F. Vestergaard, B.F. Clasen, *et al.* 2013. High-dose resveratrol supplementation in obese men: an investigator-initiated, randomized, placebo-controlled clinical trial of substrate metabolism, insulin sensitivity, and body composition. *Diabetes* **62**: 1186–1195.

32. Brasnyo, P., G.A. Molnar, M. Mohas, *et al.* 2011. Resveratrol improves insulin sensitivity, reduces oxidative stress and activates the Akt pathway in type 2 diabetic patients. *Br. J. Nutr.* **106**: 383–389.

33. Bhatt, J.K., S. Thomas & M.J. Nanjan. 2012. Resveratrol supplementation improves glycemic control in type 2 diabetes mellitus. *Nutr. Res.* **32**: 537–541.

34. Crandall, J.P., V. Oram, G. Trandafirescu, *et al.* 2012. Pilot study of resveratrol in older adults with impaired glucose tolerance. *J. Gerontol. A. Biol. Sci. Med. Sci.* **67:** 1307–1312.

35. Ghanim, H., C.L. Sia, S. Abuaysheh, *et al.* 2010. An antiinflammatory and reactive oxygen species suppressive effects of an extract of Polygonum cuspidatum containing resveratrol. *J. Clin. Endocrinol. Metab.* **95:** E1–E8.

36. Tome-Carneiro, J., M. Gonzalvez, M. Larrosa, *et al.* 2012. One-year consumption of a grape nutraceutical containing resveratrol improves the inflammatory and fibrinolytic status of patients in primary prevention of cardiovascular disease. *Am. J. Cardiol.* **110:** 356–363.

37. Magyar, K., R. Halmosi, A. Palfi, *et al.* 2012. Cardioprotection by resveratrol: a human clinical trial in patients with stable coronary artery disease. *Clin. Hemorheol. Microcirc.* **50:** 179–187.

38. Wong, R.H., P.R. Howe, J.D. Buckley, *et al.* 2011. Acute resveratrol supplementation improves flow-mediated dilatation in overweight/obese individuals with mildly elevated blood pressure. *Nutr. Metab. Cardiovasc. Dis.* **21:** 851–856.

39. Kennedy, D.O., E.L. Wightman, J.L. Reay, *et al.* 2010. Effects of resveratrol on cerebral blood flow variables and cognitive performance in humans: a double-blind, placebo-controlled, crossover investigation. *Am. J. Clin. Nutr.* **91:** 1590–1597.

40. Smoliga, J.M., O. Vang & J.A. Baur. 2012. Challenges of translating basic research into therapeutics: resveratrol as an example. *J. Gerontol. A. Biol. Sci. Med. Sci.* **67:** 158–167.

41. Perel, P., I. Roberts, E. Sena, *et al.* 2007. Comparison of treatment effects between animal experiments and clinical trials: systematic review. *BMJ* **334:** 197.

Ann. N.Y. Acad. Sci. ISSN 0077-8923

ANNALS OF THE NEW YORK ACADEMY OF SCIENCES
Issue: *Resveratrol and Health*

Therapeutic potential of resveratrol in obesity and type 2 diabetes: new avenues for health benefits?

Silvie Timmers,[1] Matthijs K.C. Hesselink,[2] and Patrick Schrauwen[1]

[1]Department of Human Biology and [2]Department of Human Movement Sciences, NUTRIM School for Nutrition, Toxicology and Metabolism, Maastricht University Medical Center, Maastricht, the Netherlands

Address for correspondence: Patrick Schrauwen, Ph.D., Department of Human Biology, NUTRIM School for Nutrition, Toxicology and Metabolism, Maastricht University Medical Center, P.O. Box 616, 6200MD Maastricht, the Netherlands. p.schrauwen@maastrichtuniversity.nl

The number of people suffering from metabolic disorders is dramatically increasing worldwide. The need for new therapeutic strategies to combat this growing epidemic of metabolic diseases is therefore also increasing. In 2003, resveratrol was discovered to be a small molecule activator of sirtuin 1 (SIRT1), an important molecular target regulating cellular energy metabolism and mitochondrial homeostasis. Rodent studies have clearly demonstrated the potential of resveratrol to improve various metabolic health parameters. To date, however, only limited clinical data are available that have systematically examined the health benefits of resveratrol in metabolically challenged humans. This short review will give an overview of the currently available clinical studies examining the effects of resveratrol on obesity and type 2 diabetes from a human perspective.

Keywords: resveratrol; sirtuins; obesity; type 2 diabetes; mitochondria

Introduction

The prevalence of metabolic disorders such as obesity and type 2 diabetes is dramatically increasing worldwide, and is reaching epidemic proportions. The WHO predicts that an alarming number of 350–400 million people will suffer from type 2 diabetes in the year 2030.[1,2] This profound increase in the number of patients diagnosed with type 2 diabetes can for the greater part be attributed to the increasing number of people dealing with obesity. The major proportion of the growing obesity problem can be attributed to changes in lifestyle, such as consumption of energy-dense/high-fat diets and the lack of physical activity.

In obesity, excessive fat accumulation in nonadipose tissues is thought to induce negative health effects. This can be illustrated by the fact that in sedentary individuals, skeletal muscle fat and liver fat accumulation is strongly associated with insulin resistance, and indeed predisposes to the development of type 2 diabetes.[3] The insulin-resistant state is furthermore also characterized by a reduced muscle mitochondrial oxidative capacity, thereby decreasing metabolic health even further. Indeed, we and others have shown that type 2 diabetic patients, as well as their nondiabetic, insulin-resistant offspring, are characterized by reduced mitochondrial function, both when measured *in vivo*[4,5] and *ex vivo*.[6–8]

In that respect, strategies aiming to improve muscle oxidative capacity, such as exercise training and calorie restriction, have proven to be highly effective in counteracting insulin resistance and type 2 diabetes. Thus, we have recently shown that a 12-week exercise training program in type 2 diabetic patients improved mitochondrial oxidative capacity, which was paralleled by improvements in whole-body insulin sensitivity.[9] Furthermore, calorie restriction for a period of six months has been shown to have beneficial metabolic effects in humans such as lowering of the metabolic rate,[10] improving insulin sensitivity,[11] increasing mitochondrial biogenesis,[12] and reducing cardiovascular risk factors.[13] However, although exercise training and calorie restriction are very effective approaches for

doi: 10.1111/nyas.12185

the prevention and treatment of type 2 diabetes, most type 2 diabetic patients—as well as people in general—may have difficulties in adhering to strict exercise training or dietary regimes. Therefore, in recent years, the search for other stimulators of mitochondrial oxidative capacity has been initiated.

Among the promising candidate mechanisms are the inducers of the mammalian sirtuins, a conserved family of NAD^+-dependent deacetylases (class III histone deacetylases) named after the founding member, the *Saccharomyces cerevisiae* silent information regulator 2 (Sir2),[14] of which the mammalian orthologue is called sirtuin 1 (SIRT1). Growing evidence has indicated that SIRT1, one of a number of proteins induced by calorie restriction, serves as a key molecule to regulate mitochondrial biogenesis, energy homeostasis, and insulin sensitivity (for review see Ref. 15). In 2003, resveratrol (3,5,4′-trihydroxystilbene) was discovered to be a potent small-molecule activator of SIRT1.[16] Resveratrol is a naturally occurring phytoalexin. The richest source of this compound is *Polygonum cuspidatum* (*Reynoutria japonica*), a plant used in oriental folk medicine. Small amounts of resveratrol are also present in, among others, grapevine products and peanuts.[16] Although data from a series of studies conducted in rodent models clearly report wide-ranging health benefits such as improvement in insulin sensitivity and glucose tolerance, a decrease in plasma lipids and liver fat, an enhancement of mitochondrial biogenesis, and a suppression of inflammation and oxidative stress,[2,17–19] only limited clinical data are available concerning its potential metabolic health effects. So many questions regarding potential health benefits of resveratrol in humans remain to be answered: important questions like, Is there sufficient evidence that all the aforementioned health benefits in rodents upon resveratrol supplementation translate into effects that are truly clinically relevant? and What are the factors determining whether resveratrol exerts a health benefit?

In this review, an overview of the currently available clinical studies examining the effects of resveratrol on obesity and type 2 diabetes will be presented and will be critically evaluated to see if there are underlying factors determining the outcome of the studies. In order to compare the genuine resveratrol effect between studies, only studies supplementing pure resveratrol (no extracts) were taken into account. Studies that used grape extracts containing small amounts of resveratrol or other formulas with multiple components were excluded.

Targets of resveratrol in obesity and type 2 diabetes

To date, the number of clinical trials that have examined the effect of resveratrol on obesity and insulin sensitivity has been limited (see Table 1 for an overview of all published peer-reviewed clinical trials on resveratrol). Several trials are currently ongoing (see clinicaltrials.gov). None of the peer-reviewed human clinical trials were designed specifically to test the hypothesis that resveratrol treatment will result in weight loss.

To date, only three clinical trials have been published examining the effects of resveratrol on whole-body energy metabolism in relation to the multiple health factors that are affected by obesity and type 2 diabetes.[20–22] Thus, we have investigated the metabolic effects of resveratrol in middle-aged, obese men with normal glucose tolerance who were not taking any medication.[21] We were able to support the notion that resveratrol might have a similar mechanism of action in obese humans as in high-fat–fed animals. Supplementation with resveratrol at 150 mg/day for 30 days resulted in stable plasma levels of resveratrol of around 183 ng/mL on average over the entire intervention period and induced health effects that mimicked the effects of calorie restriction. Resveratrol reduced sleeping and resting metabolic rate in the absence of body weight changes. Skeletal muscle mitochondrial function and fat oxidative capacity improved. Furthermore, fasting plasma glucose and insulin values were slightly decreased by resveratrol, providing us with—albeit limited—information of the effect of resveratrol on whole-body insulin sensitivity by the homeostatic model assessment of insulin resistance HOMA-IR. Gene set enrichment analysis revealed that resveratrol activated similar pathways in humans compared to mice, as mitochondrial pathways related to ATP production and oxidative phosphorylation were upregulated and inflammatory pathways were downregulated. In accordance with the rodent data, we confirmed that resveratrol supplementation induced an increase in skeletal muscle SIRT1 protein levels. These effects are encouraging since SIRT1 expression has been reported to be decreased in adipose tissue of obese women.[23]

Table 1. Summary of peer-reviewed clinical trials in the field of obesity and type 2 diabetes

Authors	Participants (*n*)	Objective	Form and dose of resveratrol	Duration	Outcome
Elliott *et al.* 2009	Type 2 diabetics	Insulin sensitivity	2.5 or 5 g	Daily for 28 days	Resveratrol decreased fasting and postprandial glucose and insulin at 5 g
Brasnyo *et al.* 2011	Type 2 diabetic men (19) on oral glucose-lowering medication	Insulin sensitivity and oxidative status	5 mg capsules in a double-blind parallel design. 10 subjects received resveratrol, 9 subjects received placebo	Twice daily for 4 weeks	Resveratrol significantly decreased insulin resistance (as measured by HOMA index), while it increased the pAkt:Akt ratio in platelets. Urinairy ortho-tyrosine (a measure of oxidative stress) decreased by resveratrol
Timmers *et al.* 2011	Healthy obese men (11)	Metabolic effects	75 mg in a randomized double-blind crossover design	Twice daily for 30 days	Resveratrol improved the metabolic profile: resveratrol reduced sleeping and resting metabolic rate. In muscle resveratrol activated the AMPK–SIRT1–PGC1α axis. Resveratrol reduced blood glucose and insulin levels, reduced liver fat, improved muscle mitochondrial function, and reduced inflammation marker in the blood
Wong *et al.* 2011	Overweight/obese men (14) and postmenopausal women (5) with untreated borderline hypertension	Acute effects on flow-mediated dilation	30, 90, or 270 mg of resveratrol or placebo in a double-blind randomized fashion	Single dose	Dose-dependent effect of resveratrol on flow-mediated dilation
Bhatt *et al.* 2012	Type 2 diabetic patients (62) on oral hypoglycemic treatment (metformin and/or glibenclamide)	Glycemic control and associated risk factors	250 mg of resveratrol in a prospective, open-label, randomized control study. The resveratrol group consisted of 28 patients (16 female and 12 male) and the placebo group consisted of 29 patients (20 female and 9 male)	Once daily for 3 months	Resveratrol improved mean HbA1c, systolic blood pressure, total cholesterol, and total protein. No changes in body weight, high-density lipoprotein, and low-density lipoprotein cholesterol were observed
Crandall *et al.* 2012	Older men (3) and women (7) with impaired glucose tolerance	Glucose tolerance, insulin sensitivity, and vascular function	1, 1.5, or 2 g of resveratrol in an open-label study	Daily for 4 weeks	Resveratrol decreased peak glucose and 3-h glucose AUC following a meal at 1.5 and 2 g. Matsuda index for insulin sensitivity improved at 1.5 and 2 g. Trend toward improved post-meal reactive hyperemia index. Weight, blood pressure, and lipids were unchanged
De Groote *et al.* 2012	Obese men (17) and obese women (15)	Oxidative stress markers	150 mg of resveratrol, 300 mg of resveratrol triphosphate, or 400 mg of catechin-rich grape seed extract	First 1 placebo capsule was given for 28 days followed by 1 capsule of resveratrol, resveratrol triphosphate or catechin-rich grape seed extract for 28 days	Resveratrol triphosphate and catechin-rich grape seed extract showed better antioxidant activities compared to resveratrol and induced important modulations in redox-related genes
Poulsen *et al.* 2013	Healthy obese men (24)	Metabolic effects	500 mg resveratrol (12) or placebo (12) in a randomized, double-blind placebo-controlled, parallel design	Thrice daily for 4 weeks	Resveratrol supplementation had no effect on insulin sensitivity (measured by a hyperinsulinemic euglycemic clamp), blood pressure, resting energy expenditure, oxidation rates of lipid, ectopic or visceral fat content, or inflammatory and metabolic biomarkers
Yoshino *et al.* 2012	Nonobese postmenopausal women with normal glucose tolerance (29)	Metabolic effects	75 mg resveratrol (15) or placebo (14) in a randomized, double-blind, placebo controlled parallel design	Once daily for 12 weeks	Resveratrol supplementation did not change body composition, resting metabolic rate, plasma lipids, or inflammatory markers. Resveratrol did not increase liver, skeletal muscle, or adipose tissue insulin sensitivity (measured by a hyperinsulinemic euglycemic clamp). Resveratrol did not affect its molecular targets including AMPK, SIRT1, NAMPT, and PGC1α in either skeletal muscle or adipose tissue

Moreover, Rutanen *et al.* reported that low adipose tissue SIRT1 expression, in insulin-resistant offspring of type 2 diabetic patients, could contribute to the disturbance in energy balance brought about by the reduction in mitochondrial function.[24]

A similar study to that of ours, also examining the metabolic effects of resveratrol in healthy obese men, using a 10-fold higher daily dose, could not confirm the health benefits of resveratrol that we observed.[20] Thus, in a parallel design, Poulsen *et al.* included 24 healthy obese males, aged between 31 and 44 years old that were not taking any prescriptive medicine and had no overt endocrine disorders, and performed extensive metabolic examinations before and after treatment with high-dose resveratrol (1500 mg/day). Subjects were advised to consume the high dose of resveratrol in three separate doses of 500 mg spread throughout the day. The pharmacokinetics of a single tablet of 500 mg was assessed in a small pilot trial and a concentration maximum between 300 and 400 ng/mL was reached 90 min after consumption. Unfortunately, no data were available on plasma resveratrol levels after multiple dosing or after the four weeks of supplementation. The authors did however measure urinary metabolites of resveratrol at week four of the intervention, which were undetectable in the placebo group. Insulin sensitivity, the primary outcome measure, was assessed by means of a hyperinsulinemic euglycemic clamp in combination with a stable ^{3}H-labeled glucose tracer infusion. Resveratrol did not induce any changes in endogenous glucose production, neither in oxidative glucose disposal nor in nonoxidative glucose disposal. Furthermore, resting energy expenditure and blood pressure were not affected by resveratrol. Ectopic (liver and skeletal muscle) and visceral fat content, measured by a combination of magnetic resonance spectroscopy and imaging, remained unaffected by the high resveratrol dose. Furthermore, resveratrol did not affect plasma biomarkers of metabolism and inflammation.

A third study, by Yoshino *et al.*,[22] also examined whether resveratrol could also exert metabolic benefits in healthy subjects. Therefore, 75 mg of resveratrol was supplemented to nonobese (BMI: ~24 kg/m^2), middle-aged (age: ~58 years old), postmenopausal women with normal glucose tolerance for a period of 12 weeks, and the effects of resveratrol on metabolism were examined. None of the participating subjects had a history or evidence of type 2 diabetes or cardiovascular disease or had been diagnosed or treated for abnormal plasma lipids or hypertension. Resveratrol supplementation did not change body composition or affect resting metabolic rate. Liver, skeletal muscle, and adipose tissue insulin sensitivity, measured by a hyperinsulinemic euglycemic clamp in conjunction with stable isotopically labeled tracers, remained unchanged by resveratrol. Also, no effect of resveratrol was seen

on plasma lipids or circulatory inflammatory markers. In fact, no evidence was found that resveratrol activated its putative molecular targets, as SIRT1 gene expression levels remained unchanged in skeletal muscle and adipose tissue, as did phosphorylation levels of AMPK in skeletal muscle. The authors did clearly show that the body was metabolizing the resveratrol. That is, total plasma resveratrol concentration increased to a maximum of around 992 ng/mL approximately 2 h after dosing and did not return to baseline levels within 6 h; the estimated half-life of elimination was estimated at 6.5 h (range: 3.5–11 h). Also, plasma resveratrol levels at the end of intervention reached a mean concentration of about 109 ng/mL in the resveratrol group, while in the placebo group resveratrol levels did not exceed the lower detection limit.

In addition to these clinical human studies with a broad focus on metabolic effects, several studies have focused on examining the insulin-sensitizing effect of resveratrol. Almost all of these studies have been performed in patients already diagnosed with type 2 diabetes, yet these studies represent considerable variety with respect to sex, body weight, and medication. Unfortunately, none of these studies measured resveratrol levels in the blood during or at the end of the intervention.

In 2009, Elliott *et al.*[25] were the first to report an effect of resveratrol in type 2 diabetic patients if dosed at 2.5 or 5 g/day for 28 days. The levels of fasting and postprandial glucose and insulin serum levels dropped significantly at a dose of 5 g/day, but few experimental details were provided, unfortunately. In 2011, another study in middle-aged type 2 diabetic men was performed by Brasnyo *et al.*[26] All patients were taking oral glucose-lowering medication and blood pressure–lowering medication (either angiotensin-converting enzyme inhibitor or angiotensin II receptor blockers). Furthermore, some of the patients included in this study suffered from diabetes-related complications such as diabetic nephropathy, diabetic neuropathy, peripheral arterial disease, angina pectoris, and IHD, or had experienced a heart attack or a stroke before the onset of the study. In a double-blind parallel design, 19 overweight, diabetic men received 5 mg of resveratrol or placebo twice daily for four weeks and insulin sensitivity and markers of oxidative stress were examined. The low dose of resveratrol improved insulin sensitivity (computed by the

Ann. N.Y. Acad. Sci. 1290 (2013) 83–89 © 2013 New York Academy of Sciences.

homeostatic model assessment of insulin resistance HOMA-IR) in the supplemented group compared to controls. Also, blood glucose levels were lowered and the peak blood glucose was lowered following a standardized meal after resveratrol. The authors suggested that decreased oxidative stress might underlie these effects, as significant reductions in 24-h urinary creatinine–normalized ortho-tyrosine concentrations and increased Akt phosphorylation in blood platelets were observed after the four weeks of resveratrol supplementation. Recently, a larger intervention trial in normal-weight males and females diagnosed with type 2 diabetes over three years ago examined the effect of resveratrol on glycemic control and associated risk factors in a prospective, open-label, randomized control fashion.[27] In this study, 62 patients, of which half were assigned 250 mg of resveratrol daily, were followed for a period of three months. Both the resveratrol group and the control group were comparable for age (around 55 years old) and gender distribution, and all patients continued to take their oral blood glucose–lowering medication (metformin, glibenclamide, or a combination of both) during the trial. Most patients in both the resveratrol group and the placebo group had hypertension as one of the comorbidities. Resveratrol did not affect fasting blood glucose levels, but did significantly lower mean HbA1c (before resveratrol: 9.99 ± 1.50%; after resveratrol: ∼9.65 ± 1.54%). Total cholesterol decreased in the resveratrol-supplemented group, which was largely explained by the decrease in LDL-cholesterol. Resveratrol did not affect HDL-cholesterol concentrations or plasma triglycerides. Systolic blood pressure was also lowered by the resveratrol supplementation, while diastolic blood pressure did not change. No changes were observed in body weight.

Furthermore, a small pilot study in subjects with impaired glucose tolerance (IGT) examined the potential of resveratrol to improve glucose tolerance and insulin sensitivity. For this intervention, Crandall *et al.*[28] studied the effects of resveratrol in older (age > 65 years old), overweight to obese men and women (BMI 29 ± 5 kg/m^2) with impaired glucose tolerance (mean fasting 110 ± 13 mg/dL and 2-h plasma glucose 183 ± 33 mg/dL) that have definite but not yet severe metabolic dysregulation, and therefore may be most amenable to intervention. After four weeks of resveratrol supplementation at a daily dose of 1, 1.5, or 2 g, post-meal plasma glucose was lowered in IGT subjects at doses between 1 and 2 g/day. Furthermore, post-meal insulin area under the curve (AUC) was significantly lowered by resveratrol, and insulin sensitivity (using the MATSUDA index) improved following treatment with resveratrol. Insulin sensitivity, computed by the HOMA-IR, was not significantly changed by resveratrol. Body weight, blood pressure, and lipids remained unchanged by resveratrol.

Taken together, so far the clinical intervention studies that have explored the therapeutic potential of resveratrol for metabolic diseases like obesity and type 2 diabetes differ tremendously in their experimental design and their outcome, making it impossible to provide an unequivocal answer whether, and under which conditions, resveratrol may exert its health benefits.

Resveratrol and vascular health

Besides a focus on insulin sensitivity, Crandall *et al.* also assessed endothelial function in their intervention.[28] Endothelial function was assessed by reactive hyperemia peripheral arterial tonometry (RH-PAT) in the fasting state and 90 min after a standard meal. Fasting RH-PAT index was essentially unchanged, but there was a trend toward improved post-meal endothelial function following resveratrol. Three other studies have also examined the effects of resveratrol on vascular health, including oxidative stress markers. It should be noted that these health parameters have been studied in a wide range of different patient groups (IGT subject, overweight to obese subjects, and type 2 diabetic subjects). Wong *et al.*[29] studied the acute effects of resveratrol on flow-mediated dilation in middle-aged, overweight to obese men and postmenopausal women with untreated borderline hypertension. At weekly intervals in a randomized double-blind, crossover comparison, subjects received a single dose of 30, 90, or 270 mg of resveratrol, or a placebo. One hour after consumption of the supplement, plasma resveratrol and flow-mediated dilation were measured. Both plasma resveratrol levels (30 mg: ∼181 ng/mL, 90 mg: ∼532 ng/mL, 270 mg: ∼1232 ng/mL) and the flow-mediated dilation of the brachial artery increased in dose-dependent fashions.

As described above, Brasnyo *et al.*[26] found a significant decrease in the concentration of the oxidative stress marker urinary creatinine–normalized ortho-tyrosine in patients with type 2 diabetes after receiving 10 mg of resveratrol for four weeks. The effect of resveratrol on oxidative stress markers was also examined in young, obese men and women.[30] In this study, the effect of resveratrol was compared to an equimolar dose of resveratrol tri-phosphate and catechin-rich grape seed extract. Resveratrol was supplemented as one capsule of 150 mg/day for a period of 28 days, and analysis of plasma total antioxidant power, lipid peroxides, and the determination of genes selected from oxidative stress–sensitive pathways by microarray was performed. Compared to resveratrol, resveratrol tri-phosphate and catechin-rich grape seed extract showed a higher biological activity characterized by increased antioxidant status, reduction of some markers of oxidative damage, and modulation of the expression of genes involved in the redox, inflammatory, and cellular response stress pathways.

New avenues for health benefits?

Taken together, there is insufficient evidence at this moment to convincingly state that resveratrol can improve overall metabolic health status in every individual who consumes it. The nine clinical intervention studies performed so far clearly illustrate divergent effects of resveratrol between the trials. Factors that may influence the outcome of the study are, among others, the dose of the resveratrol, the timing of consumption (one versus multiple doses), and the metabolic status of the subject.

The optimal dose of resveratrol is—and will remain—an important point of debate, since both the studies that did and those that did not show a positive effect of resveratrol used a similar range of resveratrol doses. In fact, the five studies that supplemented resveratrol for a period of approximately four weeks used doses from as low as 10 mg up to 5 g per day, but still report strikingly different results. For example, an improvement in markers of insulin sensitivity was reported at doses of 10 mg[26] and 150 mg,[21] but also at doses between 1.5 and 5 g.[25,28] However, one study using a dose of 1.5 g did not find any effect on insulin sensitivity.[20] Also, plasma triglycerides decreased only when a relatively low dose of resveratrol was used (150 mg),[21] but not at a high dose (1–2 g).[28]

Pharmacokinetic studies in humans have demonstrated that resveratrol is rapidly taken up after oral consumption, peaking at about 0.8–1.5 h after consumption.[31] The half-life of resveratrol increases from 1–3 h after a single dose to 2–5 h after repeated administration,[31] so one can question whether giving a single dose of resveratrol or splitting that resveratrol dose into multiple smaller doses that are being consumed throughout the day will influence the physiological outcome measures to a similar extent. Complementary to that, not all clinical studies have measured the appearance of resveratrol and metabolites in the plasma. This is considered a true limitation and further complicates the comparison of the interventions.

In animals, the main beneficial effects of resveratrol have been reported in mice on a high-fat diet,[17] suggesting that resveratrol is especially potent in reversing metabolic abnormalities. In that respect, studies that did show positive effects of resveratrol were performed in either obese subjects[21] or type 2 diabetic patients,[25–27] whereas no beneficial effects of resveratrol in healthy lean women were reported.[22] It can therefore be argued that resveratrol may only be effective when one has a certain degree of metabolic derangement, although it should be stressed that the number of studies is still too small to draw definitive conclusions.

So overall, it can be concluded that further research is still necessary at this moment before we can fully recommend the widespread use of resveratrol as a therapeutic strategy for chronic metabolic diseases. Future research should aim at trying to understand the specific determinants that influence whether resveratrol will result in a metabolic benefit (e.g., dose, timing of the day, age, extent of metabolic derangement, etc.). Furthermore, chronic intervention studies with plasma levels of resveratrol being measured are also an absolute must, as it is still unclear if long-term resveratrol treatment is beneficial to overall health status.

Conflicts of interest

The authors declare no conflicts of interest.

References

1. Wild, S., G. Roglic, A. Green, *et al*. 2004. Global prevalence of diabetes: estimates for the year 2000 and projections for 2030. *Diabetes Care* **27:** 1047–1053.
2. Baur, J.A., K.J. Pearson, N.L. Price, *et al*. 2006. Resveratrol improves health and survival of mice on a high-calorie diet. *Nature* **444:** 337–342.

3. McGarry, J.D. 2002. Banting lecture 2001: dysregulation of fatty acid metabolism in the etiology of type 2 diabetes. *Diabetes* **51:** 7–18.

4. Petersen, K.F., S. Dufour, D. Befroy, *et al.* 2004. Impaired mitochondrial activity in the insulin-resistant offspring of patients with type 2 diabetes. *N. Engl. J. Med.* **350:** 664–671.

5. Schrauwen-Hinderling, V.B., M.E. Kooi, M.K. Hesselink, *et al.* 2007. Impaired in vivo mitochondrial function but similar intramyocellular lipid content in patients with type 2 diabetes mellitus and BMI-matched control subjects. *Diabetologia* **50:** 113–120.

6. Kahn, S.E., R.L. Hull & K.M. Utzschneider. 2006. Mechanisms linking obesity to insulin resistance and type 2 diabetes. *Nature* **444:** 840–846.

7. Morino, K., K.F. Petersen, S. Dufour, *et al.* 2005. Reduced mitochondrial density and increased IRS-1 serine phosphorylation in muscle of insulin-resistant offspring of type 2 diabetic parents. *J. Clin. Invest* **115:** 3587–3593.

8. Phielix, E., V.B. Schrauwen-Hinderling, M. Mensink, *et al.* 2008. Lower intrinsic ADP-stimulated mitochondrial respiration underlies in vivo mitochondrial dysfunction in muscle of male type 2 diabetic patients. *Diabetes* **57:** 2943–2949.

9. Meex, R.C., V.B. Schrauwen-Hinderling, E. Moonen-Kornips, *et al.* 2010. Restoration of muscle mitochondrial function and metabolic flexibility in type 2 diabetes by exercise training is paralleled by increased myocellular fat storage and improved insulin sensitivity. *Diabetes* **59:** 572–579.

10. Heilbronn, L.K., L. de Jonge, M.I. Frisard, *et al.* 2006. Effect of 6-month calorie restriction on biomarkers of longevity, metabolic adaptation, and oxidative stress in overweight individuals: a randomized controlled trial. *JAMA* **295:** 1539–1548.

11. Larson-Meyer, D.E., B.R. Newcomer, L.K. Heilbronn, *et al.* 2008. Effect of 6-month calorie restriction and exercise on serum and liver lipids and markers of liver function. *Obesity* **16:** 1355–1362.

12. Civitarese, A.E., S. Carling, L.K. Heilbronn, *et al.* 2007. Calorie restriction increases muscle mitochondrial biogenesis in healthy humans. *PLoS Med.* **4:** e76.

13. Lefevre, M., L.M. Redman, L.K. Heilbronn, *et al.* 2009. Caloric restriction alone and with exercise improves CVD risk in healthy non-obese individuals. *Atherosclerosis* **203:** 206–213.

14. Brachmann, C.B., J.M. Sherman, S.E. Devine, *et al.* 1995. The SIR2 gene family, conserved from bacteria to humans, functions in silencing, cell cycle progression, and chromosome stability. *Genes Dev.* **9:** 2888–2902.

15. Yu, J. & J. Auwerx. 2009. The role of sirtuins in the control of metabolic homeostasis. *Ann. N.Y. Acad. Sci.* **1173**(Suppl 1): E10–E19.

16. Howitz, K.T., K.J. Bitterman, H.Y. Cohen, *et al.* 2003. Small molecule activators of sirtuins extend Saccharomyces cerevisiae life span. *Nature* **425:** 191–196.

17. Lagouge, M., C. Argmann, Z. Gerhart-Hines, *et al.* 2006. Resveratrol improves mitochondrial function and protects against metabolic disease by activating SIRT1 and PGC-1alpha. *Cell* **127:** 1109–1122.

18. Sun, C., F. Zhang, X. Ge, *et al.* 2007. SIRT1 improves insulin sensitivity under insulin-resistant conditions by repressing PTP1B. *Cell Metab.* **6:** 307–319.

19. Um, J.H., S.J. Park, H. Kang, *et al.* 2010. AMP-activated protein kinase-deficient mice are resistant to the metabolic effects of resveratrol. *Diabetes* **59:** 554–563.

20. Poulsen, M.M., P.F. Vestergaard, B.F. Clasen, *et al.* 2013. High-Dose Resveratrol Supplementation in Obese Men: An Investigator-Initiated, Randomized, Placebo-Controlled Clinical Trial of Substrate Metabolism, Insulin Sensitivity, and Body Composition. *Diabetes* **62:** 1186–1195.

21. Timmers, S., E. Konings, L. Bilet, *et al.* 2011. Calorie restriction-like effects of 30 days of resveratrol supplementation on energy metabolism and metabolic profile in obese humans. *Cell Metab.* **14:** 612–622.

22. Yoshino, J., C. Conte, L. Fontana, *et al.* 2012. Resveratrol supplementation does not improve metabolic function in nonobese women with normal glucose tolerance. *Cell Metab.* **16:** 658–664.

23. Pedersen, S.B., J. Olholm, S.K. Paulsen, *et al.* 2008. Low Sirt1 expression, which is upregulated by fasting, in human adipose tissue from obese women. *Int. J. Obes.* **32:** 1250–1255.

24. Rutanen, J., N. Yaluri, S. Modi, *et al.* 2010. SIRT1 mRNA expression may be associated with energy expenditure and insulin sensitivity. *Diabetes* **59:** 829–835.

25. Elliott, P.J., S. Walpole, L. Morelli, *et al.* 2009. Resveratrol/SRT-501. *Drugs Fut.* **34:** 291–295.

26. Brasnyo, P., G.A. Molnar, M. Mohas, *et al.* 2011. Resveratrol improves insulin sensitivity, reduces oxidative stress and activates the Akt pathway in type 2 diabetic patients. *Br. J. Nutr.* **106:** 383–389.

27. Bhatt, J.K., S. Thomas & M.J. Nanjan. 2012. Resveratrol supplementation improves glycemic control in type 2 diabetes mellitus. *Nutr. Res.* **32:** 537–541.

28. Crandall, J.P., V. Oram, G. Trandafirescu, *et al.* 2012. Pilot study of resveratrol in older adults with impaired glucose tolerance. *J. Gerontol. A Biol. Sci. Med. Sci.* **67:** 1307–1312.

29. Wong, R.H., P.R. Howe, J.D. Buckley, *et al.* 2011. Acute resveratrol supplementation improves flow-mediated dilatation in overweight/obese individuals with mildly elevated blood pressure. *Nutr. Metab. Cardiovasc Dis.* **21:** 851–856.

30. De Groote, D., K. Van Belleghem, J. Deviere, *et al.* 2012. Effect of the intake of resveratrol, resveratrol phosphate, and catechin-rich grape seed extract on markers of oxidative stress and gene expression in adult obese subjects. *Ann. Nutr. Metab.* **61:** 15–24.

31. Cottart, C.H., V. Nivet-Antoine, C. Laguillier-Morizot & J.L. Beaudeux. 2010. Resveratrol bioavailability and toxicity in humans. *Mol. Nutr. Food Res.* **54:** 7–16.

Ann. N.Y. Acad. Sci. ISSN 0077-8923

ANNALS OF THE NEW YORK ACADEMY OF SCIENCES

Issue: *Resveratrol and Health*

Importance of lipid microdomains, rafts, in absorption, delivery, and biological effects of resveratrol

Dominique Delmas,[1,2] Virginie Aires,[1,2] Didier J. Colin,[3] Emeric Limagne,[1,2] Alessandra Scagliarini,[1,2] Alexia K. Cotte,[1,2] and François Ghiringhelli[1,2]

[1]University of Burgundy, Dijon, France. [2]Chemotherapy, Lipid Metabolism and Antitumoral Immune Response Team, INSERM Research Center U866, Dijon, France. [3]Center for Biomedical Imaging (CIBM)–microPET Imaging Laboratory, University of Geneva, Geneva, Switzerland

Address for correspondence: Dominique Delmas, Faculty of Medicine, INSERM Research Center UMR866 "Lipids, Nutrition, Cancers," 7 Bd Jeanne d'Arc, 21000 Dijon, France. ddelmas@u-bourgogne.fr

The preventive effects of the phytoalexin *trans*-resveratrol toward cancer have been largely described at the cellular and molecular levels in both *in vivo* and *in vitro* models; however, its primary targets are still poorly identified. In this review, we show the crucial role of cell membrane microdomains, that is, lipid rafts, not solely in the initiation of the early biochemical events triggered by resveratrol leading to cancer cell death, but also in resveratrol absorption and distribution. Resveratrol accumulates in lipid rafts and is then taken up by cells through raft-dependent endocytosis. These events allow early activation of kinase pathways and redistribution of cell death receptors within lipid microdomains, events ultimately leading to apoptotic cell death.

Keywords: resveratrol; transport; cancer; rafts; apoptosis

Introduction

Resveratrol or 3,4′,5-trihydroxystilbene is a secondary metabolite produced in limited plant species and found in many natural foods (e.g., grapes, red wine, purple grape juice, and some berries).[1] In plants, resveratrol is mostly found in the *trans*-resveratrol-3-*O*-β-D-glucoside form, which is often referred to as *piceid*. Like many other plant polyphenols (i.e., flavonoids, epicatechins), resveratrol presents interesting properties against cancers. Resveratrol is able to delay or to prevent the stages of carcinogenesis.[2,3] These beneficial effects have been supported by observations at the cellular and molecular levels in both *in vitro* and *in vivo* models and reinforce the interest in grape products and dietary supplements for cancer therapy.

In the field of chemoprevention, the ability of resveratrol to prevent the occurrence of various carcinomas is related to the inhibition of the tumor cell cycle,[4,5] the activation of signaling pathways that involve kinase activations, and/or the induction of the proteolytic cascade of caspases to trigger tumor cell apoptosis.[6,7] Although the beneficial effects of resveratrol have largely been elucidated, very little is known about the mechanisms of resveratrol cellular uptake and how resveratrol initiates its biological effects. Here we review the essential role played by particular plasma membrane microdomains, also called *rafts* or *lipid rafts*, in both resveratrol absorption and distribution and in early resveratrol-induced signaling pathways leading to apoptotic cancer cell death. The last part of this review discusses the potential role of lipid rafts in resveratrol-mediated effects and in the potential restoration of tumor cell sensitivity to death receptor ligands.

Lipid rafts as dynamic membrane structures

The plasma membrane of mammalian cells is a bilayer primarily composed of thousands of types of lipids and proteins.[8] Besides delineating intra- and extracellular compartments, the plasma membrane constitutes a selective barrier through which information and matter pass. The plasma membrane structure was originally described by Singer and Nicholson in 1970 as a fluid mosaic in which

doi: 10.1111/nyas.12177

Ann. N.Y. Acad. Sci. 1290 (2013) 90–97 © 2013 New York Academy of Sciences.

inserted proteins can drift laterally and randomly in a fluid phospholipid bilayer. The current model suggests a biological membrane organized into lipid microdomains or platforms, which are distinguished from the rest of the membrane by their high content of sphingomyelin and cholesterol. This lipid raft concept was introduced to explain the generation of the glycolipid-rich apical membrane of epithelial cells.[9] In this model, two phases are distinguished. The first is the liquid-ordered L_0 raft phase, which results from the lateral association between sphingolipids in the outer leaflet and sterol in the outer and inner leaflet of the bilayer. The second phase corresponds to a liquid-disordered phase, which is nonraft in nature due to the differences in the short-ranged liquid translational and conformational order.

As mentioned, lipid rafts are ordered plasma membrane structures resulting from the preferential packing of sphingolipids and cholesterol. They are believed to cover around 35% of the cell surface. Lipid rafts are also characterized by the presence of various proteins, notably the glycosylphosphatidylinositol (GPI)-anchored proteins, which are specifically attached to membrane outer leaflet via their GPI anchor (Fig. 1, inset). In addition, these rafts are associated with dynamic structures called *caveolae*, which are plasma membrane invaginations resulting from the polymerization of the raft protein caveolin. Furthermore, rafts are highly dynamic in the sense that they can spatiotemporally recruit and localize components required for many key cellular processes, such as the intracellular transport of various molecules (e.g., viruses, xenobiotics) and the induction or response to various stimuli (e.g., xenobiotics, nutrients, and drugs).

Resveratrol uptake involves lipid raft–mediated endocytosis

Cellular uptake of xenobiotics can be achieved through passive diffusion, carrier-mediated transport, or active transport. Using radiolabeled resveratrol, we have previously shown that the polyphenol enters cells by both passive (50%) and facilitated (50%) processes based on the following observations. At 4 °C, a temperature that blocks carrier-mediated and active processes, resveratrol uptake in hepatoblastoma,[10] colon cancer, and leukemia

cells,[11] is significantly reduced relative to uptake at 37 °C. Results suggest that passive diffusion accounts for ~50% of transport. *Cis*-inhibition experiments using unlabeled resveratrol show inhibition of the total tracer uptake,[10,11] thus indicating the contribution of a carrier-mediated process.

To get insight into the nature of these carrier-mediated processes, we used pharmacological inhibitors of endocytic pathways. Pretreatment of cells with the pan-inhibitor of endocytosis monensin significantly curtailed resveratrol uptake,[11] whereas specific blockers of either clathrin- or dynamin-mediated endocytosis and macropinocytosis failed to do so. Only commonly used lipid raft disrupters (methyl-β-cyclodextrin, nystatin, and filipin) consistently impaired resveratrol uptake in colon cancer cells,[11] indicating that part of the polyphenol may use lipid rafts for intracellular penetration (Fig. 1). Lipid raft–mediated endocytosis has been described as part of the clathrin-independent endocytic pathways.[12,13] It is involved in the endocytosis of GPI-anchored proteins,[14] interleukin-2 linked to its receptors,[15] and several ether lipids (e.g., alkyl-lysophospholipid).[16] The lipophilic nature of resveratrol is consistent with its accumulation in lipid microdomains before its endocytosis (Fig. 1). Interestingly, endocytosis of resveratrol via lipid rafts was associated with an accumulation of LysoSensor™-positive acidic vesicles within cytoplasm; however, lowering intracellular pH did not modify resveratrol uptake and antiproliferative effects.[11] Yang *et al.* also suggested the involvement of lipid rafts in resveratrol uptake,[17] and they identified a specific subclass of rafts that contain caveolin-1, the main component of caveolae, which are plasma membrane invaginations implicated in various functions including endocytosis, transcytosis, and potocytosis.[18] In this study, they showed in both HepG2 cells transfected with wild-type or mutant caveolin-1 and in a hepatocellular carcinoma animal model that caveolin-1 expression increased the cytotoxic and proapoptotic activity of resveratrol in a dose- and time-dependent manner through an increase in its internalization and trafficking, as visualized with a fluorescent resveratrol derivative (dansyl-chloride resveratrol).[17] In addition, resveratrol endocytosis is not mediated by estrogen receptor (ER) α and β, as suggested by a lack of competitive inhibition by estrogen or tamoxifen.[17]

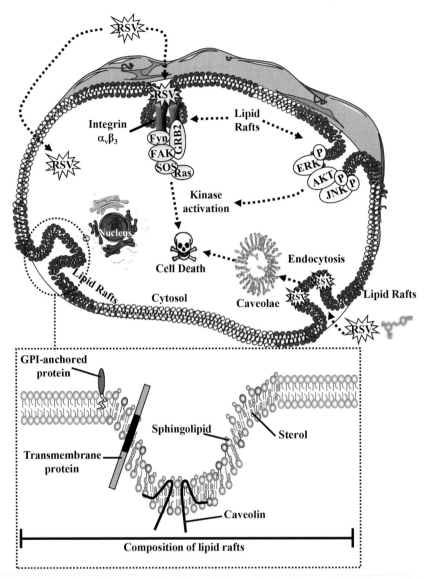

Figure 1. Lipid rafts as key players in resveratrol uptake and kinase activation. Resveratrol (RSV) accumulates in lipid rafts and enters tumor cells through lipid raft–mediated endocytosis, which is independent of clathrin. Furthermore, resveratrol binds integrin $\alpha_v\beta_3$ on the extracellular domain and promotes the formation of integrin-signaling complexes into lipid rafts, leading to the signal transduction cascade. In parallel, resveratrol induces the redistribution of various kinase proteins and their phosphorylated forms into lipid rafts that are essential to resveratrol action in cancer cells such as cell death. Inset: lipid raft composition.

Lipid raft–mediated endocytosis as a key initiator of resveratrol actions

Several studies have shown that the biological effects of various drugs, xenobiotics, or nutrients are the result of the redistribution of proteins such as receptors or other signaling proteins at the membrane level. Lipid rafts are very important in these processes, particularly in the induction or response of cells to various stimuli. Moreover, the redistribution of proteins inside or outside of rafts can cause various pathologies such as cardiovascular diseases, degenerative diseases, diabetes, obesity, inflammation, and cancers.

In fact, resveratrol accumulation in lipid rafts induces a rapid activation of various kinases, such as c-Jun NH_2-terminal kinases (JNKs); extracellular signal–regulated kinases (ERKs); and Akt in colon cancer, leukemia,[11] prostate cancer, and melanoma cells.[19] These early kinase activations are important because the presence of specific kinase inhibitors prevents resveratrol-induced apoptosis in these cells. Resveratrol-induced kinase activation is inhibited by both the pan-inhibitor of endocytosis monensin and the lipid raft disruptors methyl-β-cyclodextrin and nystatin in colon carcinoma and leukemia cells. Subsequently, this inhibition of endocytosis decreases resveratrol-induced apoptosis in cancer cells. A biochemical analysis of lipid raft content by fractionation of cell lysates on a sucrose gradient revealed that resveratrol induces the redistribution of JNKs, Akt, and ERKs (including their phosphorylated forms) into rafts (Fig. 1). As observed for kinase activation, the use of lipid raft inhibitors suppressed the resveratrol-induced redistribution of these proteins into lipid rafts. In fact, the redistribution of kinases in lipid rafts facilitates their activation and downstream induction of apoptosis.

Integrin plays a key role in resveratrol uptake and early action through lipid rafts

Rafts can be the site of interactions between receptors and their ligands: this interaction takes place first inside or outside these membrane microdomains. Once the receptors are linked to their respective ligands, intracellular transduction cascades are initiated and lead to the assembly of signaling complexes and to actin polymerization. These signaling events promote a raft migration, dependent on actin and myosin, to the site of signaling. As the different microdomain fields fuse to form macrodomains, signaling proteins that were initially in different areas find themselves in proximity to each other. Subsequently, the interactions between proteins increase, amplifying the initial signal, and therefore recruiting more rafts and more signaling proteins into these newly formed macrodomains. This process could be triggered by transmembrane glycoproteins, such as integrins, which are able to form integrin-signaling complexes that can induce a signaling transduction cascade. Indeed, the extracellular ligand–binding regions of integrins sense information relayed by the extracellular matrix and transduce these signals through their cytoplasmic domain, which interacts with the cytoskeleton. Integrins are also known to initiate cellular signaling through phosphorylation cascades, as described

for the integrin $\alpha_v\beta_3$, that can trigger extracellular signal–related kinase 1/2 (ERK1/2) signaling.[20] It has been previously shown that resveratrol can induce ERK1/2 signaling by binding the integrin $\alpha_v\beta_3$.[7,11,19,21] In this context, we also demonstrated that a prototype peptide arginine–glycine–aspartate (RGD), which is known to block integrin $\alpha_v\beta_3$, can inhibit the proapoptotic effects of resveratrol toward cancer cells.[11] Moreover, it appears that integrin $\alpha_v\beta_3$ is involved in resveratrol uptake, because the occlusion of the RGD-binding site in the integrin extracellular domain diminishes resveratrol uptake and consequently decreases resveratrol-induced apoptosis.[11] We analyzed the underlying molecular mechanisms at play, and it appears that resveratrol promotes the recruitment of the Fak, Fyn, Ras, and Grb2 proteins to form integrin signaling complexes in colon carcinoma cells.[11] This recruitment involves redistribution of these proteins and of the integrin $\alpha_v\beta_3$ into lipid rafts after exposure with resveratrol for 6 min (Fig. 1). Our data support the view that these lipid microdomains may function as microcompartments for the assembly of signaling complexes.[22] Upon integrin ligation, Fyn is activated and binds to the adaptor protein SHC via its SH3 domain. It has been previously reported that this sequence of events is necessary to couple integrins to the Ras–ERK pathway.[23] The binding of resveratrol to integrin $\alpha_v\beta_3$ has been further demonstrated by an *in silico* approach showing that it can form strong bonds with the Arg248 of the αv subunit.[24] This study also showed that the 4′-OH group of resveratrol, which is implicated in its antioxidant and antiproliferative properties, establishes bonds with Glu220 of the β3 subunit.[24]

Lipid rafts as dynamic platforms for the later effects of resveratrol

Lipid rafts also play an important role in the initiation of apoptosis in response to various molecules, such as ether lipids through the extrinsic pathway.[25] Similarly, we have previously shown that lipid rafts are implicated in the clustering or aggregation of surface receptors and adaptor molecules into membrane complexes at specific sites. These redistributions are shown to be essential for initiating signaling from a number of receptors, particularly in the initiation of Fas-mediated apoptosis during resveratrol treatment.[26] The extrinsic pathway of apoptosis is initiated by death receptors of the tumor necrosis factor (TNF) receptor superfamily. These receptors have been shown to be essential in the responses of cancer cells toward certain chemotherapeutic agents.[27] The extrinsic pathway of apoptosis primarily involves the Fas receptor (i.e., CD95, APO-1), which is the major protein for the sensing and transduction of extracellular death signals. It is mainly triggered by the ligation of Fas ligand (i.e., FasL, APO-1L, CD95L).[28,29] The transduction of the signal by ligated Fas is mediated by subsequent oligomerization of inactive caspases, resulting in their proteolytic activation. The apoptotic pathway triggered by Fas has been implicated in the anticancer response of many chemotherapeutic drugs, which underlies its critical role. The first report showing the importance of the Fas pathway in resveratrol anticancer properties described increases of FasL expression and binding to Fas.[30] However, a few other studies reported conflicting results in other cell systems. They challenged the idea of resveratrol-induced Fas-L overexpression and showed that Fas/FasL interaction is not required for resveratrol-induced apoptosis by using a blocking antibody or leukemic cells insensitive to Fas-mediated apoptosis.[31–33] Other interesting reports at this time, including our work on apoptosis, drove our subsequent studies on the mechanisms by which resveratrol triggers its proapoptotic effect. Indeed, it has been shown that chemotherapeutic agents can induce apoptosis via FADD (Fas-associated death domain) independently of FasL.[34] For instance, activation of caspase-8, which is mainly known as a consequence of death receptor–mediated apoptosis, can also occur in the amplification loop of the intrinsic apoptotic pathway. We thought that resveratrol-induced apoptosis might rely in part on such mechanisms, because caspase-8 is activated in response to the polyphenol in colon cancer cells, without ruling out a role for Fas signaling. Thus, we showed for the first time that resveratrol triggers a redistribution of Fas into the lipid rafts of the plasma membrane, but we did not find any effect on FasL expression or extracellular accumulation.[26] Other studies have confirmed the importance of the redistribution of Fas into lipid rafts in its capacity to trigger apoptosis.[35] Colocalization with the raft marker caveolin and homogenous clustering of Fas seem to be major steps in the induction of apoptosis in cancer cells in response to resveratrol.[26] Consequently, we showed that these events allow the association

of FADD and procaspase-8 in lipid rafts. Our data obtained in colon cancer cells have been confirmed recently by the team of Mollinedo in some nonsolid tumors (multiple myeloma and T cell leukemia), in which resveratrol induced clustering of Fas death receptor into lipid rafts independently of its ligand.[36] The mechanisms of receptor molecule trapping in membrane rafts are yet to be characterized. It was proposed that selective clustering of Fas involves acid sphingomyelinase-induced release of ceramide in lymphocytes or fibroblasts.[37] It could also be related to hydrophobic modifications of the receptor, associations with a partner located in lipid rafts, or an initial clustering resulting in an increase of affinity. In all these cases, we showed that Fas redistribution in the lipid rafts in response to resveratrol leads to the formation of the death-inducing signaling complex (DISC) in colon cancer cells, and consequently to the downstream events involved in the apoptotic process (i.e., Bax/Bak conformational changes and subsequent caspase-3 activation). We also demonstrated that other death receptors like DR4 and DR5 follow the same scheme of clustering and signaling in response to resveratrol.[38] These results fit with the effects of lipid ether reported in leukemia cells,[25] and highlight the role of death receptor redistribution into lipid rafts in the proapoptotic effects of resveratrol toward cancer cells.

Lipid rafts to counteract chemoresistance of tumor cells

Lipid rafts also contribute to the chemosensitization induced by various drugs through the translocation of proteins either out of (e.g., P-glycoprotein)[39] or into their structures (e.g., death receptors). Thus, we showed that in resveratrol-resistant cancer cells, a treatment with the polyphenol can enhance the cytotoxic effects of various agents, including TNF, anti-TNF receptor antibodies, and TNF-related apoptosis-inducing ligand (TRAIL).[38] Resveratrol exhibits its sensitizing properties by facilitating the formation of the DISC at the plasma membrane. It also improves apoptosis induction independently of Bax and Bak, since their knockout did not counteract its effects and Bcl-2 overexpressing cells were also affected.[40] These last observations ruled out any involvement of the mitochondria-driven intrinsic pathway in these effects. Furthermore, we demonstrated that inhibition of the redistribution of TNF-related receptors into lipid rafts

Ann. N.Y. Acad. Sci. 1290 (2013) 90–97 © 2013 New York Academy of Sciences.

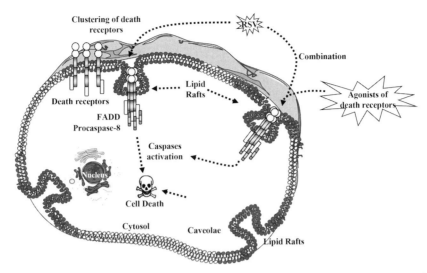

Figure 2. Lipid rafts as key players in resveratrol-induced apoptosis. Resveratrol (RSV) induces the clustering of death receptor domains (CD95, DR4, and DR5) into lipid rafts. This redistribution leads to a functional DISC, where FADD and procaspase-8 are also redistributed into lipid microdomains. These events contribute to the molecule's ability to trigger apoptosis in tumor cells, and it is an essential step for its sensitizing effect when resveratrol is used in combination with death receptor agonists.

using the raft inhibitor nystatin blocked resveratrol-sensitizing effects in these drug combinations models, which suggests that this clustering is a key event[38] (Fig. 2).

These observations highlight the potential benefit of resveratrol as an adjuvant in chemotherapy. Indeed, it is well known that antiapoptotic proteins of the Bcl-2 family are implicated in the resistance toward many anticancer agents. As we showed for TRAIL- and Fas-related therapies in colon cancer cells, resveratrol might be a useful and nontoxic means to enhance the effects of widely used cytotoxic anticancer treatments and possibly decrease the emergence of long-term resistance. Future studies in our group will test these hypotheses in preclinical *in vivo* models.

Conclusion and perspectives

In this review, we describe the importance of the membrane dynamic microdomains, dubbed lipid rafts, in resveratrol uptake, which leads to its early and later effects in cancer cells. We have highlighted the fact that lipid raft–mediated endocytosis is the early event in the molecular signaling cascade induced by resveratrol. Taken together, these findings show that accumulation of resveratrol into lipid rafts and active endocytosis are required for resveratrol to activate kinase-dependent signaling

pathways (ERKs/JNKs/Akt) and to trigger caspase-dependent apoptosis in cancer cells. A disruption of this process largely abolishes the biological effect of this polyphenol. Any residual activity observed was due to resveratrol taken up by passive diffusion. Interestingly, although resveratrol enters normal cells such as human monocytes or intestinal cells, resveratrol does not induce kinase activation, toxicity, or apoptosis.[11] All these events appear to be required for activation of downstream signaling pathways leading to cell death in tumor cells, and indicate the essential role of microdomains in the dynamics of resveratrol uptake in tumor cells and in associated biological responses.

Most of the mechanisms described in this review were obtained *in vitro*, and future works should consider them as a basis for *in vivo* preclinical studies. Thus, the link between the chemopreventive and chemotherapeutic effects of resveratrol and its integrin binding and subsequent lipid raft–mediated endocytosis should be explored further in animal studies. Such studies could be easily achieved by noninvasive molecular imaging using, for example, competitive assays with RGD-based tracers. They could also provide insight into the nature of resveratrol anticancer activity. Indeed, resveratrol might affect various tumor components through its binding to $\alpha_v\beta_3$ integrin that is found in the plasma membrane of cancer and endothelial cells. The cellular responses of these cell types to resveratrol might be mechanistically different, but they could explain its pleiotropic effects on tumors, from killing cancer cells to inhibiting angiogenesis.[41] This last effect may be comparable to promising RGD-related drug therapies.[42] Metastasis is another very important step in the development of cancer that might be targeted by resveratrol via lipid rafts. Indeed, resveratrol has been shown to increase the fluidity of the plasma membrane.[43,44] Considering that cancer cells initiate their migration/invasion by forming lipid raft–enriched invadopodia, and that this phenomenon is dependent on integrins and caveolin-1,[45] it would be interesting to check if resveratrol targets these events. Also, as the expression of caveolin-1 has been strongly correlated with chemoresistance, discovering any effect of resveratrol on the activity of this protein is important. Finally, there are still doubts about the relevance of *in vitro* studies on resveratrol since its bioavailability *in vivo* is considered poor. Indeed, it is rapidly metabolized by glucuronidation, sulfation, and hydroxylation reactions. We recently showed that sulfate derivatives of resveratrol, as well as mixtures of sulfate and glucuronide derivatives, can exert anticancer effects similar to resveratrol *in vitro.*[46] Therefore, these metabolites could account for resveratrol's properties *in vivo*. The questions posed above would benefit from a parallel analysis of the effects of resveratrol metabolites and may provide important preclinical results.

Acknowledgments

This study was supported by the Conseil Régional de Bourgogne and the Ligue Inter-régionale Grand-Est Contre le Cancer. A.S. received a postdoctoral fellowship from the Conseil Régional de Bourgogne, which supports D.D.'s group. We are grateful to Dr. J.A.H. Inkster, University of Geneva, for valuable English corrections.

Conflicts of interest

The authors declare no conflicts of interest.

References

1. Langcake, P. & R. Pryce. 1977. A new class of phytoalexins from grapevines. *Experentia.* **33:** 1151–1152.

2. Jang, M. *et al.* 1997. Cancer chemopreventive activity of resveratrol, a natural product derived from grapes. *Science* **275:** 218–220.

3. Delmas, D. *et al.* 2006. Resveratrol as a chemopreventive agent: a promising molecule for fighting cancer. *Curr. Drug Targets* **7:** 423–442.

4. Colin, D. *et al.* 2009. Effects of resveratrol analogs on cell cycle progression, cell cycle associated proteins and 5fluorouracil sensitivity in human derived colon cancer cells. *Int. J. Cancer* **124:** 2780–2788.

5. Marel, A.K. *et al.* 2008. Inhibitory effects of trans-resveratrol analogs molecules on the proliferation and the cell cycle progression of human colon tumoral cells. *Mol. Nutr. Food Res.* **52:** 538–548.

6. Delmas, D., E. Solary & N. Latruffe. 2011. Resveratrol, a phytochemical inducer of multiple cell death pathways: apoptosis, autophagy and mitotic catastrophe. *Curr. Med. Chem.* **18:** 1100–1121.

7. Lin, H.Y. *et al.* 2008. Resveratrol causes COX-2- and p53-dependent apoptosis in head and neck squamous cell cancer cells. *J. Cell Biochem.* **104:** 2131–2142.

8. Engelman, D.M. 2005. Membranes are more mosaic than fluid. *Nature* **438:** 578–580.

9. Simons, K. & G. van Meer. 1988. Lipid sorting in epithelial cells. *Biochemistry* **27:** 6197–6202.

10. Lancon, A. *et al.* 2004. Human hepatic cell uptake of resveratrol: involvement of both passive diffusion and carrier-mediated process. *Biochem. Biophys. Res. Commun.* **316:** 1132–1137.

11. Colin, D. *et al.* 2011. Endocytosis of resveratrol via lipid rafts and activation of downstream signaling pathways in cancer cells. *Cancer Prev. Res. (Phila)* **4:** 1095–1106.

12. Ikonen, E. 2001. Roles of lipid rafts in membrane transport. *Curr. Opin. Cell Biol.* **13:** 470–477.

13. Nichols, B.J. & J. Lippincott-Schwartz. 2001. Endocytosis without clathrin coats. *Trends Cell Biol.* **11:** 406–412.

14. Nichols, B.J. 2002. A distinct class of endosome mediates clathrin-independent endocytosis to the Golgi complex. *Nat. Cell Biol.* **4:** 374–378.

15. Lamaze, C. *et al.* 2001. Interleukin 2 receptors and detergent-resistant membrane domains define a clathrin-independent endocytic pathway. *Mol. Cell* **7:** 661–671.

16. van der Luit, A.H. *et al.* 2002. Alkyl-lysophospholipid accumulates in lipid rafts and induces apoptosis via raft-dependent endocytosis and inhibition of phosphatidylcholine synthesis. *J. Biol. Chem.* **277:** 39541–39547.

17. Yang, H.L. *et al.* 2009. Caveolin-1 enhances resveratrol-mediated cytotoxicity and transport in a hepatocellular carcinoma model. *J. Transl. Med.* **7:** 22.

18. Lajoie, P. & I.R. Nabi. 2010. Lipid rafts, caveolae, and their endocytosis. *Int. Rev. Cell Mol. Biol.* **282:** 135–163.

19. Lin, H.Y. *et al.* 2006. Integrin alphaVbeta3 contains a receptor site for resveratrol. *FASEB J.* **20:** 1742–1744.

20. Bergh, J.J. *et al.* 2005. Integrin alphaVbeta3 contains a cell surface receptor site for thyroid hormone that is linked to activation of mitogen-activated protein kinase and induction of angiogenesis. *Endocrinology* **146:** 2864–2871.

21. Lin, H.Y. *et al.* 2008. Resveratrol is pro-apoptotic and thyroid hormone is anti-apoptotic in glioma cells: both actions are integrin and ERK mediated. *Carcinogenesis* **29:** 62–69.

22. Baillat, G. *et al.* 2008. Early adhesion induces interaction of FAK and Fyn in lipid domains and activates raft-dependent Akt signaling in SW480 colon cancer cells. *Biochim. Biophys. Acta.* **1783:** 2323–2331.

23. Wary, K.K. *et al.* 1998. A requirement for caveolin-1 and associated kinase Fyn in integrin signaling and anchorage-dependent cell growth. *Cell* **94:** 625–634.

24. Hsieh, T.C. *et al.* 2011. Regulation of p53 and cell proliferation by resveratrol and its derivatives in breast cancer cells: an *in silico* and biochemical approach targeting integrin αvβ3. *Int. J. Cancer* **129:** 2732–2743.

25. Gajate, C. & F. Mollinedo. 2001. The antitumor ether lipid ET-18-OCH(3) induces apoptosis through translocation and capping of Fas/CD95 into membrane rafts in human leukemic cells. *Blood* **98:** 3860–3863.

26. Delmas, D. *et al.* 2003. Resveratrol-induced apoptosis is associated with Fas redistribution in the rafts and the formation of a death-inducing signaling complex in colon cancer cells. *J. Biol. Chem.* **278:** 41482–41490.

27. Krammer, P.H. 1999. CD95(APO-1/Fas)-mediated apoptosis: live and let die. *Adv. Immunol.* **71:** 163–210.

28. Smith, C.A., T. Farrah & R.G. Goodwin. 1994. The TNF receptor superfamily of cellular and viral proteins: activation, costimulation, and death. *Cell* **76:** 959–962.

29. Jiang, S. *et al.* 1999. Apoptosis in human hepatoma cell lines by chemotherapeutic drugs via Fas-dependent and Fas-independent pathways. *Hepatology* **29:** 101–110.

30. Clement, M.V. *et al.* 1998. Chemopreventive agent resveratrol, a natural product derived from grapes, triggers CD95 signaling-dependent apoptosis in human tumor cells. *Blood* **92:** 996–1002.

31. Bernhard, D. *et al.* 2000. Resveratrol causes arrest in the S-phase prior to Fas-independent apoptosis in CEM-C7H2 acute leukemia cells. *Cell Death Differ.* **7:** 834–842.

32. Dorrie, J. *et al.* 2001. Resveratrol induces extensive apoptosis by depolarizing mitochondrial membranes and activating caspase-9 in acute lymphoblastic leukemia cells. *Cancer Res.* **61:** 4731–4739.

33. Tinhofer, I. *et al.* 2001. Resveratrol, a tumor-suppressive compound from grapes, induces apoptosis via a novel mitochondrial pathway controlled by Bcl-2. *FASEB J.* **15:** 1613–1615.

34. Micheau, O. *et al.* 1999. Fas ligand-independent, FADD-mediated activation of the Fas death pathway by anticancer drugs. *J. Biol. Chem.* **274:** 7987–7992.

35. Hueber, A.O. *et al.* 2002. An essential role for membrane rafts in the initiation of Fas/CD95-triggered cell death in mouse thymocytes. *EMBO Rep.* **3:** 190–196.

36. Reis-Sobreiro, M., C. Gajate & F. Mollinedo. 2009. Involvement of mitochondria and recruitment of Fas/CD95 signaling in lipid rafts in resveratrol-mediated antimyeloma and antileukemia actions. *Oncogene* **28:** 3221–3234.

37. Grassme, H. *et al.* 2001. CD95 signaling via ceramide-rich membrane rafts. *J. Biol. Chem.* **276:** 20589–20596.

38. Delmas, D. *et al.* 2004. Redistribution of CD95, DR4 and DR5 in rafts accounts for the synergistic toxicity of resveratrol and death receptor ligands in colon carcinoma cells. *Oncogene* **23:** 8979–8986.

39. Ghetie, M.A. *et al.* 2006. Rituximab but not other anti-CD20 antibodies reverses multidrug resistance in 2 B lymphoma cell lines, blocks the activity of P-glycoprotein (P-gp), and induces P-gp to translocate out of lipid rafts. *J. Immunother.* **29:** 536–544.

40. Pohland, T. *et al.* 2006. Bax and Bak are the critical complementary effectors of colorectal cancer cell apoptosis by chemopreventive resveratrol. *Anticancer Drugs* **17:** 471–478.

41. Belleri, M. *et al.* 2008. alphavbeta3 Integrin-dependent antiangiogenic activity of resveratrol stereoisomers. *Mol. Cancer Ther.* **7:** 3761–3770.

42. Desgrosellier, J.S. & D.A. Cheresh. Integrins in cancer: biological implications and therapeutic opportunities. *Nat. Rev. Cancer* **10:** 9–22.

43. Brittes, J. *et al.* 2010. Effects of resveratrol on membrane biophysical properties: relevance for its pharmacological effects. *Chem. Phys. Lipids* **163:** 747–754.

44. Tsuchiya, H. *et al.* 2002. Membrane-rigidifying effects of anti-cancer dietary factors. *Biofactors* **16:** 45–56.

45. Murphy, D.A. & S.A. Courtneidge. 2011. The 'ins' and 'outs' of podosomes and invadopodia: characteristics, formation and function. *Nat. Rev. Mol. Cell Biol.* **12:** 413–426.

46. Aires, V. *et al.* 2013. Resveratrol metabolites inhibit human metastatic colon cancer cells progression and synergize with chemotherapeutic drugs to induce cell death. *Mol. Nutr. Food Res.* Mar 14. doi: 10.1002/mnfr.201200766. [Epub ahead of print].

Ann. N.Y. Acad. Sci. ISSN 0077-8923

Interplay between metabolism and transport of resveratrol

Alexandra Maier-Salamon,[1] Michaela Böhmdorfer,[1] Juliane Riha,[1] Theresia Thalhammer,[2] Thomas Szekeres,[3] and Walter Jaeger[1]

[1]Department of Clinical Pharmacy and Diagnostics, University of Vienna, Vienna, Austria. [2]Department of Pathophysiology and Allergy Research, Center for Pathophysiology, Medical University of Vienna, Vienna, Austria. [3]Clinical Institute for Medical and Chemical Laboratory Diagnostics, Medical University of Vienna, Vienna, Austria

Address for correspondence: Walter Jaeger, Ph.D., Department of Clinical Pharmacy and Diagnostics, University of Vienna, A-1090 Vienna, Austria. walter.jaeger@univie.ac.at

Resveratrol exhibits a variety of biological and pharmacological activities despite its extensive metabolism to sulfates and glucuronides in the intestine and liver. The metabolism of resveratrol is cell specific and strongly correlates with enzyme expression levels. However, a high rate of biotransformation, in concert with the action of the efflux transporters MRP2, MRP3, and ABCG2, reduces intracellular resveratrol concentrations, and may thereby decrease its pharmacological activity. Interestingly, biotransformation is also dependent on disease status. For example, significantly greater sulfation of resveratrol occurs in human breast tumor tissue than in adjacent nonmalignant tissue. The observed differences, however, do not correlate with the expression of sulfotransferases responsible for catalyzing resveratrol sulfation, but rather with significantly higher steroid sulfatase mRNA levels. The *in vitro* activity of resveratrol sulfates may not necessarily reflect their *in vivo* function, given the fact that ubiquitously existing human sulfatases can convert the metabolites back to active resveratrol in humans.

Keywords: resveratrol; metabolism; ABC-transporter; sulfatases

Introduction

Resveratrol (*trans*-3,4′,5-trihydroxystilbene) is a natural compound produced by more than 70 plant species, with high amounts found in grapes, berries, peanuts, and red wine. In several *in vitro* and animal models, resveratrol has been found to be active in the prevention and treatment of cancer, cardiovascular diseases, inflammation, ischemic injuries, and neurodegenerative diseases; it may also act as an antiobesity and antiaging compound. However, confirmation of these benefits in humans through randomized clinical trials has been limited, and results are moderate. One-year daily intake of resveratrol-enriched (8 mg) grape extract in hypertensive male patients with type 2 diabetes mellitus downregulated (up to 20% compared to the placebo group) the expression of the key proinflammatory cytokines CCL3, IL-1β, and TNF-α in peripheral blood mononuclear cells, but did not affect body weight, blood pressure, glucose, HbA1c, or lipids.[1] For short-term intervention studies in patients (up to one month), however, much higher resveratrol doses are necessary in order to demonstrate any pharmacological activities. Patel and coworkers demonstrated a reduced cell proliferation (5%) in tumor samples of colorectal cancer patients who consumed eight daily doses of resveratrol at 0.5 or 1.0 g for 29 days before surgical resection, indicating that resveratrol may act as a potential chemopreventive agent.[2] A recent study further investigated the anticancer activity of resveratrol in patients with chronic lymphatic leukemia. Blood samples were drawn before and four weeks after consuming resveratrol (5 g/day). Resveratrol slightly decreased *O*-linked β-*N*-acetylglucosamine protein levels in primary leukemia cells, a marker for tumor progression, resulting in reduced levels of white blood cells.[3] The moderate pharmacological effects of resveratrol in humans even at high doses may be explained by its low bioavailability following extensive intestinal and hepatic metabolism, which results in resveratrol concentrations far below the levels that have

doi: 10.1111/nyas.12198

Ann. N.Y. Acad. Sci. 1290 (2013) 98–106 © 2013 New York Academy of Sciences.

demonstrated efficacy in *in vitro* models. This discrepancy has not yet been resolved. The present review will therefore discuss the interplay between metabolism and cellular transport mechanisms as a primary factor explaining the *in vivo* activity of resveratrol.

Adverse effects of resveratrol

No adverse effects were observed in humans receiving resveratrol as a single agent at a low dose (<100 mg) in short-term and long-term (up to one year) studies. However, some side effects of resveratrol have been reported in short-term studies at doses of 1 or 1.5 g/day including mild gastrointestinal symptoms, diarrhea, and hot flashes. At and above 2.5 g/day, additional side effects include heartburn, nausea, vomiting, and abdominal pain. After administration of 5 g of a proprietary formulation containing microparticular resveratrol, renal toxicity was observed in multiple myeloma patients but not in healthy controls. There are also some literature data supporting possible resveratrol–drug interactions. In a healthy volunteer study, resveratrol (1 g/day) was shown to inhibit the cytochrome P450 isoforms CYP2C9, CYP2D6, and CYP3A4, potentially leading to increased adverse drug reactions of coadministered CYP substrates.[4] Recent *in vitro* and animal studies also showed that resveratrol enhances testosterone levels in rabbits and inhibits estradiol (E2), indicating that resveratrol may alter the homeostasis of endogenous hormones.[5,6]

Metabolism in humans and animals

The biotransformation of resveratrol is a complex process. In humans, resveratrol-3-*O*-glucuronide, resveratrol-3-*O*-sulfate, and resveratrol-4′-*O*-glucuronide are the most abundant conjugation products. In addition to these main mono-conjugates, various studies have also reported several isomers of mono- and di-conjugates.[7,8] Gut microbial metabolism of resveratrol has also been observed, resulting in the presence of dihydroresveratrol and its glucuronides and sulfates.[9] Besides these well-known metabolites, two novel resveratrol-*C/O*-conjugated diglucuronides have also been identified and quantified in plasma and urine after administration of piceid (resveratrol-3-*O*-β-D-glycoside) to healthy volunteers.[7] The degrees of glucuronidation and sulfation of resveratrol in humans, however, vary up to several fold,

possibly based on polymorphic isoforms of sulfotransferase SULT1A1 and glucuronosyltransferase UGT1A1.

The variability increases when high doses of resveratrol are administered. In a repeat-dosing study using 0.5–5 g/day of resveratrol for 29 days, the maximal plasma concentration of the resveratrol 3-*O*-glucuronide was slightly below the concentration of resveratrol-3-*O*-sulfate for low doses, whereas glucuronidation prevailed when the dose was above 2.5 g.[10] These data are in accordance with our own findings, and we have also observed that the metabolism of resveratrol strongly depends on the applied dose in human Caco-2 cells.[11] As shown in Figure 1, the amount of resveratrol that is transported across the epithelium is strongly dependent on its biotransformation. When 10 μM resveratrol was applied apically to Caco-2 cells, an *in vitro* model of the human intestinal barrier, 84% of the initial dose was metabolized, whereas only 7.6% passed the monolayer intact. Due to the observed resveratrol-3-*O*-sulfate inhibition and the saturation of the glucuronidation pathways to produce resveratrol-3-*O*-glucuronide and resveratrol-4′-glucuronide, the total amount of metabolites decreased to 7.6% when

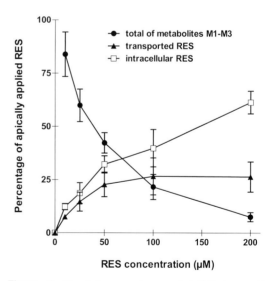

Figure 1. The influence of resveratrol-4′-*O*-glucuronide (metabolite M1), resveratrol-3-*O*-glucuronide (metabolite M2), and resveratrol-3-*O*-sulfate (metabolite M3) formation on trans-epithelial transport and intracellular accumulation of unconjugated resveratrol (RES). The data were calculated based on the percentage of the apically applied resveratrol concentration and are presented as mean ± SD (*n* = 3–6 monolayers). Data are from Ref. 11.

Table 1. Biological activities of resveratrol sulfates

Assay	Resveratrol	3-O-sulfate	4'-O-sulfate	3-O-4'-O-disulfate	3-O-5-O-disulfate
Inhibition of NF-κB	75.7 ± 2.12^a	33.0 ± 4.81^a	64.0 ± 2.26^a	53.4 ± 2.90^a	42.5 ± 4.81^a
Inhibition of COX-1	75.2 ± 4.53^a	74.3 ± 0.99^a	63.2 ± 3.39^a	23.3 ± 0.98^a	30.9 ± 2.69^a
	6.25 ± 2.50^d	3.60 ± 0.80^d	5.55 ± 1.73^d	–	–
Inhibition of COX-2	72.2 ± 4.67^a	62.0 ± 1.70^a	65.8 ± 7.64^a	16.5 ± 2.69^a	25.5 ± 5.52^a
	0.75 ± 0.52^d	7.53 ± 4.70^d	8.95 ± 1.20^d	–	–
Inhibition of NO production	71.8 ± 3.50^a	41.0 ± 0.70^a	56.8 ± 5.90^a	41.7 ± 5.50^a	4.80 ± 4.50^a
Inhibition of aromatase	34.8 ± 1.21^a	28.2 ± 1.12^a	30.4 ± 0.56^a	22.5 ± 0.64^a	20.50 ± 0.43^a
Inhibition of DPPH	65.2 ± 2.00^b	68.0 ± 1.90^b	42.8 ± 2.50^b	6.80 ± 1.00^b	14.5 ± 4.20^b
Induction of QR1	21 ± 0.46^c	2.60 ± 0.38^c	$>6.90^c$	$>10.1^c$	$>10.1^c$
Activation of SIRT1	32.2 ± 3.40^e	52.6 ± 6.60^e	36.4 ± 6.70^e	–	–
Inhibition of ROS	0.22^f	3.70^f	–	–	–

[a]Data shown as % inhibition determined at 34 μM.[13]
[b]Data shown as % inhibition determined at 340 μM.[13]
[c]Data shown as concentration to double the activity of QR1 (μM).[13]
[d]Data shown as IC_{50} (μM).[13]
[e]Data shown as K_a (μM).[14]
[f]Data shown as IC_{50} (mg/mL).[15]

200 μM resveratrol was applied to the apical side. In parallel, the total amount of unconjugated resveratrol transported from the apical chamber to the basolateral side increased to 26%. These values might be even higher considering the higher intracellular concentration of resveratrol, which accounted for 12% of total resveratrol at 10 μM and increased to 61% at 200 μM.

The metabolism of resveratrol also differs between humans and other animals. In a recent study using liver microsomes from humans, dogs, rats, and mice, we applied 100 μM resveratrol and found that rat and mouse liver microsomes had significantly higher glucuronidation activity levels than human and dog microsomes (90% of applied dose versus 65% of applied dose, respectively).[12] Distinct species-dependent differences also occurred in the stereo-selectivity of resveratrol glucuronidation. Although in human and dog liver microsomes, resveratrol-3-O-glucuronide and resveratrol-4'-O-glucuronide were generated at an average ratio of 5:1, the formation of resveratrol-4'-O-glucuronide in both rodent species was insignificant (45:1 in mouse; 50:1 in rat). Species-dependent differences were also observed in the kinetic profiles of resveratrol glucuronidation. In all of the species tested, only the formation of resveratrol-3-O-glucuronide and resveratrol-4'-O-glucuronide by dog microsomes showed a kinetic enzyme profile similar to human microsomes. Based on our results, we recommend the use of dogs rather than mice or rats as a model for resveratrol glucuronidation.

Pharmacological activity of metabolites

Currently, limited information is available regarding the possible benefits of resveratrol metabolites. Based on the current literature, sulfated conjugates are active, but it seems that their activity decreases as the degree of sulfation increases. As can be seen in Table 1, sulfated conjugates inhibit cyclooxygenase 1 and 2 (COX-1/2), α-induced NF-κB activity, aromatase, nitric oxide (NO) production, 2,2-diphenyl-1-picryl-hydrazyl (DPPH), and reactive oxygen species (ROS). Furthermore, resveratrol-3-O-sulfate mediates the induction of deacetylase sirtuin-1 (SIRT1) and quinone reductase 1 (QR1), but not quinine reductase 2 (QR2).[13–15] Interestingly, resveratrol-3-O-sulfate, in contrast to unconjugated resveratrol, was found to exert pronounced anti-estrogen activity in a yeast-hybrid system with a marked preference for the human estrogen receptors α and β.[16] Data concerning the biological activity of the resveratrol glucuronides are still scarce. Resveratrol-3-O-glucuronide exhibited only moderate inhibition of COX-1 and COX-2 (IC_{50} 150 ± 5.8 and >300 μM, respectively)[14] and was not

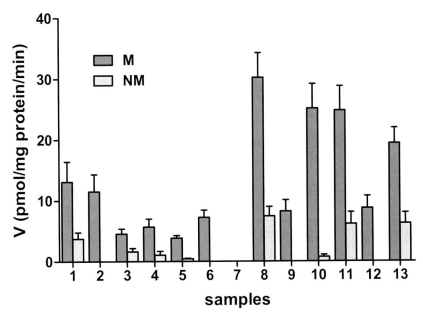

Figure 2. Formation rates of resveratrol-3-*O*-sulfate in human malignant (M) and nonmalignant (NM) breast cancer tissue samples at 1 μM resveratrol. The data represent the mean ± SD of triplicate determinations. Data are from Ref. 20.

found to possess anti-estrogen activity.[16] Recently, resveratrol-3-*O*-glucuronide and resveratrol-4′-*O*-glucuronide were found to contribute to the antiobesity effect of resveratrol, as they induced delipidating effects in maturing preadipocytes and mature adipocytes comparable to the parent drug.[17] Although cytotoxicity of resveratrol-3-*O*-sulfate, resveratrol-4′-*O*-sulfate, and resveratrol 3-*O*-4′-disulfate against hormone-dependent (MCF-7 and MDA-MB-231) and hormone-independent (ZR-75-1) breast cancer cell lines was reduced approximately 10-fold,[18] resveratrol-3-*O*-sulfate, resveratrol-3-*O*-glucuronide, and resveratrol-4′-*O*-glucuronide strongly inhibited the cell growth of the colon cancer cell lines CCL-228, Caco-2, and HTC-116, with IC_{50} values of 10.1–31.0 μM comparable to the parent compound (9.8–23.8 μM).[19] Resveratrol metabolites are therefore likely to contribute to the various health benefits that have previously been attributed only to resveratrol.

Tissue-specific metabolism of resveratrol

Only a few research groups have studied the biotransformation of resveratrol in human tissue samples. A clinical trial in colorectal cancer patients who received 0.5 or 1.0 g of resveratrol caplets daily for eight consecutive days before resection identified six metabolites in the tissue, namely resveratrol-3-*O*-glucuronide, resveratrol-4′-*O*-glucuronide, resveratrol-3-*O*-sulfate, resveratrol-4′-*O*-sulfate, resveratrol-disulfate, and resveratrol sulfate glucuronide.[2] Interestingly, in contrast to the pattern in plasma of healthy volunteers, where the sulfate glucuronide is a minor biotransformation product or, more commonly, absent,[10] it was a predominant metabolite in tumor samples from 14 out of 20 patients.

In human breast cancer cell lines and tissue samples, however, only resveratrol-3-*O*-sulfate could be detected.[20] Notably, the formation of resveratrol-3-*O*-sulfate showed a high degree of interindividual variation (Fig. 2). Resveratrol sulfation was significantly higher in 12 of 13 breast cancer tissue samples; these samples showed up to 33.5-fold higher formation rates compared with their nontumor counterparts. More significantly, the formation of resveratrol-3-*O*-sulfate was below the detection limit in 5 of the 13 corresponding tissue specimens. Uptake of dietary resveratrol in patients with little or no detectable metabolism may have increased the resveratrol concentrations in breast tumor tissues. The higher formation rates of resveratrol-3-*O*-sulfate in the tumor tissue samples led to the hypothesis that resveratrol metabolism may correlate with tissue expression of the sulfo-transferases SULT1A1, SULT1A2, SULT1A3, and SULT1E1 isoenzymes, which have been previously shown in our laboratory to catalyze resveratrol sulfation. The observed differences in resveratrol sulfation between tumor and adjacent control tissue samples, however, did not correlate with the mRNA expression levels of SULT1A2, SULT1A3, and SULT1E1. Because resveratrol sulfate may be readily hydrolyzed in tissue samples by members of the sulfatase family to regenerate the parent resveratrol, we also investigated the mRNA expression levels of arylsulfatase A (ARS-A), arylsulfatase B (ARS-B), and steroid sulfatase (STS). Using quantitative real-time reverse transcription polymerase chain reaction (RT-PCR), our studies showed significantly higher STS but not ARS-A or ARS-B mRNA levels in normal breast tissue. Notably, the level of STS mRNA expression was significantly higher in 12 of the 13 nonmalignant specimens compared to their corresponding tumor tissue samples, which could potentially explain the higher resveratrol sulfate concentrations that were observed in the breast cancer samples compared to the control breast tissue specimens. These data were confirmed by immunofluorescence staining of paraffin-embedded tissue sections of selected patients who also demonstrated more prominent localization of STS in the adjacent normal tissue.

Besides breast tissue, selective metabolism of resveratrol to resveratrol-3-*O*-sulfate also occurs in the brain, as demonstrated in the human medulloblastoma cell lines U251 and LN229.[21] The analysis of resveratrol metabolites in all target tissues is essential to better predict efficacy in clinical and epidemiological studies.

Tissue levels of resveratrol and its metabolites

Because of extensive glucuronidation and sulfation, tissue concentration of resveratrol was found to be very low or undetectable whereas maximum mean tissue concentrations of metabolites were often several-fold higher. Administration of resveratrol (1.0 g/day) for up to 29 days to patients with colorectal cancer, however, showed mean resveratrol concentrations of 674 nmoles/g in normal tissue and 94 nmoles/g in cancer specimens, respectively. Maximal mean tissue concentrations determined for resveratrol metabolites were 86 nmoles/g for resveratrol-3-*O*-glucuronide and 67 nmoles/g for resveratrol-3-*O*-sulfate.[2] These high concentrations in colorectal tissues are in excess of that required for activity *in vitro*, indicating that the colon is the preferable target organ for resveratrol. In contrast, resveratrol was detected at much lower concentrations (10.1 nmoles/g) in hepatic metastasis after oral administration (5 g/day) for up to 21 days in stage IV colorectal cancer patients.[22] Low liver levels might be explained by data from a recent pig study. Six hours after oral administration of resveratrol (6.25 mg/kg) to pigs (body weight: 80 ± 8 kg), more than 65% of the initial dose was found as resveratrol-derived metabolites (mainly as resveratrol 3-*O*-glucuronide and resveratrol-3-*O*-sulfate) in the gastrointestinal tract, 7.7% in the urine, and 1.2% in the bile. Only 0.5% of the administered dose was found in the brain, heart, lungs, kidneys, liver, pancreas, spleen, aorta tissue, urinary bladder tissue, ovaries, and uterus, strongly indicating that lack of absorption is still the main reason for insufficient resveratrol tissue levels.[23]

Cellular transport mechanisms for resveratrol and its conjugates

ATP-binding cassette (ABC) transporters are primary determinants for drug concentrations in blood and target organs, thereby strongly affecting drug response. The members relevant for drug disposition are P-glycoprotein (P-gp), the breast cancer resistance protein (BCRP; ABCG2), and the multidrug resistance-associated proteins MRP2 and MRP3. P-gp, BCRP, and MRP2 can be detected in various organs but are highly expressed in the apical membrane of villus tip enterocytes, where they facilitate the efflux of compounds back to the intestinal lumen, thus limiting oral absorption. In the gut, MRP3 is localized to the basolateral membrane and functions as a substrate pump from the intracellular compartment to the blood.

Some members of the ABC family were also involved in the secretion of resveratrol conjugates resulting from rapid intracellular metabolism. An *in vitro* study conducted in our lab using perfused isolated livers from Mrp2-competent Wistar and *Mrp2* mutant TR⁻ rats showed that the substrate specificity of resveratrol glucuronides for MRP2 was far higher than for unconjugated resveratrol (Fig. 3).[24] Although the cumulative biliary excretion

Ann. N.Y. Acad. Sci. 1290 (2013) 98–106 © 2013 New York Academy of Sciences.

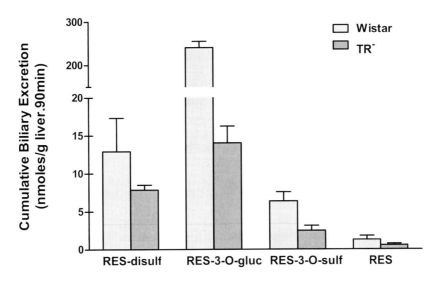

Figure 3. Cumulative biliary excretion of resveratrol-3-O-4′-disulfate (RES-disulf), resveratrol-3-O-glucuronide (RES-3-O-gluc), resveratrol-3-O-sulfate (RES-3-O-sulf), and resveratrol (RES) in control Wistar rats and mutant TR⁻ rats. The data are expressed as nmoles/g liver.90 min ± SD ($n = 3$). Data are from Ref. 24.

of resveratrol-3-O-4′-O-disulfate (M1), resveratrol-3-O-sulfate (M3), and parent resveratrol (RES) only decreased by 39%, 61%, and 56%, respectively, biliary excretion of 3-O-gucuronide (M2) dropped dramatically to 6%. Interestingly, biliary excretion of three sulfate-glucuronides was also dramatically impaired in TR⁻ rats, to amounts almost below detection limit. This finding indicates that Mrp2 almost exclusively mediates the biliary excretion of resveratrol glucuronides and sulfate-glucuronides in the rat liver but only partly mediates the biliary excretion of sulfates and of parent resveratrol. A candidate for the transport of unconjugated resveratrol and resveratrol sulfates is the BCRP (ABCG2), which plays an important role in the biliary excretion of the sulfated conjugates of steroids and various drugs. Two studies indeed demonstrated by *in vitro* and *in vivo* experiments that BCRP transports resveratrol-3-O-sulfate and, to a lesser extent, resveratrol-3-O-glucuronide.[25,26] Furthermore, they also found that MRP3 (ABCC3) transports resveratrol-3-O-glucuronide, indicating overlap in the substrate spectra of BCRP, MRP2, and MRP3.[26]

Although the biological effects of resveratrol are well described, little is known about the uptake of resveratrol and its metabolites. To quantify the cellular uptake of resveratrol in the intestine, we used Caco-2 cells as an *in vitro* model of the human intestinal barrier.[11] Based on the high and rapid permeability through Caco-2 monolayers, we conclude that passive diffusion was the major transport mechanism for unconjugated resveratrol because the transport rates were directly proportional to the amount of resveratrol applied and because the resveratrol permeability was significantly higher at 37 °C compared to 4 °C, when energy consumption is minimal. However, passive diffusion does not explain the accumulation of resveratrol to bioactive levels in targeted organs. After intravenous application of resveratrol to mice and rats, resveratrol distributes into various organs such as the liver, kidney, lungs, and spleen, whereas moderate concentrations are found in heart, testes, and brain.[27,28] Furthermore, in all of the organs analyzed, conjugated metabolites were detected at concentrations that were higher than the concentrations of the parent resveratrol, which strongly indicated active uptake transport mechanisms. This is consistent with a study by Patel *et al.*, which showed that patients with confirmed colorectal cancer who received 0.5 or 1 g of resveratrol daily for eight days before surgery could achieve resveratrol levels in the cancer tissue that were sufficient to exert antitumor activity.[2] Further studies are highly warranted to elucidate the importance of these transporters on the pharmacokinetics of resveratrol and its metabolites in humans.

Interplay between metabolism and transport

The existence of ABC transporters is not limited to the intestine and liver. On the contrary, these proteins are also found in many other tissues like the kidneys, thus affecting the distribution of many bioactive compounds. The absence of Mrp3 or Bcrp1 therefore has pronounced effects on the disposition of resveratrol *in vivo*. Mice lacking Mrp3 have substantially reduced plasma and urine levels of unmodified resveratrol and resveratrol-3-*O*-glucuronide compared with control mice after administration of parent resveratrol by gavage feeding.[26] Because resveratrol is extensively glucuronidated in the gut, the decreased plasma resveratrol-3-*O*-glucuronide level results from the absence of Mrp3 in the basolateral membrane of the enterocytes. The absence of Bcrp1, which is normally located in the apical membrane of enterocytes, leads to elevated plasma levels of all resveratrol metabolites in *Bcrp1*$^{-/-}$ mice, with the most pronounced effect on resveratrol disulfate.[26]

As both transporters are also expressed in humans, decreased expression may result in an altered tissue distribution and elimination of resveratrol from the body. Alfaras and coworkers showed a dramatic increase of resveratrol bioavailability in *Bcrp1*$^{-/-}$ mice.[29] After oral administration of 60 mg/kg resveratrol, the intestinal contents of resveratrol-3-*O*-glucuronide and resveratrol-3-*O*-sulfate decreased by 71% and 97%, respectively, indicating a lower efflux from the enterocytes.

Furthermore, the area under plasma concentration curves (AUC) for the resveratrol-3-*O*-glucuronide increased by 34%, whereas the area for resveratrol-3-*O*-sulfate increased by 392%, supporting the important role of Bcrp1 in the efflux and tissue distribution of resveratrol conjugates. The concentrations of resveratrol, resveratrol-3-*O*-glucuronide, and resveratrol-3-*O*-sulfate were also examined in the liver, kidney, lung, heart, and brain of wild-type and *Bcrp1*$^{-/-}$ mice. *Bcrp1* knockout mice showed up to three- and six-fold higher resveratrol concentrations in the liver and kidney, respectively, whereas resveratrol-3-*O*-sulfate concentrations were up to 32-fold higher in the kidney. Resveratrol-3-*O*-sulfate content in the liver was 2.6-fold higher in wild-type than in *Bcrp1*$^{-/-}$ mice. No differences in the concentrations of resveratrol, 3-*O*-glucuronide, and resveratrol-3-*O*-sulfate between wild-type and *Bcrp1* knockout mice were seen in the heart and brain.

As phase II metabolism, in concert with MRP2 and BCRP, has a major effect on oral bioavailability of resveratrol, novel formulations combining resveratrol with potent but nontoxic natural inhibitors of glucuronidation, sulfation, and efflux transporters are very likely to increase intestinal absorption, consequently leading to higher blood and tissue levels. A recent study by Fong and coworkers suggested that epicatechin, piperine, and curcumin are able to inhibit glucuronidation and sulfation in rat intestinal S9 fraction and Caco2 cell lysate.[30] As quercetin and curcumin are also known to inhibit MRP2 and

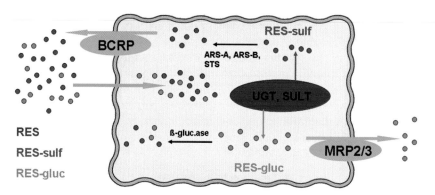

Figure 4. Interplay between cellular uptake, efflux, and metabolism of resveratrol. BCRP, breast cancer resistance protein; UGT, UDP-glucuronosyltransferase; SULT, sulfotransferase; MRP2/3, multidrug resistance proteins 2 and 3; RES-gluc, resveratrol glucuronides; RES-sulf, resveratrol sulfates; ARS-A, arylsulfatase A; ARS-B, arylsulfatase B; STS, steroid sulfatase; β-gluc.ase, β-glucuronidase.

BCRP, respectively, both compounds might be good candidates to enhance resveratrol bioavailability.

Conclusion

The so-called resveratrol paradox, that is, the relationship between resveratrol's very low bioavailability, based on its extensive metabolism, and its high bioactivity, has not yet been explained, and factors responsible for the exerted effects have not yet been identified. This review provides some strong evidence that the deconjugation of resveratrol metabolites to the pharmacologically active parent compound, in concert with the activity of efflux transporters, is at least one of the key factors that explain the observed pharmacological activities (Fig. 4). Future *in vivo* studies should therefore focus on the concentrations of resveratrol and its conjugates in target tissues, which would finally lead to better interpretations of the results obtained from clinical and epidemiological studies. In parallel, the expression levels of the various efflux and putative unknown uptake transporters and resveratrol-metabolizing enzymes, including glucuronosyltransferases and sulfotransferases but also the deconjugation enzymes β-glucuronidase and the various sulfatases, should be determined. Furthermore, possible food and drug interactions that could strongly alter the pharmacokinetics and efficacy of resveratrol metabolism have to be considered. Long-term *in vivo* studies are therefore highly warranted to determine the preventive and therapeutic efficacy of resveratrol as a dietary supplement.

Conflicts of interest

The authors declare no conflicts of interest.

References

1. Tome-Carneiro, J., M. Larrosa, M.J. Yanez-Gascon, *et al.* 2013. One-year supplementation with a grape extract containing resveratrol modulates inflammatory-related microRNAs and cytokines expression in peripheral blood mononuclear cells of type 2 diabetes and hypertensive patients with coronary artery disease. *Pharmacol. Res.* **72:** 69–82.
2. Patel, K.R., V.A. Brown, D.J. Jones, *et al.* 2010. Clinical pharmacology of resveratrol and its metabolites in colorectal cancer patients. *Cancer Res.* **70:** 7392–7399.
3. Tomic, J., L. McCaw, Y. Li, *et al.* 2013. Resveratrol has anti-leukemic activity associated with decreased O-Glcnated poteins. *Exp. Hematol.* Epub ahead of print in press.
4. Chow, H.H., L.L. Garland, C.H. Hsu, *et al.* 2010. Resveratrol modulates drug- and carcinogen-metabolizing enzymes in a healthy volunteer study. *Cancer Prev. Res.* **3:** 1168–1175.
5. Shin, S., J.H. Jeon, D. Park, *et al.* 2008. Trans-resveratrol relaxes the corpus cavernosum ex vivo and enhances testosterone levels and sperm quality in vivo. *Arch. Pharm. Res.* **31:** 83–87.
6. Ung, D. & S. Nagar. 2009. Trans-resveratrol-mediated inhibition of beta-oestradiol conjugation in MCF-7 cells stably expressing human sulfotransferases SULT1A1 or SULT2E1, and human liver microsomes. *Xenobiotica* **39:** 72–79.
7. Boocock, D.J., G.E. Faust, K.R. Patel, *et al.* 2007. Phase I dose escalation pharmacokinetic study in healthy volunteers of resveratrol, a potential cancer chemopreventive agent. *Cancer Epidemiol. Biomarkers Prev.* **16:** 1246–1252.
8. Burkon, A. & V. Somoza. 2008. Quantification of free and protein-bound trans-resveratrol metabolites and identification of trans-resveratrol-C/O-conjugated diglucuronides: two novel resveratrol metabolites in human plasma. *Mol. Nutr. Food Res.* **52:** 549–557.
9. Rotches-Ribalta, M., M. Urpi-Sarda, R. Llorach, *et al.* 2012. Gut and microbial resveratrol metabolite profiling after moderate long-term consumption of red wine versus dealcoholized red wine in humans by an optimized ultra-high-pressure liquid chromatography tandem mass spectrometry method. *J. Chromatogr. A* **1265:** 105–113.
10. Brown, V.A., K.R. Patel, M. Viskaduraki, *et al.* 2010. Repeat dose study of the cancer chemopreventive agent resveratrol in healthy volunteers: safety, pharmacokinetics, and effect on the insulin-like growth factor axis. *Cancer Res.* **70:** 9003–9011.
11. Maier-Salamon, A., B. Hagenauer, M. Wirth, *et al.* 2006. Increased transport of resveratrol across monolayers of the human intestinal Caco-2 cells is mediated by inhibition and saturation of metabolites. *Pharm. Res.* **23:** 2107–2115.
12. Maier-Salamon, A., M. Böhmdorfer, T. Thalhammer, *et al.* 2011. Hepatic glucuronidation of resveratrol: interspecies comparison of enzyme kinetic profiles in humans, mouse, rat and dog. *Drug Metab. Phamacokinet.* **26:** 364–373.
13. Hoshino, J., E.J. Park, T.P. Kondratyuk, *et al.* 2010. Selective synthesis and biological evaluation of sulfate-conjugated resveratrol metabolites. *J. Med. Chem.* **53:** 5033–5043.
14. Calamini, B., K. Ratia, M.G. Malkowski, *et al.* 2010. Pleiotropic mechanisms facilitated by resveratrol and its metabolites. *Biochem. J.* **429:** 273–282.
15. Herath, W., S.I. Khan & I.A. Khan. 2012. Microbial metabolism. Part 14. Isolation and bioactivity evaluation of microbial metabolites of resveratrol. *Nat. Prod. Res.* 1–8, iFirst.
16. Ruotolo, R., L. Calani, E. Fietta, *et al.* 2013. Anti-estrogenic activity of a human resveratrol metabolite. *Nutr. Metab. Cardiovasc.* Epub ahead of print in press.
17. Lasa, A., I. Churruca, I. Eseberri, *et al.* 2012. Delipidating effect of resveratrol metabolites in 3T3-L1 adipocytes. *Mol. Nutr. Food Res.* **56:** 1559–1568.

18. Miksits, M., K. Wlcek, M. Svoboda, *et al.* 2009. Antitumor activity of resveratrol and its sulfated metabolites against human breast cancer cells. *Planta Med.* **75:** 1–4.

19. Polycarpou, E., L.B. Meira, S. Carrington, *et al.* 2013. Resveratrol 3-O-d-glucuronide and resveratrol 4′-O-d-glucuronide inhibit colon cancer cell growth: evidence for a role of A3 adenosine receptors, cyclin D1 depletion, and G1 cell cycle arrest. *Mol. Nutr. Food Res.* Epub ahead of print in press.

20. Miksits, M., K. Wlcek, M. Svoboda, *et al.* 2010. Expression of sulfotransferases and sulfatases in human breast cancer: impact on resveratrol metabolism. *Cancer Lett.* **289:** 237–245.

21. Sun, Z., H. Li, X.H. Shu, *et al.* 2012. Distinct sulfonation activities in resveratrol-sensitive and resveratrol-insensitive human glioblastoma cells. *FEBS J.* **279:** 2381–2392.

22. Howell, L.M., D.P. Berry, P.J. Elliot, *et al.* 2011. Phase I randomized, double-blind pilot study of micronized resveratrol (SRT501) in patients with hepatic metastases-safety, pharmacokinetics, and pharmacodynamics. *Cancer Prev. Res.* **4:** 1419–1425.

23. Azorin-Ortuno, M., M.J. Yanez-Gascon, F. Vallejo, *et al.* 2011. Metabolites and tissue distribution of resveratrol in the pig. *Mol. Nutr. Food Res.* **55:** 1154–1168.

24. Maier-Salamon, A., B. Hagenauer, G. Reznicek, *et al.* 2009. Metabolism and disposition of resveratrol in the isolated perfused rat liver: role of Mrp2 in the biliary excretion of glucuronides. *J. Pharm. Sci.* **98:** 3839–3849.

25. Breedveld, P., D. Pluim, G. Cipriani, *et al.* 2007. The effect of low pH on breast cancer resistance protein (ABCG2)-mediated transport of methotrexate, 7-hydroxymethotrexate, methotrexate diglutamate, folic acid, mitoxantrone, topotecan, and resveratrol in *in vitro* drug transport models. *Mol. Pharmacol.* **71:** 240–249.

26. Van de Wetering, K., A. Burkon, W. Feddema, *et al.* 2009. Intestinal breast cancer resistance protein (BCRP)/Bcrp1 and multidrug resistance protein 3 (MRP3)/Mrp2 are involved in the pharmacokinetics of resveratrol. *Mol. Pharmacol.* **75:** 876–885.

27. Vitrac, X., A. Desmouliere, B. Brouillaud, *et al.* 2003. Distribution of [^{14}C]-trans-resveratrol, a cancer chemopreventive polyphenol, in mouse tissues after oral administration. *Life Sci.* **72:** 2219–2233.

28. Juan, M.E., M. Maijó & J.M. Planas. 2009. Quantification of trans-resveratrol and its metabolites in rat plasma and tissues by HPLC. *J. Pharm. Biomed. Anal.* **51:** 391–398.

29. Alfaras, I., M. Peruez, M.E. Juan, *et al.* 2010. Involvement of breast cancer resistance protein (BCRP1/ABCG2) in the bioavailability and tissue distribution of *trans*-resveratrol in knockout mice. *J. Agric. Food. Chem.* **58:** 4523–4528.

30. Fong, Y.K., C.R. Li, S.K. Wo, *et al.* 2012. In vitro and in situ evaluation of herb-drug interactions during intestinal metabolism and absorption of baicalein. *J. Ethnopharmacol.* **141:** 742–753.

Ann. N.Y. Acad. Sci. ISSN 0077-8923

ANNALS OF THE NEW YORK ACADEMY OF SCIENCES

Issue: *Resveratrol and Health*

Nano- and micro-encapsulated systems for enhancing the delivery of resveratrol

Mary Ann Augustin,[1] Luz Sanguansri,[1] and Trevor Lockett[2]

[1]CSIRO Preventative Health National Research Flagship and CSIRO Animal, Food and Health Sciences, Werribee, Victoria, Australia. [2]CSIRO Preventative Health National Research Flagship and CSIRO Animal, Food and Health Sciences, North Ryde, New South Wales, Australia

Address for correspondence: Mary Ann Augustin, CSIRO Animal, Food and Health Sciences, 671 Sneydes Road, Werribee, 3030 Victoria, Australia. maryann.augustin@csiro.au

There has been interest in the use of *trans*-resveratrol as a natural preventative agent for improving health and alleviating a range of diseases. However, resveratrol has low bioavailability, and this has been associated with its poor water solubility, its low stability against environmental stress, and its inability to reach a target site in the body to exert the desired health effect. Encapsulation offers a potential approach for enhancing the solubility of resveratrol, stabilizing it against *trans*-to-*cis* isomerization, and improving its bioavailability. A range of encapsulant materials, formulations, and technologies have been examined for enhancing the delivery of resveratrol. Research on the efficacy of encapsulated resveratrol formulations and relevant doses for specific applications is required before recommendations may be made for the use of these formulations for human health outcomes.

Keywords: resveratrol; encapsulation; delivery systems; stability; bioavailability

Introduction

Resveratrol (3,5,4′-trihydroxystilbene) is a phytoalexin present in natural food products such as grapes, wine, peanuts, and berries. It exists in *cis* and *trans* forms, with the *trans* form believed to be the biologically active form. In nature, it is often present as a piceid, a glucoside of *trans*-resveratrol (*trans*-resveratrol-3-*O*-β-glucoside). *Trans*-resveratrol has effects on many metabolic processes and has been suggested to modulate cardiovascular disease, inflammation, cancer, obesity, and diabetes.[1–3]

Resveratrol's low bioavailability, stemming from its low solubility in water, isomerization from the *trans* to the *cis* form in solution, and rapid clearance from the circulation, makes it difficult to maintain bioefficacious concentrations of resveratrol in the blood and target tissues of humans.[4,5] However, there is emerging evidence that biotransformation of resveratrol and other phenolic compounds by the colonic microbiota into bioactive metabolites plays an important role in the protective effects of polyphenols.[5,6]

Confronted with the problem of low oral bioavailability in a lead compound for a new drug, the pharmaceutical industry has a range of options available. These include considering whether the compound can be used as an injectable agent, application of medicinal chemistry to chemically modify the compound for improved bioavailability, formulating the compound into a modified chemical milieu that will promote its bioavailability, or a combination of these. These options are considered in the context that toxicology, human safety and efficacy studies, and regulatory approvals are all accepted parts of future drug development. A key aspect of the attraction of resveratrol as a therapeutic or chemopreventive agent is that it is a natural product with a history of being consumed by humans and has the regulatory status of being a compound that is generally recognized as safe (GRAS). To take best advantage of its GRAS status, the simplest and most cost-effective path to improving the bioavailability of resveratrol lies in the development of a delivery system that enhances its bioavailability but does not modify the compound chemically. This understanding

doi: 10.1111/nyas.12130

and the increasing evidence for a range of beneficial health properties of this bioactive stilbene underpin the increasing interest observed recently in the development of novel delivery systems for the administration of resveratrol.[7–9]

Opportunities for resveratrol delivery exist for both the pharmaceutical and food industries. It may be formulated as nutritional supplements. Alternatively, resveratrol may be carried or encapsulated by food components and/or compounds with GRAS status for incorporation into food products. We discuss the challenges in the delivery of resveratrol, with a focus on the use of carriers and novel nano- and micro-encapsulation systems to enhance the stability of resveratrol and its efficient release and uptake under *in vitro* and *in vivo* conditions.

Challenges in the delivery of phenolic bioactives

Many bioactives including phenolic compounds are unstable once they are isolated from their natural source and need to be protected from the environment and undesirable interactions with other components. They have a bitter taste, and masking the astringency of phenolic components is desirable when they are delivered orally. In addition, for a food bioactive to exert its desired physiological function, adequate concentrations of the bioactive must reach the target site in the body. However, the evidence for targeting polyphenols to a particular target tissue/cell for a specific health effect is not clear. Although circulatory levels of phenolic compounds such as resveratrol may be low after oral delivery, the influence of the gut microflora on the bioavailability of phenolic compounds should be considered. Phenolic compounds that are not taken up in the upper gastrointestinal tract are metabolized by colonic microflora into phenolic acids. Several recent reviews are available that discuss the properties of plant phenolics and their bioavailability.[10–12]

Encapsulation

Nano- and micro-encapsulation, which involve the packaging of components within a secondary material and delivering them in small particles in the nanometer to micrometer range, have the potential to enhance the delivery of bioactive compounds. Encapsulation stabilizes unstable bioactive compounds, protects them against undesirable interactions with the environment and other compo-

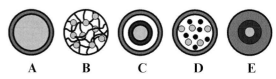

Figure 1. Morphologies of microcapsules: (A) single-core capsule, (B) dispersed core in polymer gel, (C) multilayer capsule, (D) dual-core capsule, and (E) single-core multishell capsule. Reproduced by permission of The Royal Society of Chemistry, Augustin and Hemar.[13]

nents, masks astringency tastes, and potentially targets and controls the release of the bioactive compound at a desired target tissue in the body. There are many ways of designing encapsulated formulations from systems based on the use of surfactants, lipids, biopolymers, or mixtures of these components. The designed delivery systems include simple or mixed micelles stabilized by surfactants, single bioactive cores in shell particles (e.g., emulsion droplet) or in a polymeric matrix (e.g., hydrogel and coacervates), soluble bioactive–biopolymer complexes, or the more sophisticated multiple-core and structured multilayer systems (Fig. 1). In developing a delivery system, it is essential to consider the end application and the limitations and benefits offered by encapsulation over the presentation of a neat bioactive.[13,14]

Why encapsulate resveratrol?

There are many reasons one might seek to encapsulate resveratrol. Through encapsulation, it is possible to increase resveratrol solubility in water and thereby also improve its bioavailability. Encapsulation may potentially be used to stabilize resveratrol against degradation and control its release when administered orally.[7–9] Designed oral nano- and micro-encapsulated delivery formulations containing resveratrol are an alternative to the delivery of resveratrol in tablets or hard gelatin capsules. When encapsulated with food-grade ingredients, there is the opportunity to present them in stable formats as over-the-counter nutraceutical preparations, as dietary supplements, and for incorporation into functional food products.

Delivery systems for resveratrol

A generalized approach that may be applied to designing oral formulations for stabilization, taste masking, and enhanced bioavailability of a bioactive is shown in Figure 2.[15] This approach is applicable

Ann. N.Y. Acad. Sci. 1290 (2013) 107–112 © 2013 New York Academy of Sciences.

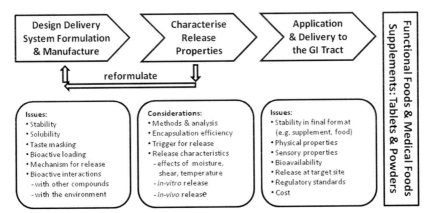

Figure 2. Generalized approach to designing formulations and processes for stabilization, taste masking, and enhanced bioavailability of a bioactive. GI tract = gastrointestinal tract. Adapted from Ref. 15.

to developing a delivery system for resveratrol. Delivery systems for resveratrol may be designed to improve resveratrol solubility, stabilize resveratrol against *trans–cis* isomerization, control its release in the gastrointestinal tract, and improve its bioavailability.

Liposomal delivery systems
Liposomes are small vesicles of amphiphilic lipids (e.g., phospholipids) that have been used by the pharmaceutical industry for carrying drugs and controlling their release at target sites in the body. Amphiphilic lipids have a bilayer membrane that encloses an aqueous core that can carry hydrophilic compounds, while lipophilic compounds can be carried within the hydrophobic region of the bilayer.

Entrapment of resveratrol in a liposomal formulation (comprising dipalmitoylphoshatidylcholine, poly(ethylene glycol)-2000-distearoylphosphatidyletanolamine, and cholesterol) has been shown to improve the solubility and the resistance of resveratrol to UV light–induced *trans–cis* isomerization.[16] Liposomal–resveratrol formulations were stable for up to three months at 4 °C. Liposomal preparations also increased resveratrol bioavailability: administration of a resveratrol–soy phosphatidylcholine complex to rats, via an enteral route, increased the levels of resveratrol in plasma and improved cardioprotective activity compared to free resveratrol administration,[17] and resveratrol entrapped in liposomes (made with enriched soy phosphatidylcholine) was superior to free resveratrol for protecting stressed cells in cell culture, and significantly increased antioxidative capability.[18]

Resveratrol–protein complexes
Proteins can serve as transporters for a number of components due to their affinity to form complexes with a variety of compounds. Various researchers have examined the interaction of resveratrol with a range of proteins and reported spontaneous resveratrol binding. Studies have shown that *trans*-resveratrol binds to bovine serum albumin ($K = 5 \times 10^4$ M^{-1})[19] and ($K = 2.5 \times 10^4$ M^{-1}),[20] collagen ($K = 5 \times 10^5$ M^{-1}),[21] fibrinogen ($K = 0.7 \times 10^4$ M^{-1}),[22] β-lactoglobulin ($K = 10^4$–10^6 M^{-1}),[23] and a range of dairy proteins (lactoferrin, hololactoferrin, apolactoferrin, whey protein isolate, and the β-lactoglobulin– and α-lactalbumin–rich fractions of whey protein isolate ($K = 1.7 \times 10^4$–1.2×10^5 M^{-1})).[24] Further, in the presence of proteins, resveratrol is more protected from *trans*-to-*cis* isomerization than when it is in the free form.[21–23] Binding of resveratrol to proteins sometimes results in a change in protein conformation, mainly in the vicinity of tryptophan residues.[22]

In more complex systems containing proteins and other components that have the ability to bind resveratrol, there can be competition for resveratrol binding. The relative affinities of resveratrol for various carriers will dictate the partitioning of resveratrol. For example, in the presence of protein (bovine serum albumin, BSA), resveratrol was extracted from the lipid bilayer and formed resveratrol–BSA complexes.[16]

Resveratrol–cyclodextrin complexes
Cyclodextrin forms complexes with resveratrol in aqueous solution. An inclusion complex is formed

where resveratrol is complexed within the hydrophobic inner cavity of cyclodextrin, forming a 1:1 complex.[25] Resveratrol is therefore protected from interacting with components in the outer aqueous environment. A complexation constant of 4,317 M^{-1} was obtained for the complex between β-cyclodextrin and resveratrol.[26] The delivery of resveratrol–cyclodextrin inclusion complexes increased the bioefficacy of resveratrol compared to delivery in its free form. For example, resveratrol solubilized by complexation with 2-hydroxyproply-β-cyclodextrin was found to be more effective than free resveratrol for preventing 7,12-dimetylbenz[a]anthrocence–induced hamster oral squamous cell carcinomas *in vitro*.[27] The improved effectiveness with the resveratrol–cyclodextrin formulation was also confirmed *in vivo* in a related hamster model.[27] An alternative method for delivery is the complexation of resveratrol with cyclodextrin-based nanosponges (nanostructured chemically hyper–cross-linked cyclodextrin), which not only stabilize resveratrol, but increase resveratrol accumulation in mucosa buccal cells (*ex vivo*) compared to free resveratrol.[28]

Solid lipid nanoparticles

Solid lipid nanoparticles comprise a solid lipid core and an amphiphilic surfactant shell. The type of lipid core and the surfactant, as well as the particle size and ζ-potential of the particle, has an influence on the properties of solid lipid nanoparticles as carriers of bioactives. The incorporation of resveratrol into solid lipid nanoparticles stabilizes resveratrol against photodegradation, and its stability is further enhanced when the solid lipid nanoparticles contain tetradecyl-γ-cyclodextrin.[29]

Studies have shown that solid lipid nanoparticles (<180 nm) are able to cross the cell membrane.[30] There was more uptake of resveratrol, and metabolic activity was increased, when cells were incubated with resveratrol-loaded solid lipid nanoparticles, compared to when the free form of resveratrol or empty solid lipid nanoparticles were used.[30]

Pectinate delivery systems

Pectinate-based delivery systems, which permit modulation of the site of release depending on the cross-linking agent used, have also been examined for the delivery of resveratrol. Resveratrol entrapped in calcium pectinate formulations was released in the small intestine, but hardening the calcium pecti-

nate beads with polyethyleneimine enabled the delivery of resveratrol to the colon *in vitro*.[31] Colon-specific delivery of resveratrol *in vivo* was achieved with the use of resveratrol-loaded zinc pectinate microparticles hardened with glutaraldehyde.[32]

Chitosan microspheres

Chitosan is a polycationic polymer that has been used for drug delivery. An approach based on emulsion cross-linking procedures was used to prepare resveratrol-loaded chitosan microspheres cross-linked with vanillin, a component with GRAS status, as an alternative to chemical cross-linking agents.[33] The vanillin cross-linked chitosan microspheres protected resveratrol against photodegradation and controlled release of resveratrol in media.[33]

Trans-resveratrol loaded into novel cationic chitosan-coated and anionic alginate-coated poly(D,L-lactide-*co*-glycolide) nanoparticles was better retained and was protected against photodegradation compared to unencapsulated resveratrol and uncoated nanoparticles. *In vitro* experiments showed that the release of resveratrol could be more effectively controlled with the coated nanoparticles.[34]

Other delivery systems

Several other approaches have been examined for stabilization and delivery of resveratrol. Examples include the encapsulation of resveratrol using water-in-oil-in-water double emulsion formulated with food grade materials[35] and in yeast cells.[36]

Encapsulated formulations containing resveratrol in combination with other bioactive compounds

There is a trend toward the delivery of combinations of bioactive compounds. Liposomal preparations containing both curcumin and resveratrol were found to be more effective for reducing prostatic adenocarcinoma *in vivo* in *Pten* knockout mice than either bioactive delivered individually.[37] Another example is a micro-encapsulated formulation containing a bioactive mixture of fish oil, tributyrin, and resveratrol within an emulsion-based system. With radioactive labeling, it was possible to conclude that micro-encapsulation did not alter transit time, but increased the levels of bioactives or their metabolites in the blood and liver in rats.[38]

Conclusion

Encapsulation overcomes some of the limitations of the low solubility, susceptibility to photodegradation, and low bioavailability of resveratrol. However, there is also a need to establish the required dose for efficacy and to ascertain the optimum site for delivery and the release kinetics required. Where resveratrol is delivered via the oral route, the effects of the food matrix on resveratrol release will need to be considered. Further research is required in enhancing the delivery and bioavailability of resveratrol to obtain the desired biological effects in humans before recommendations may be made for the use of encapsulated resveratrol formulations for target health benefits.

Conflicts of interest

The authors declare no conflicts of interest.

References

1. Chachay, V.S., C.M.J. Kirkpatrick, I.J. Hickman, *et al.* 2011. Resveratrol – pills to replace a healthy diet. *Br. J. Clin. Pharmacol.* **72:** 27–38.

2. Giovinazzo, G., I. Ingrosso, A. Paradiso, *et al.* 2012. Resveratrol biosynthesis: plant metabolic engineering for nutritional improvement of food. *Plant Foods Hum. Nutr.* **67:** 191–199.

3. Patel, K.R., E. Scott, V.A. Brown, *et al.* 2011. Clinical trials of resveratrol. *Ann. N.Y. Acad. Sci.* **1215:** 161–169.

4. Delmas, D., V. Aires, E. Limagne, *et al.* 2011. Transport, stability, and biological activity of resveratrol. *Ann. N.Y. Acad. Sci.* **1215:** 48–59.

5. Walle, T. 2011. Bioavailability of resveratrol. *Ann. N.Y. Acad. Sci.* **1215:** 9–15.

6. Gumienna, M., M. Lasik & Z. Czarnecki. 2011. Bioconversion of grapefruit and chokeberry wine polyphenols during simulated in vitro gastrointestinal digestion. *Int. J. Food Sci. Nutr.* **62:** 226–233.

7. Amri, A., J.C. Chaumeil, S. Sfar & C. Charrueau. 2012. Administration of resveratrol: what formulation solutions to bioavailability limitations? *J. Controlled Release* **158:** 182–193.

8. Neves, A.R., M. Lúcio, J.L.C. Lima & S. Reis. 2012. Resveratrol in medicinal chemistry: a critical review of its pharmacokinetics, drug-deliver, and membrane interactions. *Curr. Med. Chem.* **19:** 1663–1681.

9. Santos, A.C., F. Veiga & A.J. Ribeiro. 2011. New delivery systems to improve the bioavailability of resveratrol. *Expert Opin. Drug Deliv.* **8:** 973–990.

10. Soto-Vaca, A., A. Gutierrez, J.N. Losso, *et al.* 2012. Evolution of phenolic compounds from color and flavour problems to health benefits. *J. Agric. Food Chem.* **60:** 6658–6677.

11. Stockley, C., P.L. Teissedre, M. Boban, *et al.* 2012. Bioavailability of wine-derived phenolic compounds in humans: a review. *Food Funct.* **3:** 995–1007.

12. Bandyopadhyay, P., A.K. Ghosh & C. Ghosh. 2012. Recent developments on the polyphenol-protein interactions: effects of tea and coffee taste, antioxidant properties and the digestive system. *Food Funct.* **3:** 592–605.

13. Augustin, M.A. & Y. Hemar. 2009. Nano-structured assemblies for encapsulation of food ingredients. *Chem. Soc. Rev.* **38:** 902–912.

14. McClements, D.J., E.A. Decker, Y. Park & J. Weiss. 2009. Structural design principles for delivery of bioactive components in nutraceuticals and functional foods. *Crit. Rev. Food Sci. Nutr.* **49:** 577–606.

15. Augustin, M.A. & L. Sanguansri. 2012. Challenges in developing delivery systems for food additives, nutraceuticals and dietary supplements. In *Encapsulation Technologies and Delivery Systems for Food Ingredients and Nutraceuticals.* N. Garti & J. McClements, Eds.: 19–48. Chapter 2. Cambridge, UK: Woodhead Publishing.

16. Coimbra, M., B. Isacchi, L. van Bloois, *et al.* 2011. Improving solubility and chemical stability of natural compounds for medicinal use by incorporation into liposomes. *Int. J. Pharm.* **416:** 433–442.

17. Mukherjee, K., M. Venkatesh, P. Venkatesh, *et al.* 2011. Effect of soy phosphatidyl choline on the bioavailability and nutritional health benefits of resveratrol. *Food Res. Int.* **44:** 1088–1093.

18. Kristl, J., K. Teskač, C. Caddeo, Z. Abramović & M. Šentjurc. 2009. Improvements of cellular stress response on resveratrol in liposomes. *Eur. J. Pharm. Biopharm.* **73:** 253–259.

19. Xiao, J.B., X.Q. Chen, X.Y. Jiang, *et al.* 2008. Probing the interaction of *trans*-resveratrol with bovine serum albumin: a fluorescence quenching study with Tachiya model. *J. Fluores* **18:** 671–678.

20. Bourassa, P., C.D. Kanakis, P. Tarantilis, *et al.* 2010. Resveratrol, genistein, and curcumin bind bovine serum albumin. *J. Phys. Chem. B.* **114:** 3348–3354.

21. Zhang, J., Q. Mi & M. Shen. 2012. Resveratrol binding to collagen and its biological implication. *Food Chem.* **131:** 879–884.

22. Zhang, J., X.F. Dai & J.Y. Huang. 2012. Resveratrol binding to fibrinogen and its biological implication. *Food Biophys.* **7:** 35–42.

23. Liang, L., A. Tajmir-Riahi & M. Subirade. 2008. Interaction of b-lactoglobulin with resveratrol and its biological implications. *Biomacromolecules* **9:** 50–56.

24. Hemar, Y., M. Gerbeaud, C.M. Oliver & M.A. Augustin. 2011. Investigation into the interaction between resveratrol and whey proteins using fluorescence spectroscopy. *Int. J. Food Sci. Tech.* **46:** 2137–2144.

25. López-Nicolás, J.M., E. Núñez-Delicado, A.J. Pérez-López, *et al.* 2006. Determination of stoichiometric coefficients and apparent formation constants for β-cyclodextrin complexes of *trans*-resveratrol using reversed-phase liquid chromatography. *J. Chrom. A* **1135:** 158–165.

26. Lucas-Abellán, C., I. Fortea, J.M. López-Nicolás & E. Núñez-Delicado. 2007. Cyclodextrins as resveratrol carrier systems. *Food Chem.* **104:** 39–44.

27. Berta, G.N., P. Salamone, A.E. Sprio, *et al.* 2010. Chemoprevention of 7,12-dimethylbenz[a]anthracene (DMBA)-induced oral carcinogenesis in hamster cheek

pouch by topical application of resveratrol complexed with 2-hydroxypropyl-β-cyclodextrin. *Oral Oncol.* **46:** 42–48.

28. Ansari, K.A., P.R. Vavia, F. Trotta & R. Cavalli. 2011. Cyclodextrin-based nanosponges for delivery of resveratrol: *In vitro* characterisation, stability, cytotoxicity and permeation study. *AAPS Pharm. Sci. Tech.* **12:** 279–286.

29. Carlotti, M.E., S. Sapino, E. Ugazio, *et al.* 2012. Resveratrol in solid lipid nanoparticles. *J. Disp. Sci. Tech.* **39:** 465–471.

30. Teskač, K. & J. Kristl. 2010. The evidence for solid lipid nanoparticles mediated cell uptake of resveratrol. *Int. J. Pharm.* **390:** 61–69.

31. Das, S. & K.-Y. Ng. 2010. Colon-specific delivery of resveratrol: optimization of multi-particulate calcium-pectinate carrier. *Int. J. Pharm.* **385:** 20–28.

32. Das, S., K.-Y. Ng & P.C. Ho. 2011. Design of a pectin-based microparticle formulation using zinc ions as the cross-linking agent and glutaraldehyde as the hardening agent for colonic-specific delivery of resveratrol: *in vitro* and *in vivo* evaluations. *J. Drug Targeting* **19:** 446–457.

33. Peng, H., H. Xiong, J. Li, *et al.* 2010. Vanillin cross-linked chitosan microspheres for controlled release of resveratrol. *Food Chem.* **121:** 23–28.

34. Sanna, V., A.M. Roggio, S. Siliani, *et al.* 2012. Development of novel cationic chitosan- and anionic alginate–coated poly(D,L-lactide-co-glycolide) nanoparticles for controlled release and light protection of resveratrol. *Int. J. Nanomed.* **7:** 5501–5516.

35. Hemar, Y., L.J. Cheng, C.M. Oliver, *et al.* 2010. Encapsulation of resveratrol using water-in-oil-in-water double emulsions. *Food Biophys.* **5:** 120–127.

36. Shi, G., L. Rao, H. Yu, *et al.* 2008. Stabilization and encapsulation of photosensitive resveratrol within yeast cell. *Int. J. Pharm.* **349:** 83–93.

37. Narayanan, N.K., D. Nargi, C. Randolph & B.A. Narayanan. 2009. Liposome encapsulation of curcumin and resveratrol in combination reduces prostate cancer incidence in PTEN knockout mice. *Int. J. Cancer* **125:** 1–8.

38. Augustin, M.A., M.Y. Abeywardena, G. Patten, *et al.* 2011. Effects of microencapsulation on the gastrointestinal transit and tissue distribution of a bioactive mixture of fish oil, tributyrin and resveratrol. *J. Funct. Foods* **3:** 25–37.

Ann. N.Y. Acad. Sci. ISSN 0077-8923

ANNALS OF THE NEW YORK ACADEMY OF SCIENCES
Issue: *Resveratrol and Health*

Resveratrol-based combinatorial strategies for cancer management

Chandra K. Singh, Jasmine George, and Nihal Ahmad

Department of Dermatology, University of Wisconsin, Madison, Wisconsin

Address for correspondence: Nihal Ahmad, Department of Dermatology, University of Wisconsin, 1300 University Avenue, 423 Medical Sciences Center, Madison, WI 53706. nahmad@wisc.edu

In recent years combination chemoprevention has been increasingly appreciated and investigated as a viable and effective strategy for cancer management. A plethora of evidence suggests that a combination of agents may afford synergistic (or additive) advantage for cancer management by multiple means, such as by (1) enhancing the bioavailability of chemopreventive agents, (2) modifying different molecular targets, and (3) lowering the effective dose of agent/drug to be used for cancer management. Resveratrol has been shown to afford chemopreventive and therapeutic effects against certain cancers. Recent studies are suggesting that resveratrol may be very useful when given in combination with other agents. The two major advantages of using resveratrol in combination with other agents are synergistically or additively enhancing the efficacy against cancer and limiting the toxicity and side effects of existing therapies. However, concerted and multidisciplinary efforts are needed to identify the most optimal combinatorial strategies.

Keywords: resveratrol; cancer; chemoprevention; combination chemoprevention

Introduction

Amassed research has suggested that a number of naturally occurring agents, including those present in the human diet, may be useful against a variety of diseases including cancer. However, based on the recent literature, it is becoming increasingly clear that a single-agent approach is probably less likely to be very effective in the management of diseases including cancer. In fact, a combinatorial approach relying on a cocktail of drugs, rather than a single drug, has been in practice for disease management for a long time. As pointed out by Michael Sporn, and suggested by recent research, combination chemoprevention may be a more practical approach for cancer management.[1] In classical terms, chemoprevention is defined as a strategy to reduce the risk or delay the development or recurrence of cancer via drugs, vitamins, or other agents. However, recent studies have suggested the usefulness of a number of chemopreventive agents in therapeutic settings. Therefore, the definition of chemoprevention seems to have expanded to include the delay or even reversal of the process of carcinogenesis. It appears that combinatorial chemopreventive approaches could be effective in prevention as well as treatment of cancer. The effective combination chemopreventive approaches can make use of (1) a combination of multiple agents based on molecular targets, (2) a combination of existing drugs with chemopreventive agents, in adjuvant settings, and/or (3) a combination of agents, drugs, and life style modifications.

Resveratrol, an antioxidant present in red grapes, red wine, and a variety of other dietary sources, has been shown to possess many beneficial biological properties, including cancer chemopreventive effects. Several studies, especially in the past 15 years, have shown the cancer preventive and therapeutic potential of resveratrol in a variety of *in vitro* and *in vivo* models. In the recent past, resveratrol has arguably become one agent that holds great fascination among researchers, the news media, and the general public. Some recent studies have also evaluated the combinatorial effects of resveratrol with other naturally occurring and chemotherapeutic agents, suggesting that resveratrol can improve the efficacy of other agents.[2–8] Indeed, the strategy of using resveratrol in combination with other agents,

doi: 10.1111/nyas.12160

particularly with chemotherapeutic modalities, may hold clinical promise for cancer management. However, evidence-based scientific evaluations in appropriate models are needed to show the efficacy of resveratrol in combination with other agents. This short review provides a discussion and perspective on the potential of resveratrol-based combinatorial strategies for cancer management.

Resveratrol amid many of nature's gifts

Resveratrol, chemically known as 3,5,4'-trihydroxy-*trans*-stilbene, is a strong antioxidant that has been identified in over 70 plant species, including grape skin, raspberries, blueberries, mulberries, Scots pine, Eastern white pine, and knotweed. Resveratrol is a phytoalexin, synthesized *de novo* by plants during environmental stress and pathogenic invasion, thereby acting as a natural inhibitor of cell proliferation.[9] The use of resveratrol for health benefits can be traced back to several ancient medicine systems. For example, resveratrol is a component of darakchasava, an ancient Ayurvedic herbal formulation.[10] However, resveratrol was first isolated by Michio Takaoka from the roots of *Veratrum grandiflorum* (white hellebore) in 1940 (reviewed in Timmers *et al.*).[11] In 1963, he extracted resveratrol from the roots of the plant *Polygonum cuspidatum* (Japanese knotweed). At present, most of the commercially available resveratrol is isolated from *Polygonum cuspidatum* using high-speed counter-current chromatography.[12] The popularity of resveratrol started rising in 1992 when its occurrence was noticed in red wine and it was linked to the French paradox, the epidemiological observation that the French population possesses a lower risk of coronary heart disease despite consuming a diet rich in saturated fats.[11] Following this, scientific research on resveratrol surged at fast pace. Although resveratrol exists in both *cis-* and *trans-*stereoisomeric forms, the commercially available resveratrol is mainly the *trans*-form, which has been most extensively studied. Because of its strong antioxidant properties, resveratrol is being studied in a variety of oxidative stress–associated diseases. A number of studies have shown the benefits of resveratrol for a variety of diseases and conditions, including heart disease, neurological disorders, metabolic disorders, and degenerative conditions. Resveratrol has also been shown to improve immune function and mimic the life-lengthening effects of calorie re-

striction but without dieting. The cancer chemopreventive properties of resveratrol were first appreciated in 1997, when Jang *et al.* found that resveratrol possesses chemopreventive activity against the three major stages of carcinogenesis (i.e., initiation, promotion, and progression).[13] This was followed by an extensive effort by researchers to determine the cancer chemopreventive and therapeutic effects of resveratrol in a wide range of models.

Resveratrol for cancer management

The popularity of resveratrol in cancer chemoprevention research can be appreciated from its continuously growing number of published studies and clinical trials. Below, we have provided a very brief description on selected published studies suggesting chemopreventive/antiproliferative effects of resveratrol against some cancer types.

Studies have suggested that resveratrol could be useful against prostate cancer, which is a major neoplasm of males and represents an ideal candidate disease for chemoprevention due to its long latency and identifiable preneoplastic lesions. Resveratrol has been demonstrated to have chemopreventive effects in relevant animal models of prostate cancer. For example, Harper *et al.* have shown that resveratrol reduced the incidence by several fold of poorly differentiated prostatic adenocarcinoma in the transgenic adenocarcinoma of mouse prostate (TRAMP) model.[14] And Seeni *et al.* have demonstrated that resveratrol suppresses prostate cancer growth in the transgenic rat for adenocarcinoma of prostate (TRAP) model.[15]

The first evidence for possible skin cancer chemopreventive efficacy of resveratrol came from the study by Jang *et al.* that demonstrated chemopreventive effects of resveratrol in a classic chemical carcinogenesis model.[13] Ultraviolet (UV) light is believed to be the major cause of skin cancer; a series of studies from our laboratory demonstrated the protective potential of resveratrol against UV-mediated damage in skin (reviewed in Ndiaye *et al.*[16]). In another study using a UVB initiation–promotion protocol, we demonstrated that the topical application of resveratrol resulted in a significant inhibition in skin tumor incidence, as well as a delay in the onset of tumorigenesis, in an SKH-1 hairless mouse model.[17] Following this study, several reports demonstrated the protective efficacy of resveratrol against skin cancer (reviewed in Ref. 16). In addition, resveratrol has been shown to be effective in syngeneic melanoma mouse models.[18] Similarly, a number of studies have demonstrated the potential efficacy of resveratrol against breast cancer,[19] gastric cancer,[20] colorectal cancer,[21–23] and other cancer types such as cancers of lung, liver, pancreas, and bladder.[24–27] Thus, resveratrol, studied for cancer chemoprevention in many conditions, may have the potential to be an effective agent for cancer management. Further, resveratrol does not seem to have toxicity, as it has been shown to be reasonably well tolerated at doses of up to 5 g/day in healthy subjects without side effects.[28] However, an effective dose of resveratrol depends on disease and subject context, and remains to be thoroughly investigated.

Combination chemoprevention from ancient to modern time

Combination chemoprevention is not a new idea. Most of the world's ancient medicine systems appear to have relied on multiple agents to try to target many symptoms at the same time. Ayurveda (meaning "the science of long life" in Sanskrit), or ayurvedic medicine, an approximately 5000-year-old system of traditional medicine native to the Indian subcontinent, often uses a combination of herbs and agents for disease management. Ayurveda is still in practice in the Indian subcontinent for management of diseases including cancer.[29] There is an extensive list of herbs used, often in combinations, in the Ayurvedic management of cancer. Some of these, which have been tested and supported by modern research to have antiproliferative efficacy, include *Curcuma longa* (turmeric), *Aloe vera* (aloe), *Allium sativum* (garlic), *Abrus precatorium* (coral bead vine), *Boswellia serrata* (Indian olibanum), *Plumbago zeylanica* (leadwort), and *Vinca rosea* (periwinkle).[29] As mentioned above, the herbal Ayurvedic tonic formulation darakchasava, which is used for good health, has been shown to contain resveratrol and pterostilbene.[10] Similarly, the traditional Chinese medicine system, which also has a more than 5000-year-old history, is based on a combination approach. Traditional Chinese herbal cocktails are often used as complementary medicine approaches to manage diseases, including in cancer to diminish the side effects and/or tumor resistance to chemotherapy/radiotherapy.[30] Interestingly, a cocktail of Chinese herbs (containing spreading hedyotis herb, barbed skullcap herb, ma-yuen Job's tears

seed, *Ganoderma lucidum*, and Chinese hawthorn fruit), in conjunction with chemotherapy and radiation therapy, was shown to have favorable clinical outcome in pancreatic cancer patients with liver metastases.[31] Nature also seems to support a combinatorial approach, since food is a conglomeration of numerous beneficial ingredients. Based on emerging scientific evidence, the whole foods concept is being viewed as a better approach than a single dietary factor. It is believed that individual dietary factors in food may work additively or synergistically, to yield a better response in preventing diseases.

In modern times, the concept of multi-agent therapeutics for cancer treatment has been in practice since the 1960s, with evidence of enhanced survival in childhood leukemias and Hodgkin's disease following combination chemotherapy (compared to a single agent).[32] Currently, most cancer chemotherapeutic drugs are used in combination in order to increase efficacy and/or decrease toxicity. The rationale for recommending a multidrug regimen is to attack more than one critical function in the cancer cells, leading to improved clinical outcomes.

Thus, from ancient times to the modern era, combinatorial therapeutic strategies for disease management have been proven to be more efficacious than monotherapies. Based on recent studies and strong rationale, combination chemoprevention is being appreciated and investigated as a viable and effective strategy for cancer management.

Resveratrol-based combinations for cancer management

On the basis of recent research in a wide range of scientific disciplines, including cancer, heart diseases, metabolic conditions, and aging, resveratrol could be considered the most extensively studied flavonoid at present. Recently, researchers have begun focusing on using resveratrol in conjunction with other agents and drugs for improved response against cancer. A few examples of recent research efforts on resveratrol-based combinatorial strategies are discussed below. We have mainly focused on *in vivo* studies conducted in animal models; Table 1 provides a summary of *in vivo* studies where resveratrol-based combinations have been evaluated.

Resveratrol and piperine

A group of researchers believe that the biggest hurdle in the development of resveratrol as a drug or preventive agent is its poor bioavailability following oral ingestion, resulting from its rapid metabolism, mainly to its glucuronide and sulfate metabolites. We have recently reviewed this area of research and the different possibilities in this direction.[33] We believe that more research is needed to determine the possibility of chemopreventive efficacy of resveratrol metabolites as well as the possibility of obtaining and maintaining steady and effective *in vivo* resveratrol concentrations following chronic ingestion. However, researchers have begun to focus on different means of enhancing the bioavailability of resveratrol, as well as developing novel resveratrol analogues with superior efficacy and bioavailability. A recent study from our laboratory has shown that piperine, an alkaloid present in black pepper, can significantly enhance resveratrol levels in the blood of mice.[34] In this study, we found that addition of piperine significantly enhances the degree of exposure (i.e., AUC) to resveratrol as well as its maximum serum concentration (C_{max}) in C57BL mice.[34] Piperine has previously been shown to enhance the bioavailability of other polyphenols such as (−)-epigallocatechin-3-gallate (EGCG).[35] In another interesting recent *in vitro* study, a resveratrol and piperine combination was found to act as a sensitizer for ionizing radiation–induced apoptotic cell death.[5] Although these studies are encouraging, the effect of piperine on resveratrol bioavailability remains unknown in the human population. Further, the therapeutic efficacy of this combination in disease models needs to be assessed.

Resveratrol and quercetin

Both resveratrol and quercetin are polyphenols present in red grapes, red wine, and several other plants. However, the levels of quercetin in red wine are typically ∼10-fold higher than the resveratrol levels.[36] In a recent study, Khandelwal *et al.* showed that resveratrol and quercetin synergistically reduce the extent of restenosis (a complication of angioplasty and stenting), possibly by inhibiting vascular smooth muscle cell proliferation and inflammation.[36] Further, in a study by Zhou *et al.*, transcriptomic and metabolomic profiling revealed synergistic effects of quercetin and resveratrol supplementation in high-fat diet–fed mice.[37] It seems that additive/synergistic interactions between these two polyphenols may be one explanation for the

French paradox, especially because both of these agents are present in red wine. Thus, the combination of resveratrol and quercetin seems to have potential toward cancer management. In addition, quercetin has also been shown to inhibit sulfation of resveratrol.[38] Therefore, it is conceivable that quercetin can enhance the bioavailability, and thus therapeutic efficacy, of resveratrol by inhibiting its sulfation. However, studies are needed to explore these possibilities.

Resveratrol and melatonin

Resveratrol has also been studied in combination with the pineal hormone and known antioxidant melatonin. Kiskova *et al.* recently demonstrated that a combination of resveratrol with melatonin exerts superior chemopreventive effects in *N*-methyl-*N*-nitrosourea (NMU)–induced rat mammary carcinogenesis.[6] The data from this study showed that neither of the two agents alone had any appreciable effect on NMU-induced mammary carcinogenesis, but the combination resulted in a significant decrease in tumor incidence. Further, another study found that melatonin synergistically enhanced resveratrol-induced heme oxygenase-1, possibly through inhibition of a ubiquitin-dependent proteasome pathway.[39] The authors suggested that this combination may provide an effective means to treat neurodegenerative disorders.[39] This combination seems to have potential in cancer chemoprevention. It is possible that these two agents may target two nonoverlapping pathways. Although melatonin can function through its own receptors, resveratrol may inhibit proliferative signaling by modulating other pathways. Thus, there is a possibility that this combination may lead to a synergistic response to attenuate proliferative signaling and improve cancer chemopreventive response.

Resveratrol and tea polyphenols

In a recent study, George *et al.* determined the effect of the combination of resveratrol with black tea polyphenol in a two-stage mouse skin carcinogenesis model. It was found that the combination imparts a synergistic tumor-suppressive response, compared to either of the agents alone.[7] The authors suggested that the observed synergistic response is possibly due to a synergistic action of the two agents on same molecular targets. This is an interesting study because a synergistic action of

Ann. N.Y. Acad. Sci. 1290 (2013) 113–121 © 2013 New York Academy of Sciences.

Table 1. Studies evaluating combinations of resveratrol with other agents

Agents used in combination with resveratrol	Model system	Outcome	References
Piperine	C57BL/6 healthy mice	Piperine enhanced the serum bioavailability of resveratrol	34
Quercetin	Mice with a carotid injury	Combination synergistically reduced the extent of restenosis	36
Quercetin	High-fat diet-fed mice	Combination resulted in a restoration of high fat–induced alterations in pathways of glucose/lipid metabolism, liver function, cardiovascular system, and inflammation/immunity	37
Melatonin	NMU-induced rat mammary carcinogenesis	Combination resulted in a significant decrease in tumorigenesis	6
Black tea polyphenols	Two stage skin carcinogenesis mouse model	Combination resulted in a synergistic tumor suppressive response	7
Curcumin	BP-induced lung cancer in mice	Combination showed better chemopreventive response by maintaining adequate zinc, and modulating Cox-2 and p21 level	25
Quercetin + genistein + apigenin + EGCG + baicalein + curcumin	TRAMP mouse model of prostate cancer	All seven compounds inhibited well-differentiated carcinoma of the prostate by 58% when fed in combination as pure compounds; and 81% when fed as crude plant extracts	41
Geneistin	SV40 rat model of prostate cancer	Combination reduced the most severe grade of prostate cancer in SV40 Tag-targeted probasin promoter rat model	4
ProstaCaid	Nude mouse model of prostate cancer	ProstaCaid™, which contains a number of chemopreventive agents including resveratrol, inhibited invasive prostate cancer in a nude mouse model	42
Temozolomide	Nude mouse model of glioma	Resveratrol was found to enhance the therapeutic efficacy by inhibiting ROS/ERK-mediated autophagy and enhancing apoptosis	45
Doxorubicin (DOX)	B16/DOX mouse model of melanoma	Resveratrol was found to overcome chemoresistance by inducing cell cycle disruption and apoptosis	46
Quercitin + catechin + gefitinib	Nude mouse model of mammary cancer	Resveratrol, quercetin, and catechin combination potentiated the effects of gefitinib in inhibiting mammary tumor growth	8

multiple agents on a common pathway(s) can lead to dose-reduction of chemopreventive agents, thereby limiting the chances of side effects.

Resveratrol and curcumin

In a recent study, Malhotra *et al.* assessed the efficacy of combined supplementation of curcumin and resveratrol in benzo[a]pyrene (BP)-induced lung carcinogenesis in mice.[25] The study demonstrated that curcumin and resveratrol in combination provide a better chemopreventive response by maintaining adequate zinc levels and by modulating Cox-2 and p21.[25] Here, it is important to mention another study by Zhang *et al.*, which demonstrated that a combination of resveratrol and zinc in normal human prostate epithelial cells increased total cellular zinc and intracellular free labile zinc in the cells.[40] Since zinc is an extremely important trace element in normal prostate development as well as in prostate cancer, this finding provides a rationale to conduct further studies to evaluate the combination of zinc and resveratrol in prevention as well as treatment of prostate cancer.

Combination with other natural agents

A few other combinations containing resveratrol have also been investigated for their cancer chemopreventive effects in *in vivo* models. Slusarz *et al.* determined the preventive and therapeutic abilities of a number of agents along with resveratrol (quercetin, genistein, apigenin, baicalein, curcumin, and EGCG), *in vitro* as well as *in vivo* in TRAMP.[41] The authors found that four of the seven compounds (genistein, curcumin, EGCG, and resveratrol) inhibited Hedgehog signaling as shown by real-time reverse transcription–PCR analysis of Gli1 mRNA concentration or by Gli reporter activity.[41] The authors also found that all seven compounds, when fed in combination as pure compounds or as crude plant extracts, inhibited well-differentiated carcinoma of the prostate by 58% and 81%, respectively. In another study, resveratrol in combination with genistein provided in the diet was found to significantly reduce the most severe grade of prostate cancer in the Simian virus 40 T-antigen (SV40 Tag)–targeted probasin promoter rat model, a transgenic model of spontaneously developing prostate cancer.[4] In another study, Jiang *et al.* have shown the anticancer efficacy of the dietary supplement ProstaCaid™, which contains a number of chemopreventive agents including resveratrol,

against invasive prostate cancer in a nude mouse model.[42]

Resveratrol in combination with anticancer drugs

Plenty of *in vitro* and limited *in vivo* studies have suggested that resveratrol may enhance the antitumor effects of chemotherapeutic drugs in several cancers.[43,44] Thus, in addition to chemopreventive and cytostatic properties, resveratrol is being investigated for its potential as an adjuvant in conjunction with chemotherapeutic modalities to enhance their efficacy and/or limit their toxicities. Lin *et al.* have shown that resveratrol potentiated the therapeutic efficacy of temozolomide, an alkylating agent used in cancer therapeutics, in a mouse xenograft model of malignant glioma, through inhibiting ROS/ERK-mediated autophagy and enhancing apoptosis.[45] Resveratrol has also been shown to overcome chemoresistance in a mouse model of B16/DOX melanoma by inducing cell cycle disruption and apoptosis, leading to reduced growth of melanoma and prolonged survival of mice.[46] In a recent study, a combination of the dietary grape polyphenols resveratrol, quercetin, and catechin was shown to potentiate the effects of gefitinib in inhibiting mammary tumor growth and metastasis in nude mice.[8] These studies support the potential use of resveratrol as an adjuvant in combination with chemotherapeutic drugs for cancer management. However, a study by Fukui *et al.* suggested that resveratrol may diminish the antiproliferative effect of paclitaxel in breast cancer.[47] Therefore, more preclinical studies in appropriate models are warranted to ascertain the usefulness of resveratrol as an adjuvant.

Resveratrol in combination with other factors within its natural matrix

As discussed above, emerging evidence suggests that the whole foods concept could be a better approach than single agents due to the possibility of synergistic improvement of responses from interactions between different ingredients within a food source. For example, grapes contain several hundred compounds with health-promoting properties. These individual agents may enhance the effectiveness and bioavailability of each other. Careful studies are needed to understand and to define whether an agent(s) should be considered in isolation, in combination, or in its natural

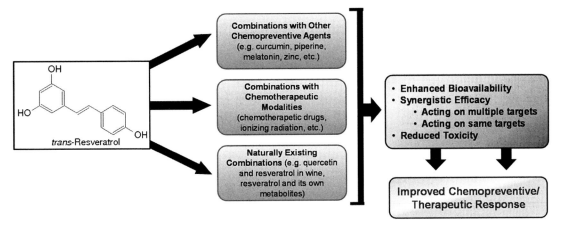

Figure 1. Resveratrol-based combinatorial strategies for cancer management.

complex form. A few examples of resveratrol-based naturally occurring combinations are provided below.

Crude extract of *Polygonum cuspidatum*, in addition to resveratrol, contains piceid (a glucoside precursor of resveratrol), polydatin (a stilbene), and emodin (an anthraquinone), among several other ingredients. All of these agents are considered to be bioactive agents with possible health-promoting effects. A study by Ghamin *et al.* assessed the effect of a *P. cuspidatum* extract (PCE) containing resveratrol on oxidative and inflammatory stress in healthy volunteers. The authors suggested that the PCE containing resveratrol had a comprehensive suppressive effect on oxidative and inflammatory stress.[48] In another phase I pilot study in colorectal cancer patients, Nguyen *et al.* found that resveratrol-containing freeze-dried grape powder inhibits the Wnt pathway, a key signaling pathway in colon cancer initiation; however, the effect was confined to the normal colonic mucosa.[49] Ortuno *et al.* conducted a pharmacokinetic study of resveratrol, in different matrices, in eleven healthy volunteers. The authors found that resveratrol was better absorbed from natural grape products than from supplements.[50] All of this evidence suggested that naturally available combinations of resveratrol and matrix of the source may be extremely important to the overall bioavailability and efficacy of resveratrol. This seems to be very important in cancer prevention settings, where chronic administration of resveratrol-containing moieties can possibly lead to an effective concentration of

resveratrol *in vivo* to provide a chemopreventive response.

Conclusions

On the basis of emerging evidence, it is becoming increasingly clear that combination chemoprevention—relying on a combination of agents with limited (nonoverlapping) toxicity, which may diminish the toxicity of each other while enhancing therapeutic efficacy—could be a very useful strategy for cancer management. It appears that resveratrol possesses a number of characteristics of an ideal chemopreventive agent, such as (1) a lack of toxicity at desired concentrations, (2) available knowledge of mechanism(s) of action, (3) human acceptability because of being a dietary ingredient, and (4) cost affordability. Recent research is focusing on resveratrol-based combinatorial strategies for the management of cancer. As discussed above and depicted in Figure 1, resveratrol-based combinations can lead to improved chemopreventive and therapeutic responses in a number of ways. On the one hand, resveratrol may be used in combination with other naturally occurring chemopreventive agents in a cancer prevention setting. On the other hand, resveratrol may be used in conjunction with existing therapeutic modalities to enhance their response and limit their toxicity. Indeed, further preclinical studies will be needed to define the most useful combinations. In addition, clinical studies are needed to ascertain the efficacy of resveratrol in adjuvant settings.

Acknowledgments

This work was partly supported by funding from the NIH (R21CA149560, R21CA176867, and R01AR059130 to NA) and the Department of Defense (W81XWH-12-1-0105 to CKS).

Conflicts of interest

The authors declare no conflicts of interest.

References

1. Sporn, M.B. *et al.* 1976. Prevention of chemical carcinogenesis by vitamin A and its synthetic analogs (retinoids). *Fed. Proc.* **35:** 1332–1338.

2. Yuan, Y. *et al.* 2012. Resveratrol enhances the antitumor effects of temozolomide in glioblastoma via ROS-dependent AMPK-TSC-mTOR signaling pathway. *CNS Neurosci. Ther.* **18:** 536–546.

3. Iwuchukwu, O.F., R.J. Tallarida & S. Nagar. 2011. Resveratrol in combination with other dietary polyphenols concomitantly enhances antiproliferation and UGT1A1 induction in Caco-2 cells. *Life Sci.* **88:** 1047–1054.

4. Harper, C.E. *et al.* 2009. Genistein and resveratrol, alone and in combination, suppress prostate cancer in SV-40 tag rats. *Prostate* **69:** 1668–1682.

5. Tak, J.K., J.H. Lee & J.W. Park. 2012. Resveratrol and piperine enhance radiosensitivity of tumor cells. *BMB Rep.* **45:** 242–246.

6. Kiskova, T. *et al.* 2012. A combination of resveratrol and melatonin exerts chemopreventive effects in *N*-methyl-*N*-nitrosourea-induced rat mammary carcinogenesis. *Eur. J. Cancer Prev.* **21:** 163–170.

7. George, J. *et al.* 2011. Resveratrol and black tea polyphenol combination synergistically suppress mouse skin tumors growth by inhibition of activated MAPKs and p53. *PLoS One* **6:** e23395.

8. Castillo-Pichardo, L. & S.F. Dharmawardhane. 2012. Grape polyphenols inhibit Akt/mammalian target of rapamycin signaling and potentiate the effects of gefitinib in breast cancer. *Nutr. Cancer.* **64:** 1058–1069.

9. Harikumar, K.B. & B.B. Aggarwal. 2008. Resveratrol: a multitargeted agent for age-associated chronic diseases. *Cell Cycle* **7:** 1020–1035.

10. Paul, B. *et al.* 1999. Occurrence of resveratrol and pterostilbene in age-old darakchasava, an ayurvedic medicine from India. *J. Ethnopharmacol.* **68:** 71–76.

11. Timmers, S., J. Auwerx & P. Schrauwen. 2012. The journey of resveratrol from yeast to human. *Aging* **4:** 146–158.

12. Yang, F., T. Zhang & Y. Ito. 2001. Large-scale separation of resveratrol, anthraglycoside A and anthraglycoside B from *Polygonum cuspidatum* Sieb. et Zucc by high-speed countercurrent chromatography. *J. Chromatogr. A* **919:** 443–448.

13. Jang, M. *et al.* 1997. Cancer chemopreventive activity of resveratrol, a natural product derived from grapes. *Science* **275:** 218–220.

14. Harper, C.E. *et al.* 2007. Resveratrol suppresses prostate cancer progression in transgenic mice. *Carcinogenesis* **28:** 1946–1953.

15. Seeni, A. *et al.* 2008. Suppression of prostate cancer growth by resveratrol in the transgenic rat for adenocarcinoma of prostate (TRAP) model. *Asian Pac. J. Cancer Prev.* **9:** 7–14.

16. Ndiaye, M. *et al.* 2011. The grape antioxidant resveratrol for skin disorders: promise, prospects, and challenges. *Arch. Biochem. Biophys.* **508:** 164–170.

17. Aziz, M.H. *et al.* 2005. Chemoprevention of skin cancer by grape constituent resveratrol: relevance to human disease? *FASEB J.* **19:** 1193–1195.

18. Bhattacharya, S., S.R. Darjatmoko & A.S. Polans. 2011. Resveratrol modulates the malignant properties of cutaneous melanoma through changes in the activation and attenuation of the antiapoptotic protooncogenic protein Akt/PKB. *Melanoma. Res.* **21:** 180–187.

19. Lee, H.S., A.W. Ha & W.K. Kim. 2012. Effect of resveratrol on the metastasis of 4T1 mouse breast cancer cells *in vitro* and *in vivo*. *Nutr. Res. Pract.* **6:** 294–300.

20. Atten, M.J. *et al.* 2005. Resveratrol regulates cellular PKC alpha and delta to inhibit growth and induce apoptosis in gastric cancer cells. *Invest. N. Drugs* **23:** 111–119.

21. Huderson, A.C. *et al.* 2012. Chemoprevention of benzo(a)pyrene-induced colon polyps in Apc(Min) mice by resveratrol. *J. Nutr. Biochem.* **24:** 713–724.

22. Juan, M.E., I. Alfaras & J.M. Planas. 2012. Colorectal cancer chemoprevention by trans-resveratrol. *Pharmacol. Res.* **65:** 584–591.

23. Patel, K.R. *et al.* 2010. Clinical pharmacology of resveratrol and its metabolites in colorectal cancer patients. *Cancer Res.* **70:** 7392–7399.

24. Athar, M. *et al.* 2007. Resveratrol: a review of preclinical studies for human cancer prevention. *Toxicol. Appl. Pharmacol.* **224:** 274–283.

25. Malhotra, A., P. Nair & D.K. Dhawan. 2011. Curcumin and resveratrol synergistically stimulate p21 and regulate cox-2 by maintaining adequate zinc levels during lung carcinogenesis. *Eur. J. Cancer Prev.* **20:** 411–416.

26. Howells, L.M. *et al.* 2011. Phase I randomized, double-blind pilot study of micronized resveratrol (SRT501) in patients with hepatic metastases: safety, pharmacokinetics, and pharmacodynamics. *Cancer Prev. Res.* **4:** 1419–1425.

27. Vang, O. *et al.* 2011. What is new for an old molecule? Systematic review and recommendations on the use of resveratrol. *PLoS One* **6:** e19881.

28. Patel, K.R. *et al.* 2011. Clinical trials of resveratrol. *Ann. N.Y. Acad. Sci.* **1215:** 161–169.

29. Garodia, P. *et al.* 2007. From ancient medicine to modern medicine: ayurvedic concepts of health and their role in inflammation and cancer. *J. Soc. Integr. Oncol.* **5:** 25–37.

30. Wang, Z. *et al.* 2012. Emerging glycolysis targeting and drug discovery from chinese medicine in cancer therapy. *Evid. Based Compl. Alternat. Med.* **2012:** 873175.

31. Ouyang, H. *et al.* 2011. Multimodality treatment of pancreatic cancer with liver metastases using chemotherapy, radiation therapy, and/or Chinese herbal medicine. *Pancreas* **40:** 120–125.

32. DeVita, V.T., Jr. & E. Chu. 2008. A history of cancer chemotherapy. *Cancer Res.* **68:** 8643–8653.

33. Ndiaye, M., R. Kumar & N. Ahmad. 2011. Resveratrol in cancer management: where are we and where we go from here? *Ann. N.Y. Acad. Sci.* **1215:** 144–149.

34. Johnson, J.J. *et al.* 2011. Enhancing the bioavailability of resveratrol by combining it with piperine. *Mol. Nutr. Food Res.* **55:** 1169–1176.

35. Lambert, J.D. *et al.* 2004. Piperine enhances the bioavailability of the tea polyphenol (–)-epigallocatechin-3-gallate in mice. *J. Nutr.* **134:** 1948–1952.

36. Khandelwal, A.R. *et al.* 2012. Resveratrol and quercetin interact to inhibit neointimal hyperplasia in mice with a carotid injury. *J. Nutr.* **142:** 1487–1494.

37. Zhou, M. *et al.* 2012. Transcriptomic and metabonomic profiling reveal synergistic effects of quercetin and resveratrol supplementation in high fat diet fed mice. *J. Proteome Res.* **11:** 4961–4971.

38. De Santi, C. *et al.* 2000. Sulphation of resveratrol, a natural compound present in wine, and its inhibition by natural flavonoids. *Xenobiotica* **30:** 857–866.

39. Kwon, K.J. *et al.* 2011. Melatonin synergistically increases resveratrol-induced heme oxygenase-1 expression through the inhibition of ubiquitin-dependent proteasome pathway: a possible role in neuroprotection. *J. Pineal. Res.* **50:** 110–123.

40. Zhang, J.J. *et al.* 2009. Effect of resveratrol and zinc on intracellular zinc status in normal human prostate epithelial cells. *Am. J. Physiol. Cell Physiol.* **297:** C632–644.

41. Slusarz, A. *et al.* 2010. Common botanical compounds inhibit the hedgehog signaling pathway in prostate cancer. *Cancer Res.* **70:** 3382–3390.

42. Jiang, J. *et al.* 2012. ProstaCaid inhibits tumor growth in a xenograft model of human prostate cancer. *Int. J. Oncol.* **40:** 1339–1344.

43. Fulda, S. & K.M. Debatin. 2004. Sensitization for anticancer drug-induced apoptosis by the chemopreventive agent resveratrol. *Oncogene* **23:** 6702–6711.

44. Gupta, S.C. *et al.* 2011. Chemosensitization of tumors by resveratrol. *Ann. N.Y. Acad. Sci.* **1215:** 150–160.

45. Lin, C.J. *et al.* 2012. Resveratrol enhances the therapeutic effect of temozolomide against malignant glioma *in vitro* and *in vivo* by inhibiting autophagy. *Free Radic. Biol. Med.* **52:** 377–391.

46. Gatouillat, G. *et al.* 2010. Resveratrol induces cell-cycle disruption and apoptosis in chemoresistant B16 melanoma. *J. Cell Biochem.* **110:** 893–902.

47. Fukui, M., N. Yamabe & B.T. Zhu. 2010. Resveratrol attenuates the anticancer efficacy of paclitaxel in human breast cancer cells *in vitro* and *in vivo*. *Eur. J. Cancer.* **46:** 1882–1891.

48. Ghanim, H. *et al.* 2010. An antiinflammatory and reactive oxygen species suppressive effects of an extract of Polygonum cuspidatum containing resveratrol. *J. Clin. Endocrinol. Metab.* **95:** E1–8.

49. Nguyen, A.V. *et al.* 2009. Results of a phase I pilot clinical trial examining the effect of plant-derived resveratrol and grape powder on Wnt pathway target gene expression in colonic mucosa and colon cancer. *Cancer Manag. Res.* **1:** 25–37.

50. Ortuno, J. *et al.* 2010. Matrix effects on the bioavailability of resveratrol in humans. *Food Chem.* **120:** 1123–1130.

Ann. N.Y. Acad. Sci. ISSN 0077-8923

An adipocentric perspective of resveratrol as a calorie restriction mimetic

Jamie L. Barger

LifeGen Technologies, LLC, Madison, Wisconsin

Address for correspondence: Jamie L. Barger, LifeGen Technologies, LLC, 510 Charmany Drive, Suite 262, Madison, WI 53719. Jamie.L.Barger@gmail.com

Adipose tissue is an active endocrine organ that responds to changes in energy balance and influences whole-body physiology. Adipose tissue dysfunction with obesity is associated with metabolic disease, neurodegeneration, inflammation, and cancer, whereas calorie restriction (CR) decreases both adiposity and disease risk. Although resveratrol does not affect obesity, it mimics long-term CR by increasing both life span in model organisms and health span in rodents. Because resveratrol's benefits in experimental animals are reminiscent of improved adipose tissue function under CR, this review synthesizes existing data to assess if resveratrol's effects may be mediated by mimicking CR in adipose tissue. In metabolically unhealthy humans, resveratrol consumption recapitulates the health benefits of CR, whereas short-term resveratrol in otherwise healthy humans mimics CR at the transcriptional, but not physiological, level. This latter observation (neutral effect of short-term resveratrol) may be protective against future disease risk; however, long-term studies in healthy humans will be needed to support this hypothesis.

Keywords: adipose tissue; calorie restriction mimetics; aging; nutrigenomics; obesity; type 2 diabetes

Relationship between adipose tissue and disease

Adipose tissue has classically been considered a relatively inert tissue that functions to store energy in anticipation of future periods of food scarcity. However, adipose tissue is now appreciated as an active endocrine organ, secreting numerous hormones, cytokines, and metabolites that are released into the blood and in turn regulate systemic physiology.[1] As the size of an adipose tissue depot increases, blood flow within the depot decreases, causing localized hypoxia that induces mitochondrial dysfunction and initiates acute immune and inflammatory responses.[2]

Interestingly, studies have shown that obesity, mitochondrial dysfunction, and inflammation are associated with a diverse array of diseases, including type 2 diabetes,[3] cardiovascular disease,[4] certain types of cancers,[5] sarcopenia,[6] and neurodegenerative disorders.[7] Because these diseases are exacerbated by an inflammatory and immune response, the available evidence strongly suggests that changes in adipose tissue bioactivity play a causative role in the pathogenesis of disease. Accordingly, therapeutic modalities that modulate adipose tissue physiology hold strong promise for the prevention and treatment of chronic disease.

Calorie restriction, adipose tissue, and disease

Long-term calorie restriction (CR), without malnutrition, increases life span in diverse species ranging from yeast, flies, and worms to mice and rats (reviewed in Ref. 8). Although studies conflict as to whether CR extends life span in nonhuman primates, a nearly universal phenomenon is an increase in health span with long-term CR, as measured by delayed onset and/or decreased risk of age-associated diseases, particularly those that have an inflammatory etiology, including cardiovascular disease,[9] cancer, type 2 diabetes, neurodegeneration,[10] and sarcopenia.[11]

Although the amount of adipose tissue and adipocyte size are increased in obesity and reduced with CR,[12] the bioactivity of adipose tissue is also influenced by diet, which may be causally linked

doi: 10.1111/nyas.12212

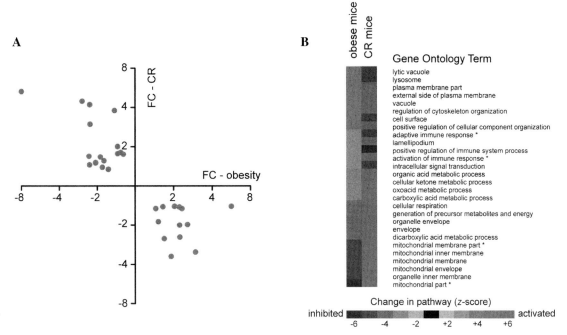

Figure 1. Calorie restriction (CR) opposes the transcriptomic pattern seen in white adipose tissue in obese mice. Analysis of previously published microarray data revealed 30 genes that were significantly ($P < 0.001$) changed in expression in obese[13] and calorie-restricted[12] mice, and the effect of CR was the opposite of that seen in obesity for all genes (A). Pathway analysis of the same data sets revealed that obesity was associated with an activation (red shading) of gene sets relating to cellular structure and the immune response and an inhibition (blue shading) of gene sets related to mitochondrial structure and metabolism; in all cases, CR opposed the obesity-related change in the activity of these gene sets (B). Asterisks in B represent pathways whereby resveratrol consumption mimicked the effect of CR in muscle of obese humans.[30] Data for individual genes are $\log_2$-adjusted fold change (FC) in expression. Each row in the pathway analysis indicates a Gene Ontology term that was significantly ($P < 0.001$) modulated in both obese and calorie-restricted mice.

to changes in whole-body physiology. The ability of CR to oppose obesity-related changes in adipose tissue activity is reflected in a reanalysis of gene expression profiling data from two independent studies of lean versus obese mice[13] and control-fed (lean) versus calorie-restricted mice.[12] There were 30 genes differentially expressed in both data sets, and the effect of CR was the opposite of obesity in all cases (Fig. 1A). To determine the biological function of genes changed by obesity and CR, pathway analysis was applied using parametric analysis of gene set enrichment[14] with gene functional categories defined by the Gene Ontology (GO) consortium (http:www.geneontology.org). This bioinformatic technique can detect modulations in predefined gene sets even when there is only a modest effect of a treatment on the expression of individual genes. Pathway analysis from obese and calorie-restricted mice showed that obesity is associated with increased activity of immune response and

inflammatory pathways as well as decreases in the activity of pathways related to mitochondrial structure and mitochondrial energy metabolism. Interestingly, CR opposed the obesity-related change in all pathways, suggesting possible mechanisms by which long-term CR protects against obesity-related disease.

Resveratrol as a CR mimetic

Despite the potent ability of long-term CR to oppose a broad spectrum of diseases, even in humans,[9] lifelong adherence to a calorie-restricted diet will not be a feasible therapy for humans. Accordingly, there has been a growing interest in identifying compounds that elicit the salutary effects of CR without requiring a reduction in calorie intake, so-called CR mimetics.[15] Although several compounds have been proposed as CR mimetics, resveratrol has received the most attention after it was shown to extend the life span of yeast,[16] flies, worms,[17]

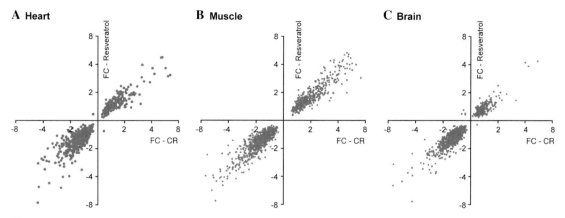

Figure 2. Gene expression profiling reveals that long-term treatment with resveratrol strongly mimics a long-term (14–30 months of age) calorie-restricted diet in multiple tissues of mice. Data are from Ref. 21. Each dot represents a gene that was significantly ($P < 0.01$) changed in expression by both CR and resveratrol (x- and y-axes, respectively; data represent $\log_2$-adjusted fold change (FC) in expression). Resveratrol mimicked 99.7%, 100%, and 99.5% of the genes changed by CR in heart, muscle, and brain (panels A, B, and C, respectively).

and fish,[18] and also improved survival, lowered inflammation, and enhanced memory in mice fed a high-fat diet.[19,20] Although resveratrol does not extend the life span of healthy mice fed a low-fat diet, there is a striking overlap between resveratrol and CR at the transcriptional level in multiple tissues of healthy mice.[21] In the heart, the expression of 747 genes was significantly changed by long-term CR and long-term consumption of a low dose of resveratrol, and resveratrol mimicked the CR effect for 745 of these genes (99.7% mimicry, Fig. 2A). Similar patterns were observed in both skeletal muscle and brain: 1164 genes were changed in expression by CR and resveratrol in muscle and the fold change was in the same direction for all genes (100% mimicry, Fig. 2B); in the brain 1134 genes were changed by both treatments with 1129 changes being in the same direction (99.5% mimicry, Fig. 2C). Resveratrol also prevented age-related changes in functional parameters in healthy mice, including motor coordination, bone mineral density, cataract formation, and cardiovascular function.[21,22]

Studies evaluating the efficacy of resveratrol in humans are emerging, though they are difficult to compare, as there are notable differences in the dose of resveratrol administered, the baseline characteristics of the subjects, and the form of resveratrol that was administered (pure resveratrol vs. resveratrol as an adjunct therapy vs. a resveratrol-containing plant extract). The dose of resveratrol consumed was low ($\leq$100 mg/day) for most studies, although

subjects in one study[23] consumed a high dose of resveratrol (1500 mg/day). For purposes of simplicity, this review will not differentiate results based on the dose administered, and will also highlight only those studies where pure resveratrol was tested as a single agent. Generally speaking, resveratrol had no effect on insulin sensitivity, glucose homeostasis, blood pressure, energy expenditure, or circulating inflammatory markers when consumed by metabolically healthy patients[23,24] (all of these measurements are positively influenced by long-term CR in humans[9]). Resveratrol did increase cerebral blood flow during a cognitive task assessment in healthy humans, although cognitive performance was not changed as a function of resveratrol.[25] In contrast, studies of patients with preexisting health conditions demonstrated that resveratrol consumption did have physiological effects, including improved endothelial function in overweight patients with elevated blood pressure,[26] improved left ventricle diastolic function in patients with stable coronary artery disease,[27] and improved markers of insulin sensitivity in patients with impaired glucose tolerance[28] or type 2 diabetes.[29] Finally, a comprehensive study of obese men showed that 30 days of resveratrol consumption strongly mimicked the health effects of a calorie-restricted diet, including decreased blood glucose and inflammatory markers, decreased blood pressure, and decreased insulin resistance (as assessed by HOMA index).[30] Although these clinical benefits of resveratrol are common to what is observed with CR in animals and humans, modulation of these surrogate markers may occur through different biological pathways. To assess whether there are mechanistic similarities between CR and resveratrol consumption, gene expression profiling was also performed in the vastus lateralis muscle, and pathway analysis revealed that resveratrol consumption decreased inflammatory gene expression and increased mitochondrial metabolism and mitochondrial structure pathways. Several of these resveratrol-sensitive pathways were also identified in the previous analysis of obesity and CR in mice (indicated by asterisks in Fig. 1B), including decreased inflammation ("adaptive immune response" and "activation of immune response") and increased mitochondrial activity ("mitochondrial membrane part" and "mitochondrial part"). Taken together, the data in humans suggest a common mechanism by which resveratrol mimics the effect of CR in humans, although the ability of resveratrol to mimic CR is most pronounced in patients with preexisting metabolic diseases.

Does resveratrol mimic CR in adipose tissue?

The balance of the available evidence in humans suggests that resveratrol improves cardiovascular, glucoregulatory, and inflammatory parameters; however, this is only observed in humans with preexisting symptoms of metabolic disease. Interestingly, similar positive health effects of resveratrol observed in metabolically compromised subjects are also observed with long-term CR (concurrent with reduced adipose tissue), thus at least some of the effects of resveratrol may be mediated though CR mimicry of adipose tissue activity. As a first step toward evaluating the ability of resveratrol to mimic CR in adipose tissue, it should first be established if long-term CR is able to oppose obesity-related changes in species other than mice (Fig. 1). Because the effect of obesity and CR in multiple species has not been examined using a consistent bioinformatic framework, we performed an analysis of published gene expression data sets in adipose tissue of obese mice,[13] obese humans,[31] calorie-restricted mice,[12] and calorie-restricted rats.[32] As seen in Figure 3, both mouse and human obesity are characterized by a marked upregulation of inflammatory/immune response pathways and downregulation in mitochondrial metabolism

pathways; moreover, CR in mice and rats consistently opposed the obesity-related changes in these pathways. Therefore, the set of biological pathways identified in Figure 3 likely represents an experimental paradigm that can be used to assess the ability of interventions to mimic CR in a manner that is protective against obesity-related diseases.

A reanalysis of gene expression data from adipose tissue of nonobese women with normal glucose tolerance[24] revealed that resveratrol consumption induced a gene expression profile opposite to mouse and human obesity and highly similar to CR in rodents (Fig. 3). A similar pattern was observed in adipose tissue of mice fed a low-fat diet containing resveratrol;[22] however, those gene expression data could not be compared in this analysis because they were performed on an experimental platform differing from the other data sets in Figure 3. Although resveratrol consumption by nonobese women with normal glucose tolerance did not improve insulin sensitivity or reduce inflammatory markers as has been reported with long-term CR (and in obese men consuming resveratrol), this is perhaps not surprising given that resveratrol consumption in young, healthy mice mimicked the gene expression pattern seen with long-term CR, but did not affect glucoregulatory parameters such as blood glucose or insulin levels.[33] Nonetheless, this analysis shows that resveratrol consumption in healthy subjects mimics the transcriptional pattern of CR in adipose tissue for those biological pathways that are conserved in diverse experimental models (mice, rats, and humans) and are relevant to obesity-related disease.

Does resveratrol exert CR mimicry by modulating obesity?

Although there are studies demonstrating that resveratrol mimics CR by attenuating adipose tissue inflammation *in vitro*,[34] other cell-culture studies report that treatment with resveratrol or resveratrol-enriched grape extracts resulted in decreased glucose uptake[35] and decreased adipocyte differentiation (adipogenesis).[36,37] The authors of these latter studies have extrapolated these limited *in vitro* results to suggest that resveratrol may hold promise as a therapy for preventing obesity. However, decreased adipogenesis is in fact a hallmark of obesity,[13] and the opposite biological effects (increased glucose uptake and increased adipogenesis)

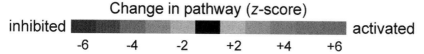

Figure 3. Resveratrol consumption by nonobese humans[24] opposes the transcriptional activity of adipose tissue seen in obesity[13,31] and mimics the effect of a calorie-restricted diet in mice[12] and rats.[32] Each row indicates a Gene Ontology term modulated in adipose tissue of (left to right) obese mice, obese humans, calorie-restricted mice, and calorie-restricted rats ($P < 0.001$ for each data set). Obesity was associated with increased activity of multiple immune response pathways and a decrease in the activity of pathways related to mitochondrial structure and mitochondrial metabolism. A calorie-restricted diet opposed these changes in mouse and rat adipose tissue, and 12 weeks of resveratrol consumption largely mimicked the effect of CR in adipose tissue of nonobese humans (nonsignificant effects indicated by black fill).

are observed in adipose tissue of mice subjected to CR[38] and under treatment with drugs used to type 2 diabetes.[39] Furthermore, there is at least one published gene expression data set describing the effect of resveratrol on adipocytes *in vitro* (http://www.ncbi.nlm.nih.gov/geo/query/acc.cgi? acc=GSE7111), and an analysis of those data revealed that the gene expression pattern of

Ann. N.Y. Acad. Sci. 1290 (2013) 122–129 © 2013 New York Academy of Sciences.

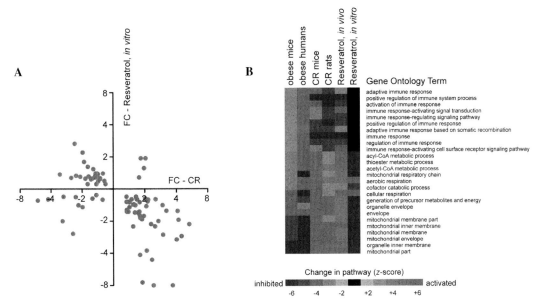

Figure 4. The effect of resveratrol on gene expression *in vitro* does not mimic either the effect of a calorie-restricted diet or the *in vivo* effect of resveratrol consumption; moreover, the transcriptional profile of resveratrol *in vitro* largely reflects the pattern seen with obesity. Analysis of previously published microarray data revealed 93 genes that were significantly ($P < 0.01$) regulated in both calorie-restricted mice and in 3T3L1 adipocytes treated with resveratrol *in vitro*; the *in vitro* effect of resveratrol mimicked the effect of CR in only 15 of 93 genes (A). Similarly, pathway analysis revealed that *in vitro* treatment with resveratrol did not modulate pathways related to the immune response (which are upregulated in obesity and downregulated by CR). In addition, *in vitro* resveratrol treatment downregulated pathways related to mitochondrial structure and function, similar to what is observed in obesity, contrasting with the effects of a calorie-restricted diet (B).

resveratrol *in vitro* is in fact opposite to that is seen with CR. This is true for both the expression of individual genes (Fig. 4A) and for biological pathways regulated by obesity, CR, and resveratrol consumption in humans (Fig. 4B). The available evidence does not suggest that resveratrol has an effect at the transcriptional level indicative of the prevention of obesity. Perhaps more importantly, the overwhelming majority of studies show no change in body weight as a function of resveratrol consumption. Therefore, it seems wise to view the results and conclusions of *in vitro* studies with caution.

Summary

Undoubtedly, diverse organ systems are necessary to coordinate and maintain health; however, the role of adipose tissue in mitigating disease is particularly compelling: obesity and adipose tissue dysfunction are associated with the incidence of many diseases, and a calorie-restricted diet (which reduces body weight and regulates adipose tissue ac-

tivity) is the most experimentally robust strategy for increasing health span by attenuating these same chronic diseases. Although CR is not a realistic therapeutic strategy for humans under free-living conditions, it does present a paradigm by which the efficacy of alternative strategies may be evaluated (including pharmaceuticals as well as natural compounds).

In short-term studies of humans with preexisting metabolic disease, resveratrol consumption improves cardiovascular parameters, positively modulates markers of insulin sensitivity, and decreases systemic inflammation. Although the amount of adipose tissue is not affected by resveratrol consumption, these physiological effects of short-term resveratrol markedly overlap with the effects of long-term CR.[12,38] Similar health benefits are observed in studies of healthy experimental animals, where long-term CR and long-term resveratrol consumption both (1) oppose the activity of adipose tissue that is observed with obesity and (2) improve diverse measurements of health span.[10,11,21,22] It should be noted that the dose of resveratrol used in these studies varies considerably, and in all cases the amount of resveratrol administered to subjects is far greater than what could be achieved through dietary means.

Although short-term resveratrol consumption in healthy nonobese women opposed the transcriptional pattern of obesity and mimicked the gene expression profile of CR in adipose tissue, we did not observe an increase in insulin sensitivity or a decrease in inflammation in healthy patients. A plausible explanation for this latter result is that these clinical parameters cannot be significantly modulated in otherwise healthy individuals. The results of this study in healthy humans are in agreement with a study in healthy mice where short-term resveratrol consumption mimicked the gene expression profile of CR, but there was no change in circulating glucose or insulin. It is tempting to speculate that the mimicry of CR in adipose tissue of healthy subjects is a component of a metabolic programming that confers protection against future disease.[40] Because the effect of resveratrol on health span in animals has only been demonstrated in long-term studies, and because *in vitro* studies of resveratrol do not appear to reflect the actions of resveratrol *in vivo*, long-term studies of resveratrol consumption in humans, while challenging, will be required to support the metabolic reprogramming hypothesis.

Conflicts of interest

The author declares no conflicts of interest.

References

1. Falcao-Pires, I. *et al.* 2012. Physiological, pathological and potential therapeutic roles of adipokines. *Drug Discov. Today* **17:** 880–889.
2. Ye, J. 2009. Emerging role of adipose tissue hypoxia in obesity and insulin resistance. *Int. J. Obes. (Lond.)* **33:** 54–66.
3. Bastard, J.P. *et al.* 2006. Recent advances in the relationship between obesity, inflammation, and insulin resistance. *Eur. Cytokine Netw.* **17:** 4–12.
4. Festa, A. *et al.* 2001. The relation of body fat mass and distribution to markers of chronic inflammation. *Int. J. Obes. Relat. Metab. Disord.* **25:** 1407–1415.
5. LeRoith, D. *et al.* 2008. Obesity and type 2 diabetes are associated with an increased risk of developing cancer and a worse prognosis; epidemiological and mechanistic evidence. *Exp. Clin. Endocrinol. Diabetes* **116**(Suppl. 1): S4–S6.
6. Jensen, G. L. 2008. Inflammation: roles in aging and sarcopenia. *JPEN J. Parenter. Enteral. Nutr.* **32:** 656–659.
7. Jagust, W. *et al.* 2005. Central obesity and the aging brain. *Arch. Neurol.* **62:** 1545–1548.
8. Weindruch, R. & R.L. Walford. 1988. *The Retardation of Aging and Disease by Dietary Restriction.* Charles C Thomas. Springfield, IL.
9. Fontana, L. *et al.* 2004. Long-term calorie restriction is highly effective in reducing the risk for atherosclerosis in humans. *Proc. Natl. Acad. Sci. USA* **101:** 6659–6663.
10. Colman, R.J. *et al.* 2009. Caloric restriction delays disease onset and mortality in rhesus monkeys. *Science* **325:** 201–204.
11. Colman, R.J. *et al.* 2008. Attenuation of sarcopenia by dietary restriction in rhesus monkeys. *J. Gerontol. A Biol. Sci. Med. Sci.* **63:** 556–559.
12. Higami, Y. *et al.* 2006. Energy restriction lowers the expression of genes linked to inflammation, the cytoskeleton, the extracellular matrix, and angiogenesis in mouse adipose tissue. *J. Nutr.* **136:** 343–352.
13. Nadler, S.T. *et al.* 2000. The expression of adipogenic genes is decreased in obesity and diabetes mellitus. *Proc. Natl. Acad. Sci. USA* **97:** 11371–11376.
14. Kim, S.Y. & D.J. Volsky. 2005. PAGE: parametric analysis of gene set enrichment. *BMC Bioinformatics* **6:** 144.
15. Minor, R.K. *et al.* 2010. Dietary interventions to extend life span and health span based on calorie restriction. *J. Gerontol. A Biol. Sci. Med. Sci.* **65:** 695–703.
16. Howitz, K.T. *et al.* 2003. Small molecule activators of sirtuins extend Saccharomyces cerevisiae lifespan. *Nature* **425:** 191–196.
17. Wood, J.G. *et al.* 2004. Sirtuin activators mimic caloric restriction and delay ageing in metazoans. *Nature* **430:** 686–689.
18. Valenzano, D.R. *et al.* 2006. Resveratrol prolongs lifespan and retards the onset of age-related markers in a short-lived vertebrate. *Curr. Biol.* **16:** 296–300.
19. Baur, J.A. *et al.* 2006. Resveratrol improves health and survival of mice on a high-calorie diet. *Nature* **444:** 337–342.
20. Jeon, B.T. *et al.* 2012. Resveratrol attenuates obesity-associated peripheral and central inflammation and improves memory deficit in mice fed a high-fat diet. *Diabetes* **61:** 1444–1454.
21. Barger, J.L. *et al.* 2008. A low dose of dietary resveratrol partially mimics caloric restriction and retards aging parameters in mice. *PLoS ONE* **3:** e2264.
22. Pearson, K.J. *et al.* 2008. Resveratrol delays age-related deterioration and mimics transcriptional aspects of dietary restriction without extending life span. *Cell Metab.* **8:** 157–168.
23. Poulsen, M.M. *et al.* 2012. High-dose resveratrol supplementation in obese men: an investigator-initiated, randomized, placebo-controlled clinical trial of substrate metabolism, insulin sensitivity, and body composition. *Diabetes* **62:** 1186–1195.
24. Yoshino, J. *et al.* 2012. Resveratrol supplementation does not improve metabolic function in nonobese women with normal glucose tolerance. *Cell Metab.* **16:** 658–664.
25. Kennedy, D.O. *et al.* 2010. Effects of resveratrol on cerebral blood flow variables and cognitive performance in humans: a double-blind, placebo-controlled, crossover investigation. *Am. J. Clin. Nutr.* **91:** 1590–1597.

26. Wong, R.H. *et al.* 2011. Acute resveratrol supplementation improves flow-mediated dilatation in overweight/obese individuals with mildly elevated blood pressure. *Nutr. Metab. Cardiovasc. Dis.: NMCD* **21:** 851–856.

27. Magyar, K. *et al.* 2012. Cardioprotection by resveratrol: a human clinical trial in patients with stable coronary artery disease. *Clin. Hemorheol. Microcirc.* **50:** 179–187.

28. Crandall, J.P. *et al.* 2012. Pilot study of resveratrol in older adults with impaired glucose tolerance. *J. Gerontol. A Biol. Sci. Med. Sci.* **67:** 1307–1312.

29. Brasnyo, P. *et al.* 2011. Resveratrol improves insulin sensitivity, reduces oxidative stress and activates the Akt pathway in type 2 diabetic patients. *Br. J. Nutr.* **106:** 383–389.

30. Timmers, S. *et al.* 2011. Calorie restriction-like effects of 30 days of resveratrol supplementation on energy metabolism and metabolic profile in obese humans. *Cell Metab.* **14:** 612–622.

31. Arner, E. *et al.* 2012. Adipose tissue microRNAs as regulators of CCL2 production in human obesity. *Diabetes* **61:** 1986–1993.

32. Linford, N.J. *et al.* 2007. Transcriptional response to aging and caloric restriction in heart and adipose tissue. *Aging Cell.* **6:** 673–688.

33. Barger, J.L. *et al.* 2008. Short-term consumption of a resveratrol-containing nutraceutical mixture mimics gene expression of long-term caloric restriction in mouse heart. *Exp. Gerontol.* **43:** 859–866.

34. Olholm, J. *et al.* 2010. Anti-inflammatory effect of resveratrol on adipokine expression and secretion in human adipose tissue explants. *Int. J. Obes. (Lond.)* **34:** 1546–1553.

35. Gomez-Zorita, S. *et al.* 2013. Resveratrol directly affects in vitro lipolysis and glucose transport in human fat cells. *J. Physiol. Biochem.* Jan 13. [Epub ahead of print].

36. Zhang, X.H. *et al.* 2012. Anti-obesity effect of resveratrol-amplified grape skin extracts on 3T3-L1 adipocytes differentiation. *Nutr. Res. Pract.* **6:** 286–293.

37. Kim, S. *et al.* 2011. Resveratrol exerts anti-obesity effects via mechanisms involving down-regulation of adipogenic and inflammatory processes in mice. *Biochem. Pharmacol.* **81:** 1343–1351.

38. Higami, Y. *et al.* 2004. Adipose tissue energy metabolism: altered gene expression profile of mice subjected to long-term caloric restriction. *FASEB J.* **18:** 415–417.

39. Fonseca, V. 2003. Effect of thiazolidinediones on body weight in patients with diabetes mellitus. *Am. J. Med.* **115**(Suppl. 8A): 42S–48S.

40. Anderson, R.M. & R. Weindruch. 2010. Metabolic reprogramming, caloric restriction and aging. *Trends Endocrinol. Metabol.: TEM.* **21:** 134–141.

Ann. N.Y. Acad. Sci. ISSN 0077-8923

ANNALS OF THE NEW YORK ACADEMY OF SCIENCES
Issue: *Resveratrol and Health*

The pig as a valuable model for testing the effect of resveratrol to prevent cardiovascular disease

Nassrene Y. Elmadhun, Ashraf A. Sabe, Michael P. Robich, Louis M. Chu, Antonio D. Lassaletta, and Frank W. Sellke

Division of Cardiothoracic Surgery, Cardiovascular Research Center, Warren Alpert School of Medicine, Brown University, Providence, Rhode Island

Address for correspondence: Frank W. Sellke, MD, Division of Cardiothoracic Surgery, Cardiovascular Research Center, Warren Alpert Medical School of Brown University, 2 Dudley Street, MOC 360, Providence, RI 02905. fsellke@lifespan.org

Resveratrol is a naturally occurring polyphenol found in the skin of red grapes, peanuts, and red wine that has been shown to modify many cardiovascular risk factors. Small animal models have been extensively used to investigate cardiovascular disease, but the results often fail to translate in clinical trials. Disease-specific pig models are emerging as clinically useful tools that may offer insight into cardiovascular disease and the effect of drugs such as resveratrol on cardiovascular health. In this paper, we discuss the advantage of using clinically relevant pig models of diabetes, hypercholesterolemia, and myocardial ischemia to investigate the role of resveratrol in cardiovascular disease prevention.

Keywords: resveratrol; myocardial ischemia; pig model; cardiovascular disease; metabolic syndrome

Introduction

Resveratrol is a naturally occurring polyphenol found in the skin of red grapes, peanuts, and red wine that has been shown to modify many cardiovascular risk factors.[1] Although resveratrol has been vigorously investigated for its apparent cardioprotective properties in animals, conclusive results in human studies are unfortunately limited. In this paper, we discuss the advantage of using clinically relevant pig models of diabetes, hypercholesterolemia, and myocardial ischemia to investigate the role of resveratrol in cardiovascular disease prevention.

Advantage of pig models in cardiovascular research

Coronary artery disease is the leading cause of death in the United States.[2] Despite major developments in diagnostics and therapies of cardiovascular disease, an estimated one in five deaths in the United States is attributed to coronary artery disease.[2] Small animal models have been extensively used in order to further develop novel therapeutic approaches for the treatment and prevention of disease.[3] However, small animal experiments often fail to translate in clinical trials.[4–6] In a review of seven leading scientific journals, Hackam *et al.* reported that only 37% of highly cited animal research trials were replicated in human randomized control trials, 18% were contradicted by randomized control trials, and 45% remained untested in human trials.[5]

Small animal and mouse models in particular have been widely used in cardiovascular research. Mouse models are appealing for a variety of reasons, including low cost, small size, readily available genetically modified strains, large litters, short reproductive cycle, and reduced ethical concerns compared to large animals.[7,8] Nonetheless, the utility of mouse models to accurately depict human disease has been called into question. In a systematic comparison of the genomic response to inflammatory disease in humans and mouse models, Seok *et al.* reported that humans have a distinctly different genomic response to acute inflammatory stresses that are not reproduced in current mouse models.[4] The disparity between the results derived from

doi: 10.1111/nyas.12216

Ann. N.Y. Acad. Sci. 1290 (2013) 130–135 © 2013 New York Academy of Sciences.

Table 1. Advantages and disadvantages of mouse and pig animal models of cardiovascular disease

	Advantages	Disadvantages
Mouse	Low cost	Inbred strains
	Easy handling	Too small invasive cardiac interventions
	Small size	Different drug doses, and drug pharmacokinetics
	Genetically modified strains	Different platelet, coagulation, and fibrinolysis
	Large litters	Many differences in physiology and pathology
	Short reproductive cycle	
	Reduced ethical concerns	
Pig	Similar cardiac anatomy	High cost
	Similar cardiac function and hemodynamics	Difficult handling
	Spontaneous atherosclerotic lesions	Labor intensive housing and feeding
	Tolerate invasive cardiac interventions	Long gestational period
	Similar drug dosing and pharmacokinetics	Late maturity (1 year)
	Clinically relevant pig models of cardiovascular disease	Ethical concerns
	Similar platelet function, coagulation, and fibrinolysis	

mouse models and human clinical trials highlights the shortcomings of mouse models in representing human disease, including the evolutionary distance between mice and humans, the inbred nature of research mouse models, and the complexity of human disease.[4] Therefore, while small animals are convenient models to investigate mechanisms of disease and test proof of concept derived from *in vitro* models, they are not always reliable as models of human disease.

Although there is no animal model that completely recapitulates human pathology, large animal models are better suited to investigate human disease (Table 1).[7] Pig models of cardiovascular disease are particularly advantageous because, similar to human hearts, pig hearts are predominately right dominant, lack preexisting collateral circulation, develop spontaneous atherosclerotic lesions, and have similar coronary circulation.[7] Pig hearts also have comparable resting left ventricular pressure and heart rate to humans, and are hemodynamically analogous to humans. Given their large size, pigs can tolerate multiple invasive cardiac interventions, including biopsy, surgery, and catheterization that is not possible in mouse models. Pigs also have similar drug pharmacokinetics, platelet function, coagulation, and fibrinolytic cascades compared to humans. The disadvantages of pig models include high cost, labor-intensive housing and feeding, and long gestational period. Pigs also do not reach ma-

turity until they are 1 year of age. And although pigs and humans have similar coagulation protein structure and maximum clot lysis, human clotting time is 2.5-fold longer than pig clotting time.[9] Notwithstanding the numerous studies demonstrating the utility of pigs as an experimental model for the study of cardiovascular disease, there are important dissimilarities and caution must be taken when extrapolating results from pig studies to humans.

Clinically relevant pig models of cardiovascular disease

Even large animal models such as the pig model need to be adapted in order to replicate human disease. Promising results in early large animal studies in chronic myocardial ischemia and angiogenesis led to great enthusiasm about their potential therapeutic implementation but failed to translate into successful phase I and phase II clinical trials, in part because patients with end-stage coronary artery disease are vastly different from the young healthy animals in which preclinical testing is performed.[10] Patients with coronary artery disease frequently have multiple comorbid conditions, including hypertension, hyperlipidemia, diabetes, and endothelial dysfunction. Therefore, our lab and others have established clinically relevant pig models to closely approximate the comorbidities frequently present in patients with chronic myocardial ischemia.

Diet-induced metabolic syndrome and type 2 diabetes

Obesity-prone Ossabaw miniswine have been shown to develop type 2 diabetes, metabolic syndrome, and coronary artery disease when fed a high-fat/high-calorie diet.[11,12] In our lab, we developed a clinically relevant animal model of metabolic syndrome and chronic myocardial ischemia by feeding Ossabaw miniswine a high-fat/high-calorie diet for 16 weeks followed by surgical placement of an ameroid constrictor to the left circumflex artery to induce chronic myocardial ischemia.[12,13] The ameroid constrictor slowly occludes the coronary artery over the course of three weeks, which simulates the gradual occlusion of a coronary artery secondary to atherosclerotic plaque.[14]

Thirteen weeks after ameroid constrictor placement, all animals are anesthetized and undergo intravenous dextrose challenge to determine glucose tolerance and insulin sensitivity.[15] Before euthanasia and tissue harvest, numerous functional parameters are measured, including heart rate, mean arterial pressure, and left ventricular pressure, using an intraaortic catheter-tipped manometer.[16] Regional contractility at rest and during demand pacing is determined by measuring longitudinal and horizontal segmental shortening by placing piezoelectric transducers in the epicardium. Myocardial perfusion is also measured by injecting microspheres into the left atrium at the time of harvest.[17] Microspheres are particles of nonradioactive metal that are injected into the left atrium at rest and during demand pacing. Microspheres lodge into perfused tissue without disrupting blood flow. After cardiac harvest, an independent laboratory counts the microspheres in each sample and calculates myocardial flow.[18] Microvascular relaxation is determined by dissecting epicardial arterioles from transmural myocardial samples. Arterioles are treated with endothelium-dependent and endothelium-independent vasodilators and microvessel relaxation is measured.[19] Capillary and arteriolar density is measured by immunohistochemical stain for CD31 and smooth muscle actin, respectively, to measure angiogenesis.

Streptozocin-induced type 1 diabetes

A type 1 diabetes pig model has also been developed by administering streptozocin, a toxin that preferentially destroys the insulin-secreting pancreatic β cells. In our lab, we developed a clinically relevant type 1 diabetes pig model by inducing type 1 diabetes at eight months of age.[16,20] Diabetic animals were split into two groups, diabetic control and insulin-treated diabetic animals. Diabetes was maintained for eight weeks before surgical intervention. All animals then underwent placement of an ameroid constrictor, and three weeks later animals underwent coronary angiography and microsphere injection at rest and with demand pacing to confirm ameroid closure and baseline myocardial perfusion. Seven weeks after ameroid constrictor placement, the animals underwent functional and hemodynamic measurements, repeat microsphere injection at rest and with demand pacing, followed by euthanasia and cardiac tissue harvest for further analysis.

Pig model of ischemia-reperfusion Injury

In addition to the ameroid-induced chronic myocardial ischemia pig models, there is an acute ischemia-reperfusion pig model. The ischemia-reperfusion model is especially useful in investigating acute myocardial infarction and prompt reperfusion as would be the case with angioplasty, thrombolytic therapy, or coronary artery bypass surgery to salvage the ischemic myocardium. In this model, all animals undergo median sternotomy and baseline hemodynamic and cardiac functional measurements. The left anterior descending coronary artery is occluded distal to the origin of the second diagonal branch using a Rommel tourniquet. After 60 min of ischemia, the tourniquet is released and the myocardium is reperfused for 120 min.[21] Indices of global and regional myocardial function are monitored and recorded at 30-min intervals for the duration of the ischemia-reperfusion experiment.[21] Left anterior descending coronary artery flow is measured using a transonic Doppler probe-reperfusion injury. At the end of reperfusion, the left anterior descending coronary artery is ligated and blue pigment is injected into the aortic root to demarcate the infarcted area. The tissue is incubated in a triphenyl tetrazolium chloride solution for 30 min and the infarct size is determined.[22] The myocardium is harvested for microvascular reactivity studies and molecular analysis. This particular animal model can be modified to study ischemia-reperfusion injury in a variety of clinically relevant scenarios. Our lab previously reported the effects of type 1 diabetes on ischemia-reperfusion

Table 2. Summary of results from resveratrol supplementation in pig models of metabolic syndrome and chronic myocardial ischemia[a]

High-dose resveratrol 100 mg/kg/day[25–29]	Low-dose resveratrol 10 mg/kg/day + VEGF pump[30]	Wine and vodka supplementation[31]
Decreased BMI	Decreased oxidative stress	Wine: improved regional contractility
Decreased serum CRP	Improved endothelial dysfunction	Wine: decreased oxidative stress
Decreased total cholesterol		Wine: improved endothelial dysfunction
Decreased LDL		Wine: improved myocardial perfusion
Decreased blood glucose		Vodka: improved myocardial perfusion
Decreased systolic blood pressure		Vodka: increased angiogenesis
Improved glucose tolerance		
Improved myocardial perfusion		
Improved endothelial dysfunction		
Increased proangiogenesis proteins		

[a]This table summarizes the key findings in three pig models of resveratrol supplementation in the setting of metabolic syndrome and chronic myocardial ischemia. BMI, body mass index; CRP, C-reactive protein; LDL, low-density lipoprotein; VEGF, vascular endothelial growth factor.

injury by injecting the animals with streptozocin before the ischemia-reperfusion experiment.[23] We have also reported the effects of type 2 diabetes and metabolic syndrome on ischemia-reperfusion injury by feeding the animals a high-fat/high-calorie diet before the ischemia-reperfusion experiment.[24]

Resveratrol in a pig model of myocardial ischemia

We conducted three studies investigating the effect of resveratrol in a pig model of diet-induced metabolic syndrome and chronic myocardial ischemia (Table 2). In the first study, animals were fed a high-fat/high-calorie diet alone or a high-fat/high-calorie diet supplemented with 100 mg/kg/day of resveratrol. Four weeks after the diet, all animals underwent placement of an ameroid constrictor and continued on their respective diets. Seven weeks after ameroid constrictor placement, all animals underwent dextrose challenge, cardiac magnetic resonance imaging, coronary angiography, microsphere injection, and tissue harvest. In the resveratrol group, there was significant improvement of glucose tolerance, myocardial perfusion, microvessel relaxation, and expression of the proangiogenesis proteins vascular endothelial growth factor (VEGF) and phosphorylated endothelial nitric oxide synthase (pENOS) compared to the control group.[25–27] The resveratrol group also had lower body mass index (BMI), serum C-reactive protein (CRP), total

cholesterol, low-density lipoprotein (LDL), blood glucose, and systolic blood pressure compared to the control group.[25,28] However, there was no difference in Rentrop collateral scores, regional myocardial function, or endothelial density.[29] This study demonstrated that high-dose resveratrol supplementation significantly improved many of the detrimental effects of metabolic syndrome, including elevated BMI, glucose intolerance, endothelial dysfunction, and hyperlipidemia, while also improving myocardial perfusion.

In a second study, animals were fed a high-fat/high-calorie diet for four weeks to induce metabolic syndrome and subsequently underwent surgical placement of an ameroid constrictor. Postoperatively, one group was supplemented with 10 mg/kg/day resveratrol and the other group continued on the high-fat/high-calorie diet alone. Three weeks after ameroid placement, all animals underwent placement of an osmotic pump to deliver VEGF to the chronically ischemic left circumflex artery territory. Seven weeks after the ameroid constrictor placement, all animals underwent myocardial perfusion analysis and tissue harvest for microvessel relaxation, protein expression and histologic analysis. Resveratrol supplementation in pigs treated with a VEGF pump had improved endothelial-dependent microvessel relaxation and decreased protein oxidative stress compared to the control. However, the addition of resveratrol abolished the improvement in myocardial perfusion and arteriolar density afforded by the VEGF treatment alone.[1,30] This study suggested that perhaps the antioxidant effects of low-dose resveratrol inhibited the oxidative stress-mediated angiogenesis in chronically ischemic myocardium.

In a third study, our lab sought to examine the effects of naturally occurring resveratrol-containing red wine and resveratrol-free vodka on the heart. Animals were fed a high-fat/high-calorie diet for four weeks to induce metabolic syndrome. All animals underwent placement of the ameroid constrictor. Postoperatively, the animals were split into three groups: one group was supplemented with red wine, the second group was supplemented with vodka, and the third group continued on the diet alone for seven weeks. Animals then underwent microsphere injection and functional myocardial measurements before euthanasia and tissue harvest. In the resveratrol-containing red wine group, there was improved regional contractility and decreased oxidative stress compared to the vodka and control group. Both the red wine and vodka groups had improved myocardial perfusion, though through two distinct mechanisms. The vodka group had increased capillary density whereas the wine group had improved microvascular relaxation: both mechanisms can improve myocardial perfusion.[31] These results corroborated our previously reported data that resveratrol-containing red wine increased myocardial perfusion, improved endothelial dysfunction, and decreased oxidative stress.

Conclusion

Although there is no ideal animal model of human pathology, disease-specific pig models are clinically useful tools that may offer insight into cardiovascular disease and the effect of drugs such as resveratrol on cardiovascular health. To date, numerous disease-specific pig models of cardiovascular disease have been developed and validated as clinically relevant animal models, which may help to bridge the disparity between the results of small animal models and clinical trials. Our lab has examined the effects of resveratrol in pig models of diet-induced metabolic syndrome and chronic myocardial ischemia. Our results suggest that resveratrol decreases the burden of chronic metabolic disease, and improves myocardial perfusion and cardiovascular health. Given the many possible benefits of

resveratrol on human cardiovascular disease, further investigation into the therapeutic applications of resveratrol is warranted in future studies.

Conflicts of interest

The authors declare no conflicts of interest.

References

1. Chu, L.M., A.D. Lassaletta, M.P. Robich & F.W. Sellke. 2011. Resveratrol in the prevention and treatment of coronary artery disease. *Curr. Atheroscler. Rep.* **13:** 439–446.
2. Thom, T., N. Haase, W. Rosamond, *et al.* American Heart Association Statistics C, Stroke Statistics Subcommittee. 2006. Heart disease and stroke statistics–2006 update: a report from the american heart association statistics committee and stroke statistics subcommittee. *Circulation* **113:** e85–e151.
3. Woodcock, J. & R. Woosley. 2008. The FDA critical path initiative and its influence on new drug development. *Annu. Rev. Med.* **59:** 1–12.
4. Seok, J., H.S. Warren, A.G. Cuenca, *et al.* 2013. Inflammation, host response to injury LSCRP. Genomic responses in mouse models poorly mimic human inflammatory diseases. *Proc. Natl. Acad. Sci. USA* **110:** 3507–3512.
5. Hackam, D.G. & D.A. Redelmeier. 2006. Translation of research evidence from animals to humans. *JAMA* **296:** 1731–1732.
6. Perel, P., I. Roberts, E. Sena, *et al.* 2007. Comparison of treatment effects between animal experiments and clinical trials: systematic review. *Br. Med. J.* **334:** 197.
7. Vilahur, G., T. Padro & L. Badimon. 2011. Atherosclerosis and thrombosis: insights from large animal models. *J. Biomed. Biotechnol.* **2011:** 907575.
8. Zaragoza, C., C. Gomez-Guerrero, J.L. Martin-Ventura, *et al.* 2011. Animal models of cardiovascular diseases. *J. Biomed. Biotechnol.* **2011:** 497841.
9. Siller-Matula, J.M., R. Plasenzotti, A. Spiel, *et al.* 2008. Interspecies differences in coagulation profile. *Thromb. Haemost.* **100:** 397–404.
10. Boodhwani, M., N.R. Sodha, R.J. Laham & F.W. Sellke. 2006. The future of therapeutic myocardial angiogenesis. *Shock* **26:** 332–341.
11. Neeb, Z.P., J.M. Edwards, M. Alloosh, *et al.* 2010. Metabolic syndrome and coronary artery disease in ossabaw compared with yucatan swine. *Comp. Med.* **60:** 300–315.
12. Lassaletta, A.D., L.M. Chu, M.P. Robich, *et al.* 2012. Overfed ossabaw swine with early stage metabolic syndrome have normal coronary collateral development in response to chronic ischemia. *Basic Res. Cardiol.* **107:** 243.
13. Elmadhun, N.Y., A.D. Lassaletta, L.M. Chu, *et al.* 2012. Atorvastatin increases oxidative stress and modulates angiogenesis in ossabaw swine with the metabolic syndrome. *J. Thor. Cardiovasc. Surg.* **144:** 1486–1493.
14. Robich, M.P., R.M. Osipov, L.M. Chu, *et al.* 2010. Temporal and spatial changes in collateral formation and function during chronic myocardial ischemia. *J. Am. Coll. Surg.* **211:** 470–480.
15. Burgess, T.A., M.P. Robich, L.M. Chu, *et al.* 2011. Improving glucose metabolism with resveratrol in a swine model of

metabolic syndrome through alteration of signaling path-ways in the liver and skeletal muscle. *Arch. Surg.* **146:** 556–564.

16. Boodhwani, M., N.R. Sodha, S. Mieno, *et al.* 2007. Insulin treatment enhances the myocardial angiogenic response in diabetes. *J. Thor. Cardiovasc. Surg.* **134:** 1453–1460.

17. Reinhardt, C.P., S. Dalhberg, M.A. Tries, *et al.* 2001. Stable labeled microspheres to measure perfusion: validation of a neutron activation assay technique. *Am. J. Physiol. Heart Circ. Physiol.* **280:** H108–H116.

18. Boodhwani, M., Y. Nakai, S. Mieno, *et al.* 2006. Hyperc-holesterolemia impairs the myocardial angiogenic response in a swine model of chronic ischemia: role of endostatin and oxidative stress. *Ann. Thorac. Surg.* **81:** 634–641.

19. Tofukuji, M., C. Metais, J. Li, *et al.* 1998. Myocardial vegf expression after cardiopulmonary bypass and cardioplegia. *Circulation* **98:** II242–II246; discussion II247–II248.

20. Boodhwani, M., N.R. Sodha, S. Mieno, *et al.* 2007. Func-tional, cellular, and molecular characterization of the angio-genic response to chronic myocardial ischemia in diabetes. *Circulation* **116:** I31–I37.

21. Sodha, N.R., R.T. Clements, J. Feng, *et al.* 2008. The effects of therapeutic sulfide on myocardial apoptosis in response to ischemia-reperfusion injury. *Eur. J. Cardio-Thorac. Surg.* **33:** 906–913.

22. Toyoda, Y., V. Di Gregorio, R.A. Parker, *et al.* 2000. Anti-stunning and anti-infarct effects of adenosine-enhanced is-chemic preconditioning. *Circulation* **102:** III326–III331.

23. Chu, L.M., R.M. Osipov, M.P. Robich, *et al.* 2010. Is hyper-glycemia bad for the heart during acute ischemia? *J. Thorac. Cardiovasc. Surg.* **140:** 1345–1352.

24. Osipov, R.M., C. Bianchi, J. Feng, *et al.* 2009. Effect of hypercholesterolemia on myocardial necrosis and apopto-sis in the setting of ischemia-reperfusion. *Circulation* **120:** S22–S30.

25. Robich, M.P., R.M. Osipov, R. Nezafat, *et al.* 2010. Resver-atrol improves myocardial perfusion in a swine model of hypercholesterolemia and chronic myocardial ischemia. *Cir-culation* **122:** S142–S149.

26. Robich, M.P., L.M. Chu, T.A. Burgess, *et al.* 2012. Resveratrol preserves myocardial function and perfusion in remote nonischemic myocardium in a swine model of metabolic syndrome. *J. Am. Coll. Surg.* **215:** 681–689.

27. Burgess, T.A., M.P. Robich, L.M. Chu, *et al.* 2011. Improv-ing glucose metabolism with resveratrol in a swine model of metabolic syndrome through alteration of signaling path-ways in the liver and skeletal muscle. *Arch. Surg.* **146:** 556–564.

28. Robich, M.P., R.M. Osipov, L.M. Chu, *et al.* 2011. Resveratrol modifies risk factors for coronary artery disease in swine with metabolic syndrome and myocardial ischemia. *Eur. J. Pharmacol.* **664:** 45–53.

29. Robich, M.P., L.M. Chu, M. Chaudray, *et al.* 2010. Anti-angiogenic effect of high-dose resveratrol in a swine model of metabolic syndrome. *Surgery* **148:** 453–462.

30. Chu, L.M., M.P. Robich, A.D. Lassaletta, *et al.* 2011. Resver-atrol supplementation abrogates pro-arteriogenic effects of intramyocardial vascular endothelial growth factor in a hypercholesterolemic swine model of chronic ischemia. *Surgery* **150:** 390–399.

31. Chu, L.M., A.D. Lassaletta, M.P. Robich, *et al.* 2012. Effects of red wine and vodka on collateral-dependent perfusion and cardiovascular function in hypercholesterolemic swine. *Circulation* **126:** S65–S72.

Ann. N.Y. Acad. Sci. ISSN 0077-8923

Resveratrol, from experimental data to nutritional evidence: the emergence of a new food ingredient

Daniel Raederstorff, Iris Kunz, and Joseph Schwager

DSM Nutritional Products, Basel, Switzerland

Address for correspondence: Daniel Raederstorff, DSM Nutritional Products Ltd., R&D Human Nutrition and Health Department, NIC-RD/HN, Building 205/018, P.O. Box 2676, CH-4002 Basel, Switzerland. Daniel.Raederstorff@dsm.com

The polyphenol resveratrol is found notably in grapes and in a variety of medicinal plants. Recently, resveratrol has been suggested to have cardioprotective effects and to improve metabolic health by mimicking the effects of calorie restriction. Numerous animal and *in vitro* studies suggest that resveratrol could improve cardiovascular and metabolic health in humans. In view of this compelling preclinical evidence, several human studies investigating the effects of resveratrol on vascular and metabolic health have been initiated. Collectively, the animal, human epidemiological, and first human intervention studies support a role of resveratrol in vascular and metabolic health. This has led to the introduction of the first supplement and food products containing resveratrol and its emergence as a promising new health ingredient. Thus, supplementation with resveratrol may be included in nutritional and lifestyle programs aiming to reduce the risk of vascular and obesity-related problems.

Keywords: resveratrol; metabolic disorders; cardiovascular; inflammation; aging

Introduction

Resveratrol, a secondary plant metabolite found in small amounts in numerous plants, has recently attracted a lot of interest among scientists, the drug and food industries, and the media. The potential health benefits have been investigated mainly with resveratrol extracted from *Polygonum cuspidatum* or synthetic, nature-identical resveratrol. Knowledge about resveratrol has been expanding rapidly in recent years; more than 5000 scientific articles describing the effects and function of resveratrol have been entered in the MEDLINE database. Resveratrol was first isolated and identified in 1940 by Michio Takaoka[1] from the dried root of white hellebore (*Veratrum grandiflorum*), but there was little interest in its biological activity for several decades. This changed in the early 1990s after it was suggested that resveratrol, one of the active polyphenols in red wine, was associated with the French paradox, which refers to the observation that people in parts of France have a relatively low incidence of coronary heart disease (CHD) mortality despite a diet rich in saturated fat.[2,3] This unex-pectedly low CHD mortality has been attributed to the regular consumption of red wine, in line with epidemiological studies suggesting that a moderate intake of wine, especially red wine, reduces the risk of cardiovascular disease.[4] *In vitro* assays showed that resveratrol may be able to protect the cardiovascular system by inhibiting platelet aggregation and LDL oxidation.[3,5] Those findings increased the awareness of resveratrol, and a number of *in vitro* and *in vivo* studies to evaluate the biological activity of resveratrol were initiated. In two seminal studies published between 2003 and 2006, resveratrol was suggested to retard the progression of the aging process by acting on sirtuins and mimicking some effects of calorie restriction (CR).[6,7] This further stimulated intense scientific interest in the pharmacological activities of resveratrol. Media coverage of the scientific findings increased awareness of the promise of resveratrol as an antiaging molecule, paving the way to the development and launch of products containing resveratrol by the food and supplement industries. Today more than 400 products containing resveratrol can be found on

doi: 10.1111/nyas.12147

the market (Mintel Global New Products Database; http://www.gnpd.com/sinatra/gnpd/frontpage/).

Background

Numerous biological activities have been attributed to resveratrol. Resveratrol has been shown to have antioxidant, anti-inflammatory, anticarcinogenic, antiaging, and cardiovascular protective properties.[7–9] The anti-inflammatory activities of resveratrol seem to be a key feature in its mode of action. In 1997, Jang *et al.*[10] suggested that the effect of resveratrol on cellular events associated with carcinogenesis, including tumor initiation, promotion, and progression, is partially attributable to its anti-inflammatory activity. This seminal paper attracted considerable interest in evaluating the anticarcinogenic effects of resveratrol (for recent reviews, see Refs. 11 and 12). The study also showed that resveratrol significantly reduced the size of edema in the carrageenan-induced rat paw edema model, a widely accepted *in vivo* model of acute inflammation. The effect size of resveratrol was similar to the anti-inflammatory drug indomethacin. The edema-suppressing activity of resveratrol was much higher than expected from the IC_{50} values observed for the *in vitro* inhibition of cyclooxygenase activity. This suggested that in addition to cyclooxygenase inhibition, resveratrol probably has anti-inflammatory activity through other mechanisms. The anti-inflammatory activity of resveratrol could be shown *in vivo* at a dose of 8 mg/kg body weight/day. This dose would correspond to a human equivalent dose of about 90 mg/day for a 70 kg human individual, using the FDA guideline recommendations to extrapolate from effective doses in animal models to human equivalent doses.[13] This inference (from animal to human studies) has also been described in detail by Reagan-Shaw *et al.* for resveratrol.[14] Those findings support the view that despite its rapid metabolism, resveratrol could have beneficial effects *in vivo* at a relatively low dose and be efficacious in humans. In the past 10 years, the mechanism of action and the health benefits of resveratrol have been extensively investigated in *in vitro* and *in vivo* systems with regard to antiaging and cardiovascular protective effects.[7,8] Moreover, resveratrol has also become a compelling topic for scientists as a molecule mimicking the effects of CR.[15] Recently, the first human studies were published,[16–22] indicating that resveratrol may have beneficial effects for humans in anti-aging, metabolic, and cardiovascular health. In this paper, we will describe in more detail the translation from the *in vitro* mechanistic findings to the effects in humans. This translational nutrition research is critical for the long-term success of a new nutraceutical, since human studies are mandatory for the substantiation of health claims.

Aging and metabolic health

Resveratrol has been found to increase the life span of different species from invertebrates to mice.[7] In mice fed a high-calorie diet, resveratrol (22 mg/kg/day) was demonstrated to prevent early mortality by suppressing obesity-related metabolic disorders.[23] Resveratrol supplementation lowered fasting glucose, improved insulin sensitivity, and prevented liver damage, in addition to improving performance in treated animals. The results suggest that despite being overweight, the resveratrol-treated mice were metabolically healthy. The aging process is complex and involves a number of pathways such as oxidative stress, cellular stress resistance, neuroendocrine systems, nutrient sensing systems, and insulin signaling.[24,25] Mechanistic studies have suggested that resveratrol acts on the aging process by targeting energy/nutrient pathways proteins such as sirtuins (SIRT1), the mammalian target of rapamycin (mTOR), and AMP-activated protein kinase (AMPK).[6,18,26] Initially, the major focus was on the effect of resveratrol on sirtuins.[7] However, it has been questioned whether sirtuins are directly or indirectly activated by resveratrol.[27] The detailed mechanisms of action of resveratrol on the aging process still need to be clarified, particularly the complex interplay between the different pathways involved. Even so, the data suggest that similarly to CR, resveratrol may act on nutrient/energy sensing systems that are considered to play key roles in the aging process. Reduced calorie intake without malnutrition has been shown to prolong lifespan in invertebrates and rodents.[25] Moreover, CR has beneficial effects on markers of diabetes, cardiovascular diseases, neurodegenerative diseases, chronic inflammation, and oxidative stress in humans.[25] In order to evaluate the long-term CR-mimicking effects of resveratrol, genome-wide transcriptional profiles were examined after supplementation of a low dose of resveratrol (4.9 mg/kg/day; corresponding to a human equivalent dose of about

30 mg/day), or CR from middle age (14 months) to old age (30 months) in mice.[28] The study showed that there was a large overlap in the change in gene expression profile during aging between the CR and the resveratrol-treated group in heart, skeletal muscle, and brain. This strongly suggested that CR and resveratrol retarded aging in similar way in those tissues. Moreover, both dietary interventions also prevented age-related cardiac dysfunction. The study indicates that resveratrol, at doses that can be readily achieved in humans, mimics some aspects of the action of CR and may be a useful micronutrient to help prevent age-related chronic diseases.

To further substantiate the role of resveratrol in the prevention of age-related metabolic and cardiovascular disturbances, several human studies have been conducted. Recently, Timmers *et al.* showed that the metabolic benefits observed in animal obesity models could also be translated into effects in humans.[18] In this randomized double-blind crossover study, resveratrol significantly reduced systolic blood pressure and improved blood glucose levels as well as insulin sensitivity in human obese men receiving 150 mg/day resveratrol for 30 days. Moreover, a significant decrease in liver fat and inflammatory markers was observed. These data indicate that resveratrol was able to mimic some aspects of CR in obese humans, as previously reported in animals.[9] Resveratrol has been shown to be beneficial with respect to insulin sensitivity and glucose metabolism in subjects with impaired glucose tolerance.[17,22,29] However, Yoshino *et al.* found that 75 mg/day of resveratrol after three months of supplementation did not improve metabolic function in nonobese healthy women with normal glucose tolerance.[20] Moreover Poulsen *et al.* observed no effect on glucose turnover and insulin sensitivity with a high dose of resveratrol (1 g/day).[21] Despite those conflicting results, most studies reported an improvement in metabolic health. Future studies need to further evaluate the effects of different doses of resveratrol and discriminate possible distinct effects in various target populations like the obese, diabetics, children, and the elderly.

Cardiovascular health

Shortly after the possible causative association of resveratrol with the French paradox, data were published that demonstrated the influence of resveratrol on markers of cardiovascular function.[3] Sub-

sequently, resveratrol has been shown to have pleiotropic effects on the cardiovascular system, including decreasing oxidative stress, inhibiting platelet aggregation and vascular smooth muscle proliferation, decreasing vascular inflammation, and improving endothelial function (for detailed reviews see, e.g., Baur *et al.*,[7] Chavay *et al.*,[8] and Schmitt *et al.*[30]). The beneficial cardiovascular effects of resveratrol are mainly ascribed to its antioxidant and anti-inflammatory properties, which preserve vascular function and retard atherosclerosis during the aging process. Thus, the effect of resveratrol on endothelial function seems to be critical for its vascular benefits. The endothelium at the interface between the blood circulation and the vascular smooth muscle plays a critical role in the regulation of vascular homeostasis. Intercellular adhesion molecule-1 (ICAM-1) and vascular cell adhesion molecule-1 (VCAM-1) are important adhesion molecules that are expressed on endothelial cells and mediate the adhesion and migration of leukocytes to the vascular endothelium, and thus might initiate inflammatory processes that eventually culminate in atherosclerotic lesions. Thus, ICAM-1 and VCAM-1 are considered as early markers of endothelial dysfunction and atherosclerosis. Resveratrol inhibited ICAM-1 and VCAM-1 expression in endothelial cells stimulated by various agonists (TNF-α, LPS) through inhibition of nuclear factor-κB (NF-κB) activation.[31,32] Moreover, resveratrol at low dose (0.1 μmol/L) significantly inhibited the adhesion of monocytes to stimulated endothelial cells, a key step in the development of atherosclerosis.[31,32] In aged rats, resveratrol (10 mg/kg/day) reversed the age-related increase in ICAM-1 gene expression, suggesting that resveratrol may limit chronic inflammation and attenuate early atherosclerotic events.[33] In addition, in a recent human *ex vivo* study, Agarwal *et al.* showed that the expression of ICAM, VCAM, and IL-8 was significantly decreased in human coronary endothelial artery cells incubated with plasma from subjects who were supplemented with 400 mg/day resveratrol (and quercetin and grape skin extract) for 30 days.[34] Vascular aging has also been associated with nuclear factor (erythroid-derived 2)-like 2 (Nrf2) dysfunction; Nrf2 transcriptionally regulates the induction of endogenous antioxidants and phase II enzymes conferring protection from oxidative damage.[35] In a recent human study,

Ghanim *et al.* showed that after a single oral dose of resveratrol (100 mg) plus a grape extract enriched in polyphenol (75 mg), the activity of Nrf2 and its downstream targets was stimulated in isolated monocytes.[36] Moreover, resveratrol has been shown to significantly increase the transcriptional activity of Nrf2 and the Nrf2 target genes in endothelial cells.[35] Resveratrol-dependent activation of Nrf2 plausibly contributes to the prevention of diet-induced endothelial dysfunction, since genetic deletion of Nrf2 in knockout animals abolished the protection. Nitric oxide (NO) is a potent vasodilator involved in the regulation of vascular homeostasis and is produced by endothelial nitric oxide synthase (eNOS). Endothelial dysfunction is reflected by reduced expression of eNOS, entailing diminished vascular NO production. Resveratrol induced a concentration- and time-dependent upregulation of eNOS mRNA in human umbilical vein endothelial cells (HUVEC). Moreover, resveratrol acutely enhanced the release of NO from endothelial cells.[37,38] Takahashi *et al.* showed that resveratrol at doses as low as 0.05 μmol/L significantly increased functional eNOS protein and NO production.[38] In spontaneously hypertensive rats (SHRs), resveratrol treatment for 10 weeks preserved vascular NO production and attenuated elevated blood pressure.[39] Endothelial-related *in vitro* and *in vivo* data indicate that resveratrol is able to reduce inflammatory stress and to promote nitric oxide biosynthesis at physiologically relevant doses. Presumably, benefits in humans are associated with this mode of action.

In 2010, Wong *et al.* published the first study showing that resveratrol was able to improve endothelial function in humans.[16] The acute effect of three single doses of resveratrol (30, 90, and 270 mg) on flow mediated dilation (FMD) of the brachial artery, a biomarker of vascular function, was assessed in the study. Plasma resveratrol levels increased dose dependently and ranged from 0.8 to 5 μmol/L. These were comparable to levels that previously have shown activity in *in vitro* model systems. Resveratrol is absorbed and rapidly metabolized to glucuronide and sulfate conjugates and distributed into tissues.[16,40–42] Recent data have shown that resveratrol metabolites remain biologically active and could eventually be converted back to free resveratrol in the tissues.[43] Measuring total resveratrol is therefore relevant to assess plasma levels after dietary intake of resveratrol. Moreover, the three doses of resveratrol significantly increased FMD by 62–91%. Thus, resveratrol could improve endothelium-dependent vasodilation at a dose of 30 mg/day in humans. In a follow-up study, daily intake of 75 mg of resveratrol over a period of six weeks produced a sustained and prolonged 23% improvement in flow-mediated dilation.[44] Magyar *et al.* showed that in patients with coronary artery diseases, resveratrol (10 mg/day) significantly improved FMD and left ventricle diastolic function over a period of three months.[19] Impaired endothelial vasodilator function may lead to the development of future CVD, and an improvement in FMD has been associated with a decrease in cardiovascular adverse events.[45] Overall, the data strongly indicate that resveratrol has beneficial effects on human circulatory function.

Conclusions

Resveratrol has received increased attention in the past decades in view of its possible beneficial effect in aging and metabolic and cardiovascular health. Those initial scientific findings have initiated a plethora of mechanistic and clinical research studies and the launch of products focusing on age-related problems and cardiovascular health. Moreover, many clinical trials investigating the beneficial effects of resveratrol are ongoing (see: www.clinicaltrial.gov database). As of April 2013, there were 15 studies in the field of metabolic health and four studies in the area of cardiovascular diseases, indicating relatively high interest. Regarding aging and metabolic problems, the experimental data indicate that resveratrol prevents pathological changes associated with high calorie intake and may thus provide a variety of beneficial health effects. Resveratrol has been shown to reduce the deleterious effects of oxidative, inflammatory, and metabolic stress. In a first human study resveratrol mimicked some aspects of CR and endurance training in obese humans. However, conflicting results on the effect of resveratrol on insulin sensitivity were observed in studies using different doses and study participants. Additional dose-response studies in different populations are needed to better define the dose and population in which subjects would benefit most from resveratrol supplementation. Regarding cardiovascular health, there is convincing *in vitro* and *in vivo* evidence suggesting that resveratrol has beneficial effects on vascular function and on early markers of atherosclerosis. Moreover, resveratrol improved endothelial function in humans at relatively low doses.

Acknowledgments

The authors would like to thank Julia Bird for critically reading the manuscript.

Conflicts of interest

The authors are employees of DSM Nutritional Products Ltd., a supplier of resveratrol.

References

1. Takaoka, M. 1940. Phenolic substance of white hellebore (*Veratrum grandiflorum* Loes fil.). III. Constitution of resveratrol. *Nippon Kagaku Kaishi* **61**: 30–34.
2. Renaud, S. & M. de Lorgeril. 1992. Wine, alcohol, platelets, and the French paradox for coronary heart disease. *Lancet* **339**: 1523–1526.
3. Frankel, E.N., A.L. Waterhouse & J.E. Kinsella. 1993. Inhibition of human LDL oxidation by resveratrol. *Lancet* **341**: 1103–1104.
4. Lippi, G., M. Franchini, E.J. Favaloro, *et al.* 2010. Moderate red wine consumption and cardiovascular disease risk: beyond the "French paradox". *Semin. Thromb. Hemost.* **36**: 59–70.
5. Bertelli, A.A.E., L. Giovannini, D. Giannessi, *et al.* 1995. Antiplatelet activity of synthetic and natural resveratrol in red wine. *Int. J. Tissue Reac.* **17**: 1–3.
6. Howitz, K.T., K.J. Bitterman, H.Y. Cohen, *et al.* 2003. Small molecule activators of sirtuins extend Saccharomyces cerevisiae lifespan. *Nature* **425**: 191–196.
7. Baur, J.A. & D.A. Sinclair. 2006. Therapeutic potential of resveratrol: the in vivo evidence. *Nat. Rev. Drug Discov.* **5**: 493–506.
8. Chachay, V.S., C.M. Kirkpatrick, I.J. Hickman, *et al.* 2011. Resveratrol—pills to replace a healthy diet? *Br. J. Clin. Pharmacol.* **72**: 27–38.
9. Timmers, S., J. Auwerx & P. Schrauwen. 2012. The journey of resveratrol from yeast to human. *Aging* **4**: 146–158.
10. Jang, M., L. Cai, G.O. Udeani, *et al.* 1997. Cancer chemopreventive activity of resveratrol, a natural product derived from grapes. *Science* **275**: 218–220.
11. Scott, E., W.P. Steward, A.J. Gescher, *et al.* 2012. Resveratrol in human cancer chemoprevention—choosing the 'right' dose. *Mol. Nutr. Food Res.* **56**: 7–13.
12. Whitlock, N.C. & S.J. Baek. 2012. The anticancer effects of resveratrol: modulation of transcription factors. *Nutr. Cancer* **64**: 493–502.
13. Center for Drug Evaluation and Research. 2005. Estimating the Maximum Safe Starting Dose in Initial Clinical Trials for Therapeutics in Adult Healthy Volunteers. U.S. Food and Drug Administration, Rockville, Maryland, USA.
14. Reagan-Shaw, S., M. Nihal & N. Ahmad. 2008. Dose translation from animal to human studies revisited. *FASEB J.* **22**: 659–661.
15. Baur, J.A. 2010. Resveratrol, sirtuins, and the promise of a DR mimetic. *Mech. Ageing Dev.* **131**: 261–269.
16. Wong, R.H., P.R. Howe, J.D. Buckley, *et al.* 2011. Acute resveratrol supplementation improves flow-mediated dilatation in overweight/obese individuals with mildly elevated blood pressure. *Nutr. Metab. Cardiovasc. Dis.* **21**: 851–856.
17. Brasnyo, P., G.A. Molnar, M. Mohas, *et al.* 2011. Resveratrol improves insulin sensitivity, reduces oxidative stress and activates the Akt pathway in type 2 diabetic patients. *Br. J. Nutr.* **106**: 383–389.
18. Timmers, S., E. Konings, L. Bilet, *et al.* 2011. Calorie restriction-like effects of 30 days of resveratrol supplementation on energy metabolism and metabolic profile in obese humans. *Cell Metab.* **14**: 612–622.
19. Magyar, K., R. Halmosi, A. Palfi, *et al.* 2012. Cardioprotection by resveratrol: a human clinical trial in patients with stable coronary artery disease. *Clin. Hemorheol. Microcirc.* **50**: 179–187.
20. Yoshino, J., C. Conte, L. Fontana, *et al.* 2012. Resveratrol supplementation does not improve metabolic function in nonobese women with normal glucose tolerance. *Cell Metab.* **16**: 658–664.
21. Poulsen, M.M., P.F. Vestergaard, B.F. Clasen, *et al.* 2013. High-dose resveratrol supplementation in obese men: an investigator-initiated, randomized, placebo-controlled clinical trial of substrate metabolism, insulin sensitivity, and body composition. *Diabetes* **62**: 1186–1195.
22. Crandall, J.P., V. Oram, G. Trandafirescu, *et al.* 2012. Pilot study of resveratrol in older adults with impaired glucose tolerance. *J. Gerontol. A Biol. Sci. Med. Sci.* **67**: 1307–1312.
23. Baur, J.A., K.J. Pearson, N.L. Price, *et al.* 2006. Resveratrol improves health and survival of mice on a high-calorie diet. *Nature* **444**: 337–342.
24. Martin, G.M. 2011. The biology of aging: 1985–2010 and beyond. *FASEB J.* **25**: 3756–3762.
25. Fontana, L., L. Partridge & V.D. Longo. 2010. Extending healthy life span–from yeast to humans. *Science* **328**: 321–326.
26. Liu, M., S.A. Wilk, A. Wang, *et al.* 2010. Resveratrol inhibits mTOR signaling by promoting the interaction between mTOR and DEPTOR. *J. Biol. Chem.* **285**: 36387–36394.
27. Park, S.J., F. Ahmad, A. Philp, *et al.* 2012. Resveratrol ameliorates aging-related metabolic phenotypes by inhibiting cAMP phosphodiesterases. *Cell* **148**: 421–433.
28. Barger, J.L., T. Kayo, J.M. Vann, *et al.* 2008. A low dose of dietary resveratrol partially mimics caloric restriction and retards aging parameters in mice. *PLoS ONE* **3**: e2264.
29. Bhatt, J.K., S. Thomas & M.J. Nanjan. 2012. Resveratrol supplementation improves glycemic control in type 2 diabetes mellitus. *Nutr. Res.* **32**: 537–541.
30. Schmitt, C.A., E.H. Heiss & V.M. Dirsch. 2010. Effect of resveratrol on endothelial cell function: molecular mechanisms. *Biofactors* **36**: 342–349.
31. Ferrero, M.E., A. E. Bertelli, A. Fulgenzi, *et al.* 1998. Activity in vitro of resveratrol on granulocyte and monocyte adhesion to endothelium. *Am. J. Clin. Nutr.* **68**: 1208–1214.

32. Csiszar, A., K. Smith, N. Labinskyy, *et al.* 2006. Resveratrol attenuates TNF-alpha-induced activation of coronary arterial endothelial cells: role of NF-kB inhibition. *Am. J. Physiol. Heart Circ. Physiol.* **291:** H1694–H1699.

33. Ungvari, Z., Z. Orosz, N. Labinskyy, *et al.* 2007. Increased mitochondrial H2O2 production promotes endothelial NF-kappaB activation in aged rat arteries. *Am. J. Physiol. Heart Circ. Physiol.* **293:** H37–H47.

34. Agarwal, B., M.J. Campen, M.M. Channell, *et al.* 2013. Resveratrol for primary prevention of atherosclerosis: clinical trial evidence for improved gene expression in vascular endothelium. *Int. J. Cardiol.* In press.

35. Ungvari, Z., Z. Bagi, A. Feher, *et al.* 2010. Resveratrol confers endothelial protection via activation of the antioxidant transcription factor Nrf2. *Am. J. Physiol. Heart. Circ. Physiol.* **299:** H18–H24.

36. Ghanim, H., C.L. Sia, K. Korzeniewski, *et al.* 2011. A resveratrol and polyphenol preparation suppresses oxidative and inflammatory stress response to a high-fat, high-carbohydrate meal. *J. Clin. Endocrinol. Metab.* **96:** 1409–1414.

37. Wallerath, T., G. Deckert, T. Ternes, *et al.* 2002. Resveratrol, a polyphenolic phytoalexin present in red wine, enhances expression and activity of endothelial nitric oxide synthase. *Circulation* **106:** 1652–1658.

38. Takahashi, S. & Y. Nakashima. 2012. Repeated and long-term treatment with physiological concentrations of resveratrol promotes NO production in vascular endothelial cells. *Br. J. Nutr.* **107:** 774–780.

39. Bhatt, S.R., M.F. Lokhandwala & A.A. Banday. 2011. Resveratrol prevents endothelial nitric oxide synthase uncoupling and attenuates development of hypertension in spontaneously hypertensive rats. *Eur. J. Pharmacol.* **667:** 258–264.

40. Walle, T., F. Hsieh, M.H. DeLegge, *et al.* 2004. High absorption but very low bioavailability of oral resveratrol in humans. *Drug Metab. Dispos.* **32:** 1377–1382.

41. Vitrac, X., A. Desmouliere, B. Brouillaud, *et al.* 2003. Distribution of [14C]-trans-resveratrol, a cancer chemopreventive polyphenol, in mouse tissues after oral administration. *Life Sci.* **72:** 2219–2233.

42. Lin, S.P., P.M. Chu, S.Y. Tsai, *et al.* 2012. Pharmacokinetics and tissue distribution of resveratrol, emodin and their metabolites after intake of *Polygonum cuspidatum* in rats. *J. Ethnopharmacol.* **144:** 671–676.

43. Hoshino, J., E.J. Park, T.P. Kondratyuk, *et al.* 2010. Selective synthesis and biological evaluation of sulfate-conjugated resveratrol metabolites. *J. Med. Chem.* **53:** 5033–5043.

44. Wong, R.H., N.M. Berry, A.M. Coates, *et al.* 2012. Sustained improvement of vasodilator function by resveratrol in obese adults. *J. Hypertens.* **30:** e70.

45. Shechter, M., A. Issachar, I. Marai, *et al.* 2009. Long-term association of brachial artery flow-mediated vasodilation and cardiovascular events in middle-aged subjects with no apparent heart disease. *Int. J. Cardiol.* **134:** 52–58.